Health Maintenance Organizations

The Milbank Readers
John B. McKinlay, general editor

Health Maintenance Organizations

Milbank Reader 5

edited by John B. McKinlay

The MIT Press
Cambridge, Massachusetts
London, England

Printed and bound in the United States of America

Library of Congress Cataloging in Publication Data

Main entry under title:
Health maintenance organizations.

 (The Milbank reader series ; 5)
 Bibliography: p.
 Includes index.
 1. Health maintenance organizations—United States—Addresses,
essays, lectures. 2. Health maintenance organizations—Addresses, essays,
lectures. I. McKinlay, John B. II. Series. [DNLM: 1. Health maintenance
organizations—United States—Collected works. W 275 AA1 H438]
RA413.5.U5H39   362.1'0425   81–12387
ISBN 0–262–63081–8 (pbk.)   AACR2
      0–262–13180–3 (hard)

Contents

Foreword

During 1973–74, the Milbank Memorial Fund, in conjunction with
Prodist (New York), produced four edited volumes that drew together and organized published papers from the well-known and
respected *Milbank Memorial Fund Quarterly*. In producing these
four initial resource books (*Research Methods in Health Care, Politics
and Law in Health Care Policy, Economic Aspects of Health Care*, and
Organizational Issues in the Delivery of Health Services), the Fund had
attempted to respond to heavy and continuing requests for accessibility and economy of the Milbank papers. The success of the
four books exceeded even the most optimistic expectations, and all
are now, unfortunately, out of print. They were adopted as course
texts by many different health-related disciplines, were used
widely throughout North America and abroad, were acquired by
many university and professional libraries and were favorably reviewed in internationally respected professional journals.

The foreword to the earlier series noted that we always "planned
to keep this series active and responsive to changing needs. Suggestions for future volumes will be welcome." Since their release,
there have been numerous inquiries, requests, and suggestions for
further volumes dealing with new and emerging issues concerning
health care and social policy. The titles included in this second
wave of edited volumes attempt to respond again to this widespread enthusiasm and need.

A venture of this nature has several obvious limitations. First of
all, the universe from which the contributions were selected was
limited to the *Milbank Memorial Fund Quarterly/Health and Society*,
and to several books produced by the Fund as a result of round-
table meetings on particular health-care issues. However, more
than enough rich material by eminent scholars was available for at
least the present volumes. For the editor, a major problem was to
decide which of several excellent papers had to be omitted (for
reasons of economy, coverage, datedness, etc.) rather than what
was available for inclusion in each volume. It should be emphasized that all of the authors represented here have progressed in
their thinking and have advanced their work in other journals and

books since original publication of the papers. Some have altered their theoretical orientation and some even their substantive interests. Wherever possible the editor has selected contributions published since the early 1970s. Indeed, most of the articles were first published within the last three or four years. Articles that were widely recognized as classic statements were selected from earlier years. Finally, several contributions dealt with a breadth of issues and were of sufficient quality to warrant their inclusion in more than one volume. Since each volume is likely to appeal to somewhat different readerships, this duplication was not considered problematic but rather enhanced the treatment of some health-care issues and the value of each volume.

It is hoped that this new series will help teachers, researchers, policymakers, public administrators, and especially students to overcome an ever-increasing problem: namely, how to gain easy and economical access to the rich resources contained in recent Milbank Memorial Fund publications.

Introduction

When Health Maintenance Organizations (HMOs) were first debated and then introduced only a decade ago, no one predicted that their number would increase so rapidly so as to become one of the major forms of health care delivery in the United States. This relatively unique form of health care organization and financing raises some profound policy issues many of which are addressed in this volume.

The four papers in the first section consider the development of HMOs. Ernest Saward and Mervyn Greenlick provide an interesting discussion of some of the concerns and issues influencing the early development of HMOs. They considered the emergence of HMOs as a rather classic example of federal policy making in health. From their vantage point nearly a decade ago, they considered the likelihood of widespread implementation doubtful, not because the HMO was without merit, but because the fee-for-service pattern was left intact with most of the rewards and few of the constraints. It is certainly useful to reflect on their discussion in light of what has transpired over the intervening decade.

Richard McNeil and Robert Schlenker consider the role of three forces that seemed to influence the development of HMOs during the early 1970s. They suggest that the rapid increase in the number of HMOs during the 1970s was primarily due to favorable market conditions in certain areas of the country combined with a highly encouraging federal policy towards HMOs. Contrary to earlier beliefs, legal restrictions do not appear to have been a serious barrier to HMO development. In 1973–74, new legislation was enacted at both the federal and state levels ostensibly to encourage HMO development. The authors' review of this particular legislation suggests that while it certainly did remove many of the old legal requirements that apparently were not serious barriers to HMO development, it also imposed a host of new conditions and requirements on HMO participation in the health care marketplace. Ironically, it appears that some of these new features impeded the operation of the very market forces that encouraged the earlier HMO growth. John Iglehart's paper discusses the federal government's interest in promoting the development of HMOs as a unique experiment in venture capitalism. HMOs involve an activity that requires some reconciliation of the sometimes competing goals and procedures of government and private business. Within the context of the Department of Health and Human Services that appears to favor regulatory approaches, the Office of Health Maintenance Organization (OHMO) suggests some marketplace solutions to problems in the production, distribution and financing of health care. Donald Moran considers the recent policy fad that seeks to inject competition into the market for health care financing. He argues that pushing procompetition legislation through Congress may have unanticipated consequences for its proponents. Given these and several other political considerations, Moran suggests that it may be preferable to turn to an accommodation of interests that provides some contraints on adverse selection and free riders, some contraints on plan innovation and product differentiation, some bias against fee-for-service solo practitioners, and some risk that the American people, left to themselves in an open system, may spend more rather than less on health care.

Some determinants of choice with respect to HMOs are discussed in the two papers in the second section. Richard Tessler and David Mechanic examine the basis for the selection of prepaid group practice in a dual choice situation and the social, attitudinal and health characteristics of populations choosing prepaid programs in contrast to other plans. In response to open-ended questions concerning reasons for the decisions they made, those selecting prepaid group practice most frequently referred to the more comprehensive coverage provided and to the fact that, at the time of choice, they lacked a continuing or adequate relationship with a physician. Enrollees in the prepaid program appeared to be better educated and, contrary to some previous findings, more likely to be uninsured. There was little evidence that these enrollees brought distinctive attitudes and orientations toward illness and medical care with them. They did, however, tend to report more chronic conditions than persons who declined to enroll in the prepaid program. On a number of other indicators of health status, the prepaid program enrollees were comparable to those retaining an alternative health insurance option. Berki and Ashcraft review a range of studies conducted in recent years concerning the determinants of choice by enrollees of HMO versus other provider systems. They find that breadth of coverage, lower cost and assured access to benefits are key elements anticipated in the choice, but so too are the perceived limitations inherent in selection of a physician within a closed panel plan and the inconvenience of centralized sites.

Now that we have about ten years of experience with HMOs, we can turn to the third section that focuses on the actual performance of HMOs. Some early evidence is discussed by Milton Roemer and William Shonick. They suggest that the prepaid group practice model of HMO yields lower hospital use, relatively more ambulatory and preventive services, and lower overall costs (counting both premiums and out-of-pocket expenditures) than conventional open market fee-for-service patterns. Although economies of scale in group practice are not proved, the evidence suggests that this is at least a theoretical possibility. Data also point to reduced disability from the prepaid group practice type of HMO, as well as to more favorable consumer attitudes (based mainly on the economic advantages in spite of certain impersonalities of clinics) than exist towards conventionally insured private solo practice. The authors are alert to HMO hazards of underservicing and distorted risk selection, but believe that with appropriate public monitoring, HMOs constitute an approach to health planning stressing local initiatives, competition and incentives to self-regulation. The paper by Harold Luft updates evidence on aspects of the performance of HMOs. Total costs for HMO members are shown to be lower than for those enrolled in conventional insurance plans. It is argued that this cannot be accounted for solely by matters of efficiency, quality, consumer self-selection, or physician satisfaction. While there is some optimism in policy circles that HMOs will encourage beneficial competitive responses by traditional health care providers, too little is known at present to determine whether this is in fact occurring.

Frederic Wolinsky, in a broad ranging review of nine studies of the performance of HMOs, suggests that the following five points are now generally agreed upon: hospitalization rates in HMOs are up to 45% lower than those in conventional insurance systems; total costs are less in HMOs than in conventional insurance systems; seemingly higher levels of preventive care utilization in HMOs may actually be a reflection of the more extensive coverage that they offer in comparison with conventional health insurance plans; HMO enrollees tend to be more satisfied with the technical aspects of the medical care they receive than are those in conventional insurance plans, but the conventionally insured are more satisfied with their patient/practitioner relationships; although the evidence is certainly not complete, the quality of care received in HMOs appears to be at least equal to, if not better than, that received in the average conventional insurance plans. Wolinsky finds that the most important and agreed-upon point is that although reduced costs and lower hospitalization rates in HMOs are now rather well documented, we still remain uncertain as to how these are actually achieved. He goes on to identify the incentive and disincentive structures operating in HMOs and discusses some of the methodological problems associated with evaluating their performance. He then analytically reviews recent literature.

Emil Berkanovic and his colleagues report data from a larger study in which a prepaid medical foundation was compared with a non-prepaid fee-for-service system as to how health care is perceived by both Medicaid recipients and physicians. The data employed are confined to the issue of the impact of prepayment on Medicaid recipients' perceptions of their access to health care. Few differences were found between the two forms of health care delivery as regards accessibility or acceptability. The authors suggest that the fears of some critics of the HMO concept with respect to prepayment creating incentives for the denial of services are not supported by their data. They conclude that the organizational features of medical practice which affect access are actually quite similar for the two systems studied. Finally, Mark Blumberg considers some of the speculations on the causes of the frequently observed lower rates of hospital use and group practice, or HMO, members than by persons covered by other health care arrangements. The assertion that this is because HMO enrollees are a self-selected healthier population, or that hospital utilization is not fully recorded is challenged in a major Californian study on the *actual* health and hospital use of a representative sample of persons under 65 years of age. Blumberg's paper provides a useful background to several of the papers that follow.

A range of other pertinent issues presented by and affecting HMOs are discussed in the fourth section. James Hester suggests that much of that already written about the concept, operation and performance of HMOs—their use of resources compared with other health service systems—masks the real differences among HMOs themselves. It is maintained that investigation of discrete units within a unified HMO program actually shows a surprising diversity. There is reason to believe that the HMO concept may be particularly suited to the area of dental care. According to Max Schoen, the principal dental diseases, caries and periodontal disease, affect almost the entire population and result in considerable pain and discomfort with eventual tooth loss if untreated. These disorders can either be prevented or their effects minimized through dental intervention so that intact functioning dentitions can be maintained. Despite the fact that enough practicing dentists probably exist in the United States to achieve these results, the majority of the population lose all of their natural teeth if they live out their normal life spans. The solo practice fee-for-service system, even with third party payment, may reduce the difficulties somewhat, but cannot solve the problem. Prepaid dental group practice, either independently or as part of a general health care system, has the potential of virtually eliminating edentulism in the population.

Although not directly concerned with HMOs, the paper by Richard Scheffler on pricing behavior of medical groups has important implications for policy concerning HMOs. His data, collected by mail survey from medical groups in North Carolina, suggest that the prices charged by medical groups are positively influenced by the per capita income of the county in which the group is located and the per physician utilization of medical, technical and officer personnel. The study also suggests that a non-physician manager, and a non-salaried system of remuneration to member physicians, are negatively related to the price of medical services. The paper by Eliot Freidson considers the organizational influences on both consumer and provider behavior. He discusses some ways in which a prepaid service contract and closed panel practice brings a new dimension to the consumer/practitioner relationship, and how physicians respond to it. Unable to manage "unreasonable demands for service" by use of a fee barrier or encouragement to "go elsewhere," as in traditional solo fee-for-service practice, physicians were disturbed by a new type of demanding patient who claimed services on the basis of contractual rights and threatened appeal to higher bureaucratic authority. The new form of organization and financing afforded by Health Maintenance Organizations therefore appears to profoundly influence patient behavior and the work of health professionals.

Finally, Carl Stevens considers medical malpractice in relation to HMOs. The many problems associated with medical malpractice have led to advocacy of abandoning the fault finding and litigation approaches to the problem. Stevens believes that Health Maintenance Organizations afford unique institutional settings for developing appropriate alternatives. Explicit contracts between provider managers and member patients can allow consumers to determine how much risk prevention and overall quality they are prepared to invest in. Not just principles of economic efficiency, but also of distributional equity can inform HMO performance standard contracts; and arbitration may be the best mode for managing disputes arising from them.

John B. McKinlay

I The Development of HMOs

HEALTH POLICY AND THE HMO

ERNEST W. SAWARD

AND

MERWYN R. GREENLICK

Policy making is fraught with difficulty. The long-range results are often far afield from the original expectation. This, of course, has been conspicuous in such fields as defense, foreign affairs and economics. Serious attempts to formulate a national policy for the delivery of medical services are relatively new for the United States. Foreseeing the ultimate result of any policy decision is quite difficult. It was certainly not perceived that the laudable Flexner reform of medical education, aided and implemented by the support of medical education through research funds from the federal government, would ultimately create a crisis in the access to primary medical care. The reforming of medical education to change and shorten the medical curriculum, the creation of a "specialty" of primary family practice and the genesis of new health professionals, such as the nurse practitioner and the physician's assistant, are all attempts to ameliorate the effects of a policy decision made sixty years ago. This is not to say that the policy decision was wrong; the inference is that the ultimate results were difficult to foresee.

The past seven years have seen much activity at the federal level in attempts to make health policy. The dominant event is, of course, the modifications of the Social Security Act creating the Medicare and Medicaid programs in 1965. The size of these programs was matched by the size and acrimony of the debate

Milbank Memorial Fund Quarterly, April, 1972

preceding its passage. Parts of the Act creating these programs reflect the thoughts of those who were in advocacy, and indeed, parts of the Act reflect the thoughts of those who were in opposition. It was, in great part, an Act of compromise. Being of very broad scope, many of the provisions were without significant precedent. Many of the decisions about specific items were made with only fragmentary information, for the data were not at hand on which to base policy in a more predictive fashion. The crisis in health care followed quite promptly.

The amendments of the Economic Opportunity Act of 1966 established the authority for the comprehensive Neighborhood Health Center component of the Office of Economic Opportunity. The success or failure of this policy decision over the past five years is not at issue. However, the amount of information available to forecast the results of this innovative series of demonstrations was small indeed, and it is doubtful that what little existed was significantly taken into account in formulating the policies.

The Regional Medical Programs, as envisioned in the De-Bakey Committee Report, bear only faint resemblance to the resultant Act (PL 89–239). The Act itself, with its admonishing stricture against changing the organization of the delivery of health services, stands in contrast to the main thrust of the present program, which is, indeed, to change the organization of the delivery of health services. The Partnership for Health, Comprehensive Health Planning Act (PL 89–749), also displays a significant disparity between the intent of the original health policy and the program practice after a five-year period.

All of these programs, each a major policy decision, each problem-ridden in its execution, were entered upon with high intent but with a very small information base on which to make a decision. There are many more examples. Even a superficial review points up that the data available for decision making are not only scarce but of widely varying quality. This state of affairs leads to assertion, strong advocacy and equally strong denial. Social policy is inevitably based on ideology and not on information. Perhaps this situation is inevitable. Nevertheless, the thought recurs that perhaps more adequate sources of information about health services would lead to the formulation of more accurately predictive policy in this crisis-ridden field.

The size of the stake is huge and is rapidly increasing. The estimates made of the cost of Medicare and Medicaid prior to its implementation in 1966 and the subsequent cost overruns cannot help but remind one of the defense industry. The effect on state budgets of Medicaid has provoked a crisis in local financing and political recriminations that extend far beyond the health field. Some of the remedies advocated, such as institutional price controls and peer review organizations for professionals, would seem to be derived from the homeopathic philosophy.

The nation is at the beginning of a major new thrust in health policy—the era of the Health Maintenance Organization. It has been widely heralded for the past two years. It is one of the policy issues on which the President and his administration, Wilbur Mills and the House Ways and Means Committee, and Senator Kennedy all agree! Although imminent, the Congress has not yet acted on any of the many related proposals.

The name Health Maintenance Organization (HMO) is new in the past two years. Considering the state of the art, it must be considered a politicized euphemism. The vast majority of the work of any such organization that fulfills the requirements being laid down will be sickness care; and, indeed, on the assumption that man is mortal, it will probably remain so into the future. However, with that caveat, the HMO is intended to provide the inherent motivation for any prevention and any cost-effective disease detection that exists.

Inasmuch as the term Health Maintenance Organization is not self-revealing as to the concepts implied, it is necessary to make them more explicit. The noun in the term Health Maintenance Organization is "organization," and the first provision is that there be an organization of comprehensive medical services with the understanding of a guaranteed access to these services in relation to medical need. The second provision is that of an enrolled population that has had a choice of systems of medical care and has voluntarily chosen the HMO.

Finally, the costs of all care are to be mutualized among the defined population so that a total budget is funded. The budget is then paid by contract to the providers of care, both professional and institutional, who, in turn, agree to deliver their respective services for an agreed-upon-in-advance capitation. The resultant dynamic is to convert morbidity from its usual status as an asset of the providers to the status of a liability to them. Hence, the provider, like the consumer, has his economic interest in morbidity prevention. Thereby the rather optimistic name of Health Maintenance Organization.

The President, in his health message of November 18, 1971, states:[1]

> In recent years, a new method for delivering health services has achieved growing respect. This new approach has two essential attributes. It brings together a comprehensive range of medical services in a single organization so that a patient is assured of convenient access to all of them. And it provides needed services for a fixed-contract fee which is paid in advance by all subscribers.
>
> Such an organization can have a variety of forms and names and sponsors. One of the strengths of this new concept, in fact, is its great flexibility. The general term which has been applied to all of these units is HMO—Health Maintenance Organization.
>
> The most important advantage of Health Maintenance Organizations is that they increase the value of the services a consumer receives for each health dollar. This happens first because such organizations provide a strong financial incentive for better preventive care and for greater efficiency.
>
> Under traditional systems, doctors and hospitals are paid, in effect, on a piecework basis. The more illnesses they treat—and the more service they render—the more their income rises.
>
> This does not mean, of course, that they do any less than their very best to make people well. But it does mean that there is no economic incentive for them to concentrate on keeping people healthy.

A fixed-price contract for comprehensive care reverses this illogical incentive. Under this arrangement, income grows not with the number of days a person is sick but with the number of days he is well. HMO's therefore have a strong financial interest in preventing illness, or, failing that, in treating it in its early stages, promoting a thorough recovery and preventing any reoccurrence. Like doctors in ancient China, they are paid to keep their clients healthy. For them, economic interests work to reinforce their professional interests.

And the House Committee on Ways and Means in its report to the Congress states:[2]

Your committee believes that a serious problem in the present approach to payment for services in the health field, either by private patients, private insurance or the government, is that, in effect, payment is made to the provider for each individual service performed, so that other things being equal, there is an economic incentive on the part of those who make the decisions on what services are needed to provide more services, services that may not be essential and even unnecessary services.

A second major problem is that, ordinarily, the individual must largely find his own way among various types and levels of services with only partial help from a single hospital, a nursing home, a home health agency, various specialists and so on. No one takes responsibility, in a large proportion of the cases, for determining the appropriate level of care in total and for seeing that such care, but no more, is supplied.

The pattern of operation of Health Maintenance Organizations that provide services on a per capita prepayment basis lends itself to a solution of both these problems with respect to the care of individuals enrolled with them. Because the organization receives a fixed annual payment from enrollees regardless of the volume of services rendered, there is a financial incentive to control costs and to provide only the least expensive service that is appropriate and adequate for the enrollee's needs. Moreover, such organizations take responsibility for deciding which services the patient should receive and then seeing that those are the services he gets.

Secretary Elliot Richardson, in the White Paper of May, 1971, after reiterating in similar words the idea and motivation of HMO's, describes the findings that interest the government in this form of organization.[3]

> In contrast with more traditional and alternative modes of care, HMO's show lower utilization rates for the most expensive types of care (measured by hospital days in particular); they tend to reduce the consumer's total health-care outlay; and—the ultimate test—they appear to deliver services of high quality. Available research studies show that HMO members are more likely than other population groups to receive such preventive measures as general checkups and prenatal care, and to seek care within one day of the onset of symptoms of illness or injuries.

The sources cited for these conclusions are from the studies of Denson, *et al.,* and Shapiro, *et al.,* and from the Social Security Administration, Office of Research and Statistics on the Medicare Program.

In his remarks before the American Hospital Association in Chicago on August 24, 1971, the Secretary stated: "I am firmly convinced that at this time, no alternatives are superior to ours in the strength of their base of knowledge. . . ."[4] The Secretary, however, clearly pointed out the state of the art in this manner:[5]

> I should like to say, however, in passing, that our proposals evolved out of an examination of literally hundreds of options. And one of our judgmental criteria was: how far may we go with an option given our state of knowledge.
>
> In some instances, we found the knowledge to be extensive, sufficiently so to propose sweeping changes. In other instances, we were brought up sharply by the taut reins of ignorance. We were wary then, and are wary now, of panaceas calling for universal and abrupt changes, where the base of knowledge is so fragile it can support little more than fancy.

The American Medical Association is, however, unconvinced. In its publication on Health Maintenance Organizations of May, 1971, quoting its testimony before the Senate finance Committee on H.R. 17550, the Association states:[6]

> We believe that cost and utilization data should first be developed with control demonstrations testing the capability of such a

program to accomplish its purpose. There are questions regarding in-fact cost savings, as well as the quality of health care which may be provided when there are economic incentives to providers to reduce utilization.

These statements, that of Secretary Richardson as to no alternatives being superior in regard to the strength of the base of knowledge, and the American Medical Association's forthright skepticism, rather well stake out the ground of debate on the validity of the HMO strategy. Many secondary grounds of debate concern financing, tactics of promotion, what manner of organizations might qualify and many other derivative issues, but all pend on the nature of evidence that the HMO is, indeed, a better way.

As previously mentioned, the name Health Maintenance Organization in its present connotation is new in the past two years. However, the notions that lie behind the name are not new. It is always hard to say when ideas originate, and, in fact, they often keep being reinvented. The President, in his health message, cited the idea's being present in ancient China, and inasmuch as this has been oft cited over the years, there may be some substance to it. A Chinese scholar, however, and one professionally engaged in working with these concepts, has stated that he has had great difficulty authenticating any widespread use of the notion in ancient China.[7] Medical mutuals and "Friendly Societies" with similar ideas did indeed exist in the nineteenth century in Europe and the lands that had been colonized by Europeans.

The most significant, reasoned and detailed approach in the United States stems from the series of reports of the Committee on the Cost of Medical Care, reporting from 1927 to 1932, that advocated prepayment and group practice as specific policies for rationalizing the American medical care system.[8] The professional founder of the Kaiser Foundation Medical Care Program, which dates back to 1933, has reported that he was not influenced by this report, inasmuch as it did not come to his attention until many years after the program he founded was already successful.[9] Perhaps this offers a lesson for those who spend considerable portions of their time sitting on committees studying health policy. Theoretical hypotheses are often of little avail without viable examples.

Most of the prototype organizations that now would qualify as HMO's had their origins in the 1930's and 1940's, and most of the evidence in regard to cost and utilization comes from those organizations. They have been known as prepaid group practices. Each was involved in controversy from its origin. Organized medicine, which would now like to develop controlled demonstrations, originally was restrained from annihilating them only by federal and state Supreme Court decisions. The American Medical Association arrived at an alleged neutral position with the Larson Committee Report of 1959.[10] Many of the constituent medical societies, however, have taken much longer to arrive at such a neutral position, if indeed they have.

None of this long debate appeared to influence the federal government in arriving at a Health Maintenance Organization policy. It was only with medical care cost escalation and the resultant budgetary dilemmas, particularly as they affected the Medicare and Medicaid programs, that the executive and legislative branches of the government became sensitized and aware of any options.

The Medicare law, as passed in 1965, mentioned prepaid group practice and capitation payment as a result of the prepaid group practice organizations' efforts to modify the law to allow their usual manner of program function. However, to this day, and despite several modifications of the law, the prepaid group practice programs remain functioning on a cost reimbursement basis, a process quite at variance with prospective budgeting.

The attempts, however, to make the Social Security Administration and the Congress aware of these difficulties and the resultant data comparing the health care utilization of the elderly under these programs with the national averages proved to be a very salutary exercise. It is largely on the basis of these data and the data flowing from the Federal Employees Health Benefits Act of 1959 that the federal government became aware of its option. Reports of various study groups and commissions have underlined these differences,[11] but if it were not for the involvement of the Congress with the funding of its own creations, sensitivities to such reports would be markedly less.

As these data developed year after year, together with conceptual arguments to elucidate why such data resulted from these programs,[12] government authorities became progressively more interested. When, finally, in July of 1969, the President proclaimed a health crisis and called for significant innovation in the health care system, the examination of options became inevitable. The approach of the prepaid group practices was clearly being advocated as the solution to the American health care crisis. What was the information on hand at that time concerning prepaid group practices on which sufficient judgments about HMO's could be made? What was the quality of the data? What information might have been available, considering the state of the art, and in what way might the state of the art be advanced in a practical manner to significantly contribute to policy making? Examining the state of the art relative to social policy concerning the HMO is instructive in assessing data needs in health policy generally. Certainly many of the questions are the same and many of the data are equally available.

Evaluating the effectiveness of a medical care form, such as prepaid group practice, requires the measuring of that form's performance against its stated goals.[13] In medical care the goals are to reduce morbidity, minimize disability and avoid premature death. Measuring effectiveness has two components. The first is the measurement of the technical performance of the system. The second assessment relates to measuring the form's acceptance; how well, for example, prepaid group practice has gained acceptance by the population and by the providers of care. Unfortunately, research in each of these areas has been limited, and it has been difficult to draw any definitive conclusions.

Donabedian indicates that the evaluation of quality can proceed by evaluating the structure, process and outcome of the medical care system.[14] It is possible to use this framework in the assessment of effectiveness of prepaid group practice. This type of evaluation does not answer specific questions about the health of the populations of prepaid group practice programs. Rather, it asserts that when an appropriate structure and an appropriate process are developed and certain outcomes can be observed, these outcomes will affect positively the health of the population. This approach seems reasonable, but the ultimate evaluation, of course, must determine if belonging to a prepaid group practice program improves the health status of the population enrolled. Little evidence exists that personal health services provided in any current system materially affect the health status of populations. The scientific problems of measurement and the difficulties of experimental design in medical care are constraints.

We are left with the assessment of structure, process and a limited outcome in evaluating prepaid group practice relative to the remaining medical care systems. For example, it has been argued that integrating care in a hospital-based system, providing the centralization inherent in the use of a single medical record and making available all needed resources under central administrative control provide the potential for making appropriate services available at all times. If there are no financial barriers to care and if all appropriate services are available, an increased probability exists that care will be of adequate quality.

Further, it is argued that the medical care system can be organized to minimize the motivation for physicians to proceed inappropriately. It can avoid, for example, providing financial incentives to unnecessarily hospitalize patients or to perform unnecessary surgery. In prepaid group practice the relation between the financing system and the organization of medical care is critical in structuring the environment to avoid motivtion for such undesirable behavior. The capitation payment to physicians, by providing the group a fixed income for each person enrolled in the system, is designed to facilitate use of appropriate service.

It has been asserted that in prepaid group practice the colleague interaction is an important determinant of quality, even though little experimental evidence exists concerning this point. Such factors as the ready availability of all specialties, the ease of consultation and the easy exchange of information can be viewed as positively influencing the quality of care. On the other hand, it has been argued that social pressure can be applied for inappropriate behavior as well as appropriate behavior in an organized situation. In the highly structured situation of group practice organizations, attitudes, good or bad, concerning quality and appropriate utilization of services will be reflected in the practice pattern of physicians.

In a tightly knit prepaid group practice structure, it is simple to institute peer review on the behavior of individual physicians. The providers of care have to use and see each other's work because of the unit medical record. It is assumed that this unit record leads to better quality. In the unorganized system, records are maintained by one man and are not subject to the critical review of general use, except in the hospital. The contemporary demand for peer review has caused county medical societies throughout the country to attempt to develop peer review mechanisms in the solo practice, fee-for-service system.

Differential outcomes resulting from the process and structural differences in prepaid group practice systems appear as utilization pattern differences. In particular, there is a reduction in surgery on patients of prepaid group practice physicians and some increases in the use of preventive services. Donabedian, for example, has concluded that tentative evidence indicates that unjustified surgery tends to be less frequent in a prepaid group practice program.[15] He refers particularly to the much lower tonsillectomy rates in prepaid group practice in the federal employees health benefit program. He cites differences in overall hospitalization rates and in rates for surgical procedures among group practice patients. He further cites data indicating that preventive services are used more frequently by members of prepaid group practice programs, particularly higher utilization for cervical cytology examination and more appropriate use of general and prenatal checkups among members of the group practice plans. A higher proportion of group practice members make contact with a physician each year, thereby increasing the probability of preventive care. Data are limited in these areas, however, both with regard to behavior within the prepaid group practice program and to data deriving from the solo practice, fee-for-service system.

As has been mentioned many times, most Kaiser physicians are either board certified or board eligible and the system's hospitals are all approved by the Joint Commission for the Accreditation of Hospitals. This is true to a varying degree in other group practices. These are structural features generally considered to be related to quality. Also, Kaiser, HIP and increasingly other prepaid group practice plans have research units that continually assess various aspects of system performance and feed results back into the system. Such systematic research is rarely attempted in other segments of the medical care system because neither a defined population base nor an integrated unit record system are available. This type of research provides at least the potential for assessing and therefore affecting quality.

In evaluating the effectiveness of the prepaid group practice organizations, assessment of the acceptance factors is certainly indicated. How does participation in this system affect satisfaction with medical care by both the patients and the providers of care? Evidence on consumer and professional satisfaction is fairly scanty, although work has proceeded since Friedson's classic work.[16] It is possible, however, to make two broad generalizations about this question of consumer satisfaction. First, the great majority in any medical care system appear to be fairly well satisfied with the health services they have. In addition, there appears to be a hard core of the dissatisfied, perhaps as high as ten per cent, who dislike many things about the medical care system in which they participate.[17]

The major problem in evaluating consumer satisfaction with prepaid group practice programs is the difficulty of answering the question: Compared to what? Significant dissatisfaction with the arrangements of medical care is being expressed throughout the United States. Significant numbers have no arrangements. Various consumer-oriented groups have been attacking much of the medical care system, but, particularly, they have been raising questions concerned with participant satisfaction.

The statement has been made that members of the Kaiser Foundation Medical Care Program are generally satisfied with their medical care system. The system serves more than two million members, having had a very high growth rate. The dual or multiple choice requirement of the Kaiser Program indicates this growth is based on periodic individual decisions and not on majority action of groups. On the other hand, prepaid group practice programs have not attained this high growth rate in some parts of the country.

A survey recently completed on a sample of the Kaiser membership in Portland indicates significant general satisfaction with the medical care system, but also indicates the pervasiveness of certain typical criticisms.[18] A large proportion of people interviewed recalled they joined Kaiser because of recommendations from friends or relatives. Generally the participants' motivation for joining Kaiser was financial rather than a view that the organization of care was significantly better than care in the community in general. These data may indicate that the total coverage of services at a reasonable premium is the prime attraction of the system. After receiving service in the system, the members appeared relatively satisfied with the quality of care, the cost, the facilities and the physician characteristics generally, but appear to express some dissatisfaction with particular system characteristics, including waiting time for an appointment. Less than six per cent suggested that Kaiser physicians were not as good as physicians outside of Kaiser, whereas nearly twenty per cent felt they were better. The majority said they were about the same.

The above data are generally consistent with Donabedian's conclusions that the majority of subscribers to group practice plans are satisfied with their plan in spite of the substantial differences in the various plans. He points out that the subscribers who complain about medical care have a great many things about which to complain. He states that an appreciable proportion of complaints made by subscribers of prepaid group practice plans are applicable to medical care generally.[19]

The existence of an organized system provides the capability of changing the factors causing unhappiness among consumers of care. The Group Health Cooperative in Seattle, for example, is controlled by an active consumer board that is greatly concerned with matters of consumer satisfaction. The role of the consumer in the development of this prepaid group practice program has been well detailed by MacColl.[20]

The basic belief in the consumer's right to purchase his preference has been put forth as important in controlling provider behavior. However, because the supply of medical care practitioners is relatively tight, the right to withhold his dollar from the providers of services if dissatisfied is a very weak control. The potential exists for organized consumer groups to influence the behavior of the medical care system and to increase satisfaction within the system. This is one of the goals of health maintenance organization development. The federal legislation pending is likely to have mandates for consumer involvement in the planning and provision of services in HMO's.[21] Consumer control has been more or less implemented in the Office of Economic Opportunity (OEO) Neighborhood Health Center projects, but the score has not yet been tallied on the relation between consumer satisfaction and the degree of consumer influence and control in the system. It is possible that the level of patient satisfaction is no different in organizations controlled by consumers than in organizations controlled by the suppliers of care.

Data are almost nonexistent concerning the satisfaction of physicians in prepaid group practice, and it is nonexistent concerning the relative satisfaction of the other personnel in the system. Some feel that, in general, physicians participating in prepaid group practices are satisfied with this type of arrangement. Conceptually, at least, group practice is designed to increase physician satisfaction. The freedom from concern with the mundane business operations of medical practice, the ability to arrange hours and to limit the excessive burdens of long night and weekend calls, the ready availability of various fringe benefits and the easy access and social support of working with a group of esteemed colleagues combine to make group practice an apparently favorable work environment. Whereas the reports from medical directors of prepaid group practice organizations in the 1950's and early 1960's reflected the difficulties of recruiting adequate physicians,[22] recent reports indicate recruiting is only difficult because of the present inadequate supply of physicians in certain specialty fields of practice. Recruitment of physicians for prepaid group practice programs has become relatively successful.

Published data, again from the Kaiser-Permanente medical care system, indicate a low turnover rate for physicians once they become involved with the program. The Kaiser medical care system is organized by contracting for medical services with autonomous partnerships of physicians, the various Permanente Medical Groups. The partnerships hire new physicians as salaried employees for periods from two to three years. At the end of this probationary period, acceptable physicians are taken into the partnership. Data for the years 1966 through 1970 from the Permanente Medical Group indicate an average turnover rate of less than ten per cent per year for employed physicians in the probationary period and less than two per cent per year for the partners.[23]

A recent study published by Smith is one of the few to even explore the attitudes of other personnel in prepaid group practice programs.[24] This study does not provide the basis for comparison, but there is little reason to believe that personnel would be any less satisfied working in hospitals or ambulatory care facilities associated with prepaid group practice programs. Certainly the availability of pension and other benefits and the stability of working in a large organization might increase satisfaction for most.

In general, much work remains to be done in assessing acceptance factors. Particular attention should be paid to the concomitant relation between satisfaction and the behavior of patients and providers within the system. It might be possible to evaluate the acceptance factors of prepaid group practice programs and other medical care systems, differentiating those factors that relate to the financing of the system from those that relate to the organization of care.

Much of the social policy discussion concerning the HMO is brought about because of asserted economic advantages of the prepaid group practice arrangements. These arguments can only be assessed in light of the evaluation of the efficiency of this form of organization. In a review of economic research in group medicine, Klarman points out that the expected savings from group practice medicine might include two major components: economies of scale in the production of services and a lower rate of hospital utilization widely associated with the prepaid form of group practice.[25] However, to adequately evaluate the efficiences of prepaid group practice, it is necessary to assess the total input needed to produce required services for a population of given characteristics. Prepaid group practice should be viewed as a medical care delivery system that accepts responsibility for the organization, financing and delivery of health care services to a defined population. The attainment of this definition ought to set the bounds for this evaluation.

There is little reason to believe that the contributions of prepaid group practice in the efficiency of medical care would be from efficiencies of scale. Efficiencies of scale, deriving from internal operating efficiencies of a medical care organization, ought not be expected to provide a significant magnitude of savings even if they do exist. For example, there is no reason to believe that a prepaid group practice system could produce a single unit of hospital care more economically than another hospital of the same size. Nor is there even reason to believe that the prepaid group practice system could produce any single doctor office visit more cheaply than other practitioners.

Nevertheless, the expenditures for producing medical care services for a total population covered by prepaid group practice programs are less than the expenditures for care to similar populations covered in the traditional solo fee-for-service system. These expenditure differences arise from what can properly be called the "system efficiencies" of prepaid group practice. The reductions in expenditure for the care of total populations derive from many sources. It is clear that the populations covered by prepaid group practice programs use fewer days of hospital care per person in the population than do similar populations in the community system, even when utilization outside of the system is taken into account.

The organization of the total medical care system, including financing factors, medical practice factors, facility supply factors, all act in the same direction to maintain the lower use of hospitals by the total population. By integrating fiscal responsibility with the organization of medical care, prepaid group practice can reduce incentives for the physician or the population to prefer that inappropriate services be provided on an inpatient basis. Services in or out of hospital are financed in the same manner. The full range of services can be made available within a prepaid group practice program, so that physicians and population find inpatient, ambulatory care, diagnostic and most other services equally available.

The impact of these phenomena can be seen in historical data from Kaiser, Portland.[26] As the cost per day of hospitalization rose in the Kaiser Hospital in Portland from $13.23 per patient day in 1950 to $54.80 per day in 1966, paralleling the national increase, the cost of hospitalization per member year increased from $12.53 in 1950 to $27.31 in 1966. A four-fold increase per patient day was reflected as a two-fold plus increase in cost per member per year because the use of hospital days per person per year in the population decreased concurrently. It is this difference in the rate of increase in cost per day and cost per person per year that accounts for the difference in the cost of hospitalization for the Kaiser-Portland population relative to the remainder of the community.

A similar perspective must be taken to evaluate the potential of prepaid group practice programs for appropriate use of manpower in the United States. Bailey questions the relative efficiency of group practice in the production of medical services by relating the number of ancillary personnel per physician and the number of visits per physician in various sizes of group practice.[27] However, the more relevant measure, and the one that really defines the impact of the system efficiencies, is the number of physicians and other personnel required to provide the total medical care services for a population.

Stevens has estimated the number of physicians that would be needed to provide medical care to the American population, other things being equal, if the relative ratio of physicians to population for the United States totally was equal to that of Kaiser-Portland.[28] He estimates the need to be ten per cent fewer physicians than were, in fact, available in the United States.

These data were not meant to imply that it would have been possible to provide care for the total population of the country in a Kaiser-like system, but rather to point out the possibility of other solutions to the problem of the current disequilibrium in physician services other than simply increasing the number of physicians. The study is cited here to point out the difference between Bailey's approach of evaluating efficiency by looking at efficiencies of scale and Stevens' approach of assessing "system efficiencies." Stevens asks, "What are the inputs necessary to provide service to the entire population?" and not, "What are the inputs necessary to produce a given unit of service?"

Data are now available that bear on the magnitude of outside utilization in Kaiser, and particularly in Kaiser in Portland. The above-mentioned survey of members of the Health Plan in Portland gathered information on the outside utilization of members. Preliminary tabulations of these data indicate that about ten per cent of the population had at least one use of outside medical care services in the twelve months preceding the interview. A characteristic use was for the member new to the system to use his old source of service for a minor problem. These services accounted for considerably less than ten per cent of the total services used by the population, and a significant portion was for services paid for by and known to the medical care system.

Critics have asserted that the use of hospitalization in prepaid group practice programs represents an underutilization of hospital services. Considering that the technology has not yet been developed to appropriately measure differences in health status in populations, it can only be said that the population using medical care services in prepaid group practices with a hospital base of two beds per 1,000 does not appear to be any less healthy or appear to have any higher mortality rates, than do populations receiving hospital care in a system utilizing four hospital beds per 1,000. In contradiction to more equating with better, one must be cognizant of the risk of iatrogenic, hospital-based disease.

It is quite clear that two different forms of organization are envisaged in the Health Maintenance Organization concept. Prepaid group practice is obviously the dominant idea, and the data derived to support the HMO have been derived from prepaid group practice, as seen in the Secretary's White Paper.[29] Further, in speaking of the HMO concept, the President has referred to "one-stop shopping" as part of it. Obviously, "one-stop shopping" in regard to the HMO can only mean the centralized, integrated, organized group practice model.

However, another model is extant—the medical foundation, or decentralized model, in which services are rendered in each individual physician's office. The medical foundation model quite clearly stems from experience of the San Joaquin Medical Foundation. This program, founded by the San Joaquin Medical Society under the leadership of Dr. Donald Harrington, dates from 1954. Part of the impetus for its creation stems indirectly from prepaid group practice. The International Longshoremen's and Warehousemen's Union on the Pacific Coast had initiated a coastwise contract for prepaid group practice for its members who lived in areas where prepaid group practice was available (the major West Coast ports) with service starting in January, 1950.

After a few years' experience the Union was more satisfied with the medical care provided in those areas that had prepaid group practice. In response to the Kaiser Program's being urged by the Union to extend its services to the inland Sacramento River ports in 1954, the San Joaquin Medical Society arranged the prototype of the present foundation program with representatives of this union and the employer association. The program was then extended to other groups who wished to enroll. An insurance carrier served as the intermediary, setting the premium rates and underwriting the liability.

The principles of the foundation methodology, as they evolved, included an insistence upon broad, comprehensive coverage, so that the appropriate services could be used; a fixed fee schedule acceptable to all participating physicians as full payment; and peer review of the medical performance of the collaborating physicians so that quality could be reviewed. Quality, in this context, was defined as appropriateness of the medical care process for the presumed diagnosis. Claims for services that were judged inappropriate were to be denied.

The medical foundation concept at this stage of development lacked one of the elements considered essential to the HMO concept. It had no prospective budget or capitation in which the providers are put at risk for the responsibility for the delivery of comprehensive services. There has been an experiment with this approach for "MediCal" in the past two years, with asserted cost savings to that program. On the basis of this limited operational experience as underwriters, the medical foundations have become the decentralized model of HMO. The active role of advocacy of the HMO option by the medical foundations has gained wide Congressional support.

One of the repeated statements of the administration is that there are to be possible many innovative forms of HMO. Almost every form put forward so far has been a variant of the prepaid group practice or medical foundation model, with some that seem to be combinations of the two. No totally new idea has come forward. It should be emphasized that neither prepaid group practice nor the medical foundation is a monolithic concept,[30] there being a wide range of varieties of each.

Countervailing forces are at work in the federal government in sponsorship of the HMO option. Foremost, perhaps, is the urgency to implement such a program so that this choice will be available to a significant portion of the American public in a significant number of places in this decade. This is a monumental task, and some of the difficulties have been detailed elsewhere.[31] The opposing tendency on the part of the government is to make rules and regulations sufficiently constraining so that this new system cannot be abused. The potential for abuse is significant. The abuses that have occurred within the Medicare and Medicaid programs have been well publicized, and the administrators of these programs have felt the heat of Congressional investigation. They are naturally inclined to protect themselves by creating rules and regulations that would provide meaningful control to prevent such abuse. H.R. 11728, the Health Maintenance Act of 1971, submitted by Congressman William Roy of Kansas, is quite precise in defining an HMO.[32]

The paradox, of course, is that the professional providers of health service outside of HMO's find themselves under very little control and constrained by very few rules and regulations.

In general, there is an open-ended payment system, where each piece of work performed has a "usual and customary" price tag, and the manner of enterprise is quite free indeed. The only constraint is against fraud. The providers are being asked to take advantage of the health maintenance option under detailed constraints. They are being asked to underwrite the risk financially with a prospective budget, with which most have had very little experience. Although interest is high in the HMO concept, it should not be expected that this phenomenon, like Asian flu, will sweep the country within a few months.

The public may be strongly motivated to want this type of access to organized services on a budgeted basis. But what of the incentives to the provider, particularly the professional provider, who at present has very few constraints, in either the way he practices or the way he is rewarded? Marginal economic incentives, depending on his underwriting risk, may be enough to arouse his curiosity and even enough to move professionals to apply for planning grants for HMO's. But when the totality of constraints and their implication become clear, the enthusiasm for operations may diminish.

Certainly, to many in the profession the decentralized model of HMO, the medical foundation, seems a much less radical transformation of their present way of practice. However, a hard look at past experiences in this realm is not encouraging. The Medical Service Bureaus in the Pacific Northwest were prototype HMO's created in response to the depressed financial circumstances of the 1930's. Underwriting commonly resulted in the payment of a pro rata reduction of the nominal fee schedule. This made for unhappy physicians. The physician tended to distinguish the patients who paid him a full fee from those who returned to him a pro rata reduction or discounted fee. Characteristically the latter fee was distinguished as a second-class fee, and, hence, the patient became, pari passu, a second-class patient. This made for unhappy patients as well as unhappy physicians. Although these early models were not exact prototypes of the present day HMO, their operational similarity was close enough to be a warning as to the generalization of this phenomenon.

It has been often asserted that these medical care systems cater essentially to the working populations; that the socio-economic population distribution is truncated because the very poor and the wealthy are not included. Particularly if poor populations are excluded, HMO's are not likely to have widespread significance in solving the problems in universal access to medical care.

Population groups covered by most group practice programs in the United States were enrolled through occupational groups. Since 1950, health care entitlement has usually been a fringe benefit of employment. The early history of most of the prepaid group practices in existence is dominated by the enrollment of large groups that formed the nucleus for the growth of that program. HIP was stimulated almost entirely by enrollment of city employees in New York. The Kaiser Foundation Health Plan of Oregon was dominated early by its relation with the longshoremen's union; Community Health Association in Detroit by the United Auto Workers, and the Group Health Association of Washington, D. C., by the federal employees.

Although most of the prepaid group practice programs have diversified their memberships and now provide service to members of all of the socioeconomic classes, the distribution of members is not yet equivalent to the general community distribution. Those without entitlement by employment are underrepresented. This, of course, is true of all health insurance in this country.

The prepaid group practice programs gained experience in dealing with federal funding agencies because of Medicare. A significant proportion of the membership of various programs was over 65 years of age, and it was necessary to develop a modus operandi for collecting governmental payments for the provision of services. The process was initially difficult, as previously mentioned, because the federal government could not deal with capitation payments.[33]

When the amendments to the Economic Opportunity Act were passed in 1966, establishing authority for the Neighborhood Health Center component of OEO, two prepaid group practice programs, the Medical Foundation of Bellaire, Ohio,[34] and Kaiser, Portland,[35] were funded as OEO Neighborhood Health Centers. These group practice programs offered the poor an opportunity to participate in established medical care systems already delivering health services to a diverse group in the same geographic area.

This approach was significant because it obviated the time, expense and complexity of building, staffing and organizing new and segregated medical care facilities for the poverty group. The group practice organizations indicated that facilities already existed in many poor areas that could be utilized for the provision of health care services for the indigent. These programs demonstrated the feasibility of organizing and delivering health care through existing medical care systems although it was necessary to finance care from the public sector.

The two programs appeared to succeed in their objectives,[36] and other prepaid group practice programs have developed ways to provide medical care to poverty groups, including the Group Health Cooperative of Seattle, the Kaiser Foundation of Southern California and Hawaii, the Group Health Association of Washington, D. C., the Community Health Association of Detroit, the Harvard Community Health Foundation, and HIP. There is little reason to believe that the prepaid group practice programs cannot accept a proportionate share of the indigent population into their system. What appear necessary are financing mechanisms that are flexible enough to deal with the capitation form of payment and stable enough to produce continuity of membership.

A genuine concern of the medical foundation type of HMO is its ability to deliver health services to the urban poor. The centralized prepaid group practice model of the HMO quite clearly can create a Neighborhood Health Center and organize services to be delivered to whatever population lives in proximity, and this has been demonstrated, although on a limited scale because of the inability to obtain the financing for a massive test.[37] The problem with the decentralized foundation model is that the individual physicians have largely left the ghetto area in which the urban poor reside, and therefore physical access to the physicians, who are in numbers in suburbia, has little practicality for this population.

For HMO's in general the critical deficit of the poor is their lack of effective entitlement. The nature of Medicaid financing, creating large local tax burdens, constrains the program from implementing the original intent of Title 19. If the costs of the population to be served in an HMO must be mutalized on an equitable basis and the Title 19 mechanism is inadequate, the disadvantaged will be excluded. Only by falling back upon the much larger base of direct federal revenues can the poor effectively participate in HMO programs.

For an HMO to function on a forecast budget and make comprehensive services available on a continuous basis to those who recognize themselves as members of such a program, there cannot be any "on-again-off-again" eligibility status. Eligibility and membership must be on the same basis as most negotiated groups and the federal employees, with the opportunity for enrollment and disenrollment being usually no greater than annual. The difficulties cited, which are formidable, stand in the way, at this time, of general implementation of the HMO option for the impoverished, either in the form of prepaid group practice or in the form of medical foundations, unless there is, by legislation, new federal entitlement.

These options, therefore, are not completely feasible without a form of national health insurance that provides adequate financing for comprehensive medical care and provides it in such a way that eligibility is continuous and without categorization. Furthermore, the incentives for HMO's, at present, in view of the simultaneous constraints as cited above, are not so great as to produce significant change. A form of national health insurance that truly provides equal sums of monies for equal numbers of people of the same characteristics may lead to a reasonably rapid reorganization of the delivery of health services. But to expect one group of providers to accept risk, regulation and a closed-end financial system while leaving others in an unregulated, open-ended system is unreasonable.

It is interesting to contemplate the special dilemma of the medical schools and their interest in the HMO option.[38] In summary, the schools are seriously underfunded. They are dissatisfied with their organization of ambulatory care and ambulatory care teaching. On initial study of these factors, the HMO option appears as a solution to both problems. However, most schools, by tradition and location, are involved with indigent populations with inadequate entitlement. Furthermore, there is inherently little faculty dedication to the responsibilities of continuous primary care. If an HMO is to be voluntary as to membership and self-sustaining as to premiums, how are the teaching costs to be paid, in view of the competitive nature of the option? These issues have been explored elsewhere.[39]

It is clear that we need to know much more about how all HMO's operate, particularly from the consumer viewpoint. Much of the information could be gathered from the presently operating examples. Federal funding for this practical research has not been forthcoming. No agency seems to feel primarily responsible for funding such studies. But when this is accomplished in depth across large samples of the various delivery systems, policy making will be on a firmer base.

The HMO policy is thus a rather classic example of federal policy making in health. Considerable reliance is being placed on this alternate form of health services delivery system to contain the costs of health care. But the likelihood of widespread successful implementation under present circumstances is doubtful. This is not because the HMO does not have merit, but because the present fee-for-service pattern is left with most of the rewards and few of the constraints.

The total national expenditures on health care from all sources for the federal fiscal year 1974 are officially forecast at $105,400,000,000, if no new legislation is enacted.[40] All proposed new legislation increases this huge total. This is one dollar of each thirteen in the projected GNP. More people will be involved in "providing health" than in growing food. Despite the size and scope of this expenditure, it is not uncommon for physicians to express the wish that medical care were not such a political issue! It is evident that any activity taking one dollar in thirteen will remain in the forefront of political action regardless of the kind of legislation passed or not passed. An analogy may be made with agriculture. Ever since the Secretary, Henry Wallace, asked that the little pigs be destroyed, there has never ceased to be a controversy about the farm policy in Congress and in the nation, and never has a policy been produced that pleased all. Because of its size and its personal significance, "health care" will repeat this process with even greater intensity and acrimony.

Medical care research, under these circumstances, must inevitably grow and develop new sophistication and productivity. If the product of the medical care process is to be better health, then health must be defined in a way that can be better measured. A generally accepted yardstick or index of this state would be a significant advance. Measuring the outcome in terms of health by examining various medical care processes has been extraordinarily difficult. Counting the pieces of the process, the dollars, the manpower, the days of hospitalization, the office visits, the technical tests performed and so forth, has been an inadequate substitute for outcome measurement, but unfortunately reflects the state of the art.

The National Center for Health Services Research and Development, an agency of the Department of Health, Education, and Welfare, was created in 1967 to serve the nation in the function its name implies. It is apparently not a field in which quick results are to be expected. Edgar Trevor Williams, the Secretary of the Rhodes Trust of Oxford, in a speech[41] at Chicago, reviewed the role the Nuffield Foundation had played in the United Kingdom in relation to the National Health Service. It had been the sponsor of research, and then demonstration, on a scale just large enough to be significant, testing the interjection of new ideas and processes into the National Health Service. The result often so clarified an issue that it led the bureaucracy into implementing the reform on full national scale. Our National Center has not yet played this role, if this is even an expected part of its mission.

It may remain for private funds to undertake this risk-laden role. It is probably much more than coincidence that the current presidents of some of the major American foundations have been drawn from the physician leaders of medical care administration. It may be that with their support of health care research, health policy can be made from a much more secure information base in the future.

REFERENCES

[1] United States Congress, House Document No. 49, 92nd Congress, Health, message from President of United States relative to building national health strategy, February 18, 1971.

[2] ———, House, Committee on Ways and Means, *Social Security Amendments of 1971; Report on H.R. 1,* House Report No. 92-231, 92nd Congress, 1st Session, 1971, p. 89.

[3] United States Department of Health, Education, and Welfare, *Towards a Comprehensive Health Policy for the 1970's, A White Paper,* Washington, D. C., United States Government Printing Office, May, 1971, p. 32.

[4] Richardson, E. L., Remarks before the American Hospital Association, Chicago, Illinois, August 24, 1971, p. 2 (of mimeograph copy).

[5] *Ibid.,* pp. 1, 2.

[6] American Medical Association, Division of Medical Practice, *HMO's as Seen by the AMA: An Analysis,* May, 1971, p. 6.

[7] Chu, P., personal communication.

[8] Committee on the Costs of Medical Care, MEDICAL CARE FOR THE AMERICAN PEOPLE, the Final Report, adopted October 31, 1932, Chicago, The University of Chicago Press, reprinted by the U. S. Department of Health, Education, and Welfare, Public Health Service, Health Services and Mental Health Administration, Community Health Service, 1970.

[9] Garfield, S. R., personal communication.

[10] Larson, Leonard W., et al., Report of the Commission on Medical Care, JAMA, Special Edition, January 17, 1959.

[11] National Advisory Commission on Health Manpower, REPORT, Washington, United States Government Printing Office, 1967, Volumes 1 and 2.

[12] Saward, E. W., The Relevance of Prepaid Group Practice to the Effective Delivery of Health Services, The New Physician, 18, January, 1969.

[13] Greenlick, R., The Impact of Prepaid Group Practice on American Medical Care: A Critical Evaluation, Annals of the American Academy of Political and Social Science; The Nation's Health: Some Issues, 399, 100–113, January, 1972.

[14] Donabedian, A., An Evaluation of Prepaid Group Practice, Inquiry, 6, 3–27, September, 1969; , A REVIEW OF SOME EXPERIENCES WITH PREPAID GROUP PRACTICE, Bureau of Public Health Economics, Research Series No. 12, Ann Arbor, Michigan, The University of Michigan, School of Public Health, 1965.

[15] Donabedian, Inquiry, op. cit.

[16] Freidson, E., PATIENTS' VIEWS OF MEDICAL PRACTICE, New York, Russell Sage Foundation, 1961.

[17] Donabedian, Inquiry, op. cit.

[18] Pope, C. R. and Greenlick, M., Determinants of Medical Care Utilization: Selected Preliminary Tables from Household Interview Survey, unpublished report presented to Kaiser Foundation Oregon Region Research Policy Committee, San Francisco, California, June 21, 1971.

[19] Donabedian, Inquiry, op. cit.

[20] MacColl, W., GROUP PRACTICE AND PREPAYMENT OF MEDICAL CARE, Washington, D. C., Public Affairs Press, 1966.

[21] United States Congress, House, H.R. 11728, 92nd Congress, 1st Session, A Bill to Amend the Public Health Service Act to Provide Assistance and Encouragement for the Establishment and Expansion of Health Maintenance Organizations, and for Other Purposes, 1971.

[22] Saward, E. W., Experience with the Recruitment of Physicians to Prepaid Group Practice Medical Care Plans, unpublished presentation to the American Public Health Association, 90th Annual Meeting, Miami, Florida, October 17, 1962.

[23] Cook, W. H., Profile of the Permanente Physician, in Somers, A. R. (Editor), THE KAISER-PERMANENTE MEDICAL CARE PROGRAM: A SYMPOSIUM, New York, The Commonwealth Fund, 1971, p. 104.

[24] Smith, D .B. and Metzner, C. A., Differential Perceptions of Health Care Quality in a Prepaid Group Practice, Medical Care, 8, 264–275, July–August, 1970.

[25] Klarman, H. E., Economic Research in Group Medicine, NEW HORIZONS IN HEALTH CARE: PROCEEDINGS OF THE FIRST INTERNATIONAL CONGRESS ON GROUP MEDICINE, Winnipeg, Wallingford Press Ltd., 1970, pp. 178–193.

[26] Saward, E. W., Blank, J. D. and Greenlick, M., Documentation of Twenty Years of Operation and Growth of a Prepaid Group Practice Plan, *Medical Care*, 6, 231–244, May–June, 1968.

[27] Bailey, R. M., Economies of Scale in Medical Practice, in Klarman, H. (Editor), EMPIRICAL STUDIES IN HEALTH ECONOMICS, Baltimore, The Johns Hopkins Press, pp. 255–273.

[28] Stevens, C. M., Physician Supply and National Health Care Goals, *Industrial Relations, A Journal of Economy and Society*, 10, 119–244, May, 1971.

[29] United States Department of Health, Education, and Welfare, *op. cit.*

[30] Steinwald, C., *Foundations for Medical Care*, Blue Cross Reports, Research Series 7, Chicago, Blue Cross Association, August, 1971.

[31] Saward, E. W., The Relevance of the Kaiser-Permanente Experience to the Health Services of the Eastern United States, *Bulletin of the New York Academy of Medicine*, 46, 707–717, September, 1970.

[32] United States Congress, House, H.R. 11728, *op. cit.*

[33] Wolkstein, I., Incentive Reimbursement and Group Practice Prepayment, PROCEEDINGS OF THE 19TH ANNUAL GROUP HEALTH INSTITUTE, Washington, D. C., Group Health Association of America, 1969, pp. 92–100; West, H., I. Group Practice Prepayment Plans in the Medicare Program, *American Journal of Public Health*, 59, 624, April, 1969; Newman, H. F., II. The Impact of Medicare on Group Practice Prepayment Plans, *American Journal of Public Health*, 59, 629, April, 1969.

[34] Goldstein, G., Paradise, J., Neil, M. and Wolfe, J., Experiences in Providing Care to Poverty Populations, PROCEEDINGS OF THE 19TH ANNUAL GROUP HEALTH INSTITUTE, *op. cit.* p. 74.

[35] Colombo, T., Saward, E. and Greenlick, M., The Integration of an OEO Health Program into a Prepaid Comprehensive Group Practice Plan, *American Journal of Public Health*, 59, 641, April, 1969.

[36] Greenlick, M., Medical Service to Poverty Groups, in Somers, *op. cit.*, p. 138.

[37] Colombo, Saward and Greenlick, *op. cit.*, pp. 641–650.

[38] Danielson, J. M., Director, Department of Health Services and Teaching Hospitals, Association of American Medical Colleges, personal communication, July 14, 1971.

[39] Saward, E. W., Some Caveats for Medical Schools, in Somers, *op. cit.*, pp. 183–188.

[40] United States Department of Health, Education, and Welfare, A STUDY OF NATIONAL HEALTH INSURANCE PROPOSALS INTRODUCED IN THE 92ND CONGRESS: A SUPPLEMENTARY REPORT TO THE CONGRESS, Washington, D. C., July, 1971.

[41] Williams, E. T., speech given at the American Hospital Association Convention in Chicago, Illinois, August, 1971.

HMOs, Competition, and Government

RICHARD McNEIL, Jr.

ROBERT E. SCHLENKER

This article considers the role of three sets of forces affecting the development of health maintenance organizations (HMOs) during the early 1970s: legal restrictions, market conditions, and the federal government's policy stance. Our review of the evidence suggests that the rapid increase in the number of HMOs during this period was primarily due to favorable market conditions in certain areas of the country combined with a highly encouraging federal policy toward HMOs. Legal restrictions do not appear to have been as serious a barrier to HMO development as was earlier believed.

In 1973–74, major new legislation was enacted at both the federal and state levels, ostensibly to encourage HMO development. Our review of this legislation suggests that, while it removes many of the old legal requirements which apparently were not serious barriers to HMO development, the new legislation imposes a host of new conditions and requirements on HMO participation in the health care marketplace. Ironically, some of these new features may impede the operation of the very market forces which encouraged the earlier HMO growth.

In 1970 the term Health Maintenance Organization (HMO) was coined, and HMOs were loudly and widely proclaimed as a major component of a new federal initiative to "restructure" the medical care delivery system.[1] Much of the HMO concept's appeal was based on evidence that HMOs could offer their members comprehensive care at lower costs than conventional fee-for-service

---

[1] The sine quà non of an HMO is prepayment for medical care in contrast to the fee-for-service mode's use of postpayment. More specifically, we define an HMO as an organization which accepts contractual responsibility to assure the delivery of a stated range of health services, including at least ambulatory and in-hospital care, to a voluntarily enrolled population in exchange for an advance capitation payment, where the organization assumes at least part of the financial risk or shares in the surplus associated with the delivery of medical services. This definition includes many of the so-called "foundation-type HMOs." The federal HMO strategy was officially unveiled in a March 1970 statement by Robert H. Finch, then Secretary of HEW (Lavin, 1970). President Nixon's February 1971 Health Message to Congress strongly reinforced the HMO strategy as a major federal initiative. Later that year, an HEW White Paper called for a national goal of 1,700 HMOs in operation by 1980 (HEW, 1971:37).

M M F Q / Health and Society / *Spring 1975*

providers.[2] But just as important, HMOs were also seen as offering benefits extending beyond their membership in the form of a strong competitive stimulus for improved performance by the traditional fee-for-service sector. Competition from HMOs would, it was asserted, improve the efficiency of health care delivery and help contain rapidly rising medical costs for everyone. By the same token, most HMO advocates recognized (Havighurst, 1970; Ellwood et al., 1971) that effective competition from fee-for-service providers would be an important incentive for HMOs to maintain high-quality standards.

From the vantage point of the early 1970s the outlook for HMO development was mixed. On the one hand the cost and price record of the "prototype HMOs" relative to the fee-for-service delivery method indicated HMOs could compete effectively in the health care market. Yet on the other hand, the establishment of HMOs appeared to be blocked in many areas by consumer ignorance of the HMO concept, provider hostility, and what were thought to be serious legal barriers to HMO development created by various state and federal laws and practices.

In this article we examine two aspects of HMO development. First, we note the rapid recent growth in the number of HMOs and attempt to determine the relative importance of *market, legal*, and *policy* conditions in influencing this rapid HMO growth during the 1970–73 period.[3] We find that the available evidence is consistent with the hypothesis that the number of HMOs has grown primarily in response to favorable market conditions and high-level-policy encouragement from the federal government. Legal conditions, with two exceptions, do not appear to have greatly retarded HMO formation.

Second, in light of these results, we evaluate the major changes in legal conditions which occurred during 1973 and 1974.

[2]These contentions were supported by data on "prototype" HMO-like organizations such as the Kaiser Foundation Health Plan, the Health Insurance Plan of Greater New York (HIP), Group Health Cooperative of Puget Sound, and the Foundation for Medical Care of San Joaquin County. See, for example, Donabedian (1969) and Greenberg and Rodburg (1971); the most recent comprehensive review of HMO performance is by Roemer and Shonick (1973).

[3]Our definitions of "*market, legal,* and *policy* conditions" are given in the text which follows.

We conclude that while most of these new laws—ostensibly aimed at encouraging HMOs—do remove some legal barriers, they replace them with new ones. Paradoxically, the new laws intended to encourage HMOs may ultimately be more detrimental than those they replace.

HMO Growth in the Early Seventies[4]

As a starting point in examining HMO development, Table 1 summarizes our estimates of the increasing number of operational HMOs in recent years. In this table, in most of the data which follow, California is distinguished to highlight special trends in that state.[5] Table 1 shows that the number of operational HMOs has increased dramatically since the end of 1969. For the country as a whole, the number of HMOs increased fivefold in just five years. This precociousness is even more impressive in light of the length of time involved in starting an HMO. InterStudy's survey data indicate that for HMOs becoming operational during 1970–73, this process took about two and a half years.

Total HMO enrollment in the country was around five million in mid-1974, of which nearly 70 percent was in the two largest organizations, the Kaiser Foundation Health Plan and the Health Insurance Plan of Greater New York (HIP). Almost half the HMOs had fewer than 5,000 enrollees. Thus, while enrollment trends will become a major indicator of HMO success or failure over the long run, at this stage we feel it most appropriate to focus on the growth in the *number* of HMOs.

[4]Much of the information for this article (InterStudy, 1973–74; Schlenker, Quale, and McNeil, 1973; Schlenker, Quale, Wetherille, and McNeil, 1974; and Schlenker, 1974) is taken from InterStudy's ongoing program of HMO research.

[5]California's uniqueness stems, among other things, from a long history of HMO presence in the state (notably Kaiser) and from its Medicaid (Medi-Cal) policy which, in contrast to other states, encourages recipients to obtain their medical care from HMOs (or, as they are called under Medi-Cal, Prepaid Health Plans, PHPs). Considerable controversy surrounds this aspect of Medi-Cal, and many contend the program lacks appropriate safeguards for both the Medi-Cal recipients and the state. Supporters maintain (Medical Care Review, 1973) the program has been very successful in restraining the previously uncontrolled costs of the program.

TABLE 1

Estimated Number of Operational HMOs
(at End of Each Year)

	1969	*1970*	*1971*	*1972*	*1973*	*1974*
Total						
Number of HMOs	37	41	52	79	133	183
Percentage increase over previous period	—	11	27	52	68	38
Total excluding California						
Number of HMOs	21	25	34	51	75	102
Percentage increase over previous period	—	19	36	50	47	36
California						
Number of HMOs	16	16	18	28	58	81
Percentage increase over previous period	—	—	13	56	107	40

Conditions Influencing Recent HMO Growth

Although the number of HMOs has grown rapidly, Table 1 masks considerable variation across geographical areas. We have attempted to analyze these variations to assess the relative importance to HMO development of various legal, market, and policy forces. Because of the time lag involved in HMO start-up, we concentrated on conditions in existence around 1970–71.

Legal Conditions

As of August 1973, 25 states had one or more HMOs in operation. We compared this group of states to the 25 states without HMOs for those laws usually cited as barriers to HMO development. Since very few states changed these laws prior to 1973 (and many states still have not changed), a comparison of the two groups of states should give some indication of the influence of these state laws on HMO development. Table 2 shows that while there are some differences in legal conditions between the HMO and non-HMO state groups, there are no clear differences in the frequency

TABLE 2

State Laws Affecting HMOs[a]

	Strict insurance regulation	Some insurance regulation	Physician control	Open physician panel	Nonprofit only	Advertising prohibited	Professional corporate restriction	Certificate of need: outpatient	Certificate of need: inpatient
Total number of states with provision	3	33	14	9	40	15	3	11	20
By subgroup:									
25 states with HMOs	0	18	6	2	22	8	2	8	14
25 states without HMOs	3	15	9	7	19	7	1	3	6

[a]These laws are those usually cited as legal barriers to HMO development. "Insurance regulation" requires HMOs to meet various financial reserve requirements, although, in contrast to insurance companies, HMOs provide services and not dollar payments. "Physician control" refers to laws which require that physicians constitute all or a part of an HMO's controlling body. "Open physician panel" provisions are a part of some states' Blue Cross enabling act and require an HMO to allow the participation of any physician in the HMO. "Nonprofit only" indicates a requirement that a key component of the HMO (usually the plan entity) be organized on a nonprofit basis. "Advertising prohibited" indicates that the HMO cannot advertise its benefit package and rates. "Professional corporate restriction" indicates a restrictive application to HMOs of laws controlling the incorporation of physician groups. "Certificate of need" laws are discussed later in the text; basically, they require governmental approval prior to certain changes in services or expansion in facilities. For more details, see Schlenker et al. (1973: Chapter III).

with which the laws thought to severely restrict HMOs appear in the two groups.

This table shows that HMOs succeeded in becoming operational in states with every legal barrier except "strict insurance regulation." (We found only three states which we considered as having such regulation, Alaska, Nebraska, and North Carolina. As we shall see, other conditions could well be responsible for the absence of HMOs in these states at the time of the study.) State laws requiring "physician control" and "open physician panel" are the only legal conditions which seem to associate with complete HMO absence.[6]

InterStudy's mid-1973 survey of operational HMOs also indicates that these legal conditions are less important in limiting

[6]State legal conditions could, of course, slow the growth in the number of HMOs and affect their organizational form; and this would not be revealed by our comparison. For example, InterStudy's mid-1973 survey suggests that HMOs adopt special organizational forms to avoid laws against for-profit operation. Nearly half the HMOs indicated they were "nonprofit" but had for-profit subsidiaries.

HMO formation and development than originally believed. We asked HMO administrators to cite the factors they perceived as significant barriers to their HMO's formation and growth. Three-fourths saw gaining access to employer and other potential member groups as their most serious formation and growth problem. The second most serious formation barrier was opposition from other providers, followed by problems of obtaining financial support. For growth barriers, obtaining financial support was second, and provider opposition third. The fourth most serious barrier for both formation and growth was expanding physician staff. A legal barrier was, in general, felt by HMOs to be only the fifth most serious formation or growth barrier they faced.

Market Conditions

In contrast to legal conditions, market conditions seem strongly related to the presence or absence of HMOs in a state. The HMO and non-HMO state groups reveal striking differences in a number of variables indicating demand, supply, and price conditions in the medical care marketplace. Table 3 presents the averages of a group of these variables for the two groups of states. The data indicate that states with HMOs, as compared to the states without HMOs, tend to have higher incomes, larger and more urbanized populations, more physicians per capita, higher hospital costs per day and per capita, and greater public and private insurance expenditures. While such differences are, of course, far from conclusive, they are consistent with the hypothesis that HMOs will locate where they can best compete with the conventional medical care delivery system, and that they can best compete where consumers spend considerable amounts on medical care (and especially on hospital care) through insurance, out-of-pocket expenses, and taxes for government medical assistance programs.

Legal and Market Conditions in Urban Areas

State data provide only gross measures of conditions affecting HMO development. Local area conditions may be much more important. To explore this issue we have made a preliminary examination (Schlenker, 1974) of both legal and market conditions during the 1971–73 period in Standard Metropolitan Statistical

TABLE 3

HMO and Non-HMO State Group Comparison
for Selected Market-Related Variables

Variables	Average for HMO States	Average for Non-HMO States
Demographic-Economic[a]		
1. Total population, 1970	5.3 million	2.8 million
2. Population density per square mile, 1970	225	64
3. Percent of population in urbanized areas, 1970	59	30
4. Mean family income, 1969	$11,341	$9,570
Health Resources and Expenditures[b]		
5. Patient-care physicians per 100,000 persons, 1970	126	93
6. Short-term hospital beds per 1,000 persons, 1971	4.1	4.5
7. Hospital costs per day, 1971	$84	$67
8. Hospital costs per person, 1971	$94	$77
9. Insurance premium per person under 65, 1970	$105	$90
10. Medicare payments per enrollee, 1970	$328	$277
11. Medicaid payments per inhabitant, fiscal 1971	$27	$16

[a]These data are all from the 1970 U.S. population census.

[b]The physician data are from *Distribution of Physicians in the U.S., 1970* (American Medical Association, 1971); the hospital data are from *Hospital Statistics, 1971* (American Hospital Association, 1972) and the *U.S. Statistical Abstract 1972;* insurance data are from the *1972-73 Source Book of Health Insurance Data* (Health Insurance Institute); Medicare data are from *Medicare; Reimbursement by State and County, 1970* (HEW, SSA, Office of Research and Statistics, 1973); and Medicaid data are from *Medicaid and Other Medical Care Financed from Public Assistance Funds: Fiscal Year 1971* (HEW, SRS, National Center for Social Statistics, 1972).

Areas, SMSAs. A comparison of averages for SMSAs with HMOs versus those without revealed the same general pattern for legal and market variables as just presented for the state comparisons.[7] Further, regression analysis indicated that SMSA population size and hospital expenses per patient day were highly significant and positively related to the probability of both HMO presence and new HMO formations in an SMSA. At the same time the legal

[7]Legal conditions, of course, continued to be measured at the state level; each SMSA therefore took on the values of the legal variables of its state.

variables indicating open-physician-panel and control requirements were significant and negatively related to these probabilities. These results are consistent with our earlier findings; in particular, the strong relationship between hospital costs and HMO presence and formation supports the hypothesis that HMOs thrive where they can best compete with other providers by reducing the use of high-cost hospital care.

The regression analysis also indicated the importance of HMO presence in an SMSA prior to 1972 as a predictor of new HMO formation during 1972–73. In other words, once one or two hardy HMOs broke the ice, others tended to follow. Three quarters of the HMOs formed in 1972–73 located in SMSAs which already had one or more HMOs at the end of 1971. This phenomenon of innovation followed by imitation is quite common in a competitive market economy and was noted long ago by Schumpeter (1934). The new HMOs might have followed older ones because conditions favorable to the early HMOs also appealed to later entrants (perhaps more so because of the earlier HMOs' success in overcoming initial obstacles). Or, new HMOs might have followed because the early HMOs posed a competitive threat to other providers, causing them to retaliate by forming their own HMOs. In either case, the phenomenon of innovation followed by imitation lends support to the hypothesis that the pattern of HMO development represents a response to salient conditions in the marketplace.

Other data also support the "market response" explanation of HMO growth. InterStudy's 1973 survey of HMOs revealed, for example, a significant increase in the frequency of Blue Cross/Blue Shield sponsorship of HMOs over the 1970–73 period. This suggests that during this period the Blues may have been "testing the water" with HMOs and responding to a perceived competitive threat from HMOs to their traditional market position. Also, the sponsorship of HMOs by private corporations increased during the same period and this too could be interpreted as a response to market incentives by a group which was in the past usually outside the health care delivery field but tends to respond to market incentives. Finally, physician groups became increasingly involved in HMO sponsorship, especially during 1972–73, perhaps partly in response to the competitive threat posed by new HMOs sponsored by others.

Policy Conditions

Of the conditions which we examined as potential influences on HMO development, "policy conditions" are the most difficult to specify. By that term we mean the posture, other than as expressed in law, which government adopts toward HMOs within its jurisdiction. We distinguish "policy conditions" from "legal conditions" because "policy" is not always embodied in law, especially in the case of a new phenomenon such as HMOs. As we use the term, "policy conditions" indicates a general "governmental acceptance factor" which in turn is indicated by, for example, funding, promotional efforts, and speeches and writings by governmental authorities.[8]

An examination of the status of state and federal policy toward HMOs during the period of rapid HMO development in the early seventies suggests that federal policy probably had a very encouraging effect on HMO development, and that state policy, except in California, probably had very little influence on HMO development.

Federal policy. A federal policy of HMO encouragement manifested itself in two ways during 1970–73. The first was strong public statements endorsing the HMO concept. As noted above, the administration first officially outlined its HMO strategy in March 1970 and reinforced this in 1971 with presidential message and an HEW White Paper. These actions prompted wide discussion of the HMO strategy in the professional literature, (see Lavin, 1970; Ellwood et al., 1971; Saward and Greenlick, 1972). This rhetorical initiative undoubtedly raised the legitimacy of HMOs and suggested that more substantive federal assistance would soon be forthcoming.

The second manifestation of the positive federal policy toward

---

[8]It is also convenient to distinguish between "legal" and "policy" conditions because we are considering both state and federal government. State government has until recently had very little "policy" toward HMOs in the sense of a considered stance toward encouraging or discouraging HMO development. Yet as we have seen above, a number of states had laws which affected HMOs, even though those laws were typically enacted for other purposes. In contrast to the states' "law without policy," the federal government initially had a considered, coherent policy of encouraging HMOs but only limited federal law affecting HMOs.

HMOs during 1970–73 was modest funding. From fiscal year 1971 to 1973 the federal government expended $28 million in grants and contracts related to HMO development (HEW, 1974b). Of this amount, $12 million was used to finance resource development and technical assistance for organizations not directly involved in the provision of prepaid health services. The remaining $16 million went to direct planning and development grants to 79 organizations, of which 17 were operational by March 1974. Also during fiscal years 1971–73, ten additional operational HMOs received some form of technical assistance from HEW. The direct impact of these funds was modest. Federally funded HMOs account for only a small part of the HMO growth over those years, and the funded HMOs' existence cannot be attributed in most cases solely to federal funding. However, the funding and highly visible oratorical activity together were taken by many to presage greater federal encouragement of and assistance to HMOs in the future, and many organizations were thereby prompted to go ahead with HMO development.

State policy. In contrast to the clearly favorable federal policy, it is difficult to identify a state policy toward HMOs, much less to evaluate its influence. With the exception of California noted above, most states do not seem to have had a "policy" toward HMOs until at least 1973. As we have seen, most states have applied certain laws to HMOs which were thought to hamper HMO development. But the piecemeal application of these laws— which had been typically enacted much earlier with far different organizations in mind—hardly indicated anything as organized and coherent as the term "policy" implies. If anything, these laws suggest that until very recently most states have not had a "policy" of encouraging or discouraging HMO development.

HMO Development in 1970–73, in Summary

The main conclusion we derive from the legal, market, and policy data is that HMO formation and growth during 1970–73 was primarily a response to favorable market and federal policy conditions. In short, federal policy provided an encouraging backdrop, and HMO development then proceeded in those areas where HMOs could best compete with other providers.

This is not to say that legal conditions were unimportant, but they do not appear to have been as detrimental to HMO formation as was initailly assumed. However, in late 1973 and early 1974 major legal changes occurred at both the federal and state levels, heralding a new phase in HMO development. We turn now to consider these new legal conditions in light of the 1970–73 experience.

New Laws Affecting HMOs

Nineteen seventy-three and early 1974 brought much new HMO legislation at both the federal and state levels. Given the importance of market conditions which seems indicated by the evidence just presented, the standards for evaluating this new legislation must, in our view, also be market-related. Our concern is not simply whether these new laws will encourage or discourage HMO development, but whether these new laws will encourage or discourage *fair market competition* in the medical care delivery system by allowing HMOs and the fee-for-service mode to compete on equal footing and without compromising medical care quality. The basic principle underlying a fair-market-competition standard is that obstacles which unfairly bar HMO entry into the medical care market should be removed, but that HMOs should not receive any special advantages (such as undue subsidization) relative to the rest of the medical care delivery system. This standard has been well articulated in the recent policy statement on HMOs by the Institute of Medicine of the National Academy of Sciences (1974).

Certainly, "fair market competition" is not a completely objective standard. Reasonable people can differ as to whether specific laws are preferential to one group or not. In our estimation, most new HMO legislation reflects the view that competitive market forces cannot be relied on to ensure adequate medical care quality from HMOs. To varying degrees, the new laws constrain the HMO's cost-containment incentives in an attempt to protect the consumer against quality reductions. The evidence on this point to date is mixed, but suggests the danger is minimal. Studies of prototype HMOs have not found inferior medical care, and have often found the opposite (Roemer and Shonick, 1973). On the other hand, allegations of poor quality do surround some of the new

California PHPs. As the discussion below suggests, in our view most of the new legislation sacrifices too much in potential cost containment to gain quality safeguards, many of which may be either unnecessary of ineffective. The primary effects of many of these so-called safeguards may be, unfortunately, to slow the process of HMO formation and to raise the cost of HMO care (perhaps above competitive levels for a large segment of the market) without significantly increasing the consumer's protection against inferior medical care.

A further drawback of many of the new laws is that the beneficial requirements they do impose on HMOs are not also imposed on their competitors (insurers and providers). We hope, however, this imbalance will only be temporary, and future programs such as national health insurance will require all health care insurers and providers to adhere to minimal-quality and consumer-safeguard standards.

The discussion below considers first, at the state level, HMO enabling acts, certificate-of-need laws, and Medicaid. We will then turn to federal laws, specifically to Medicare and the HMO Act of 1973.

State HMO Enabling Acts

As pointed out earlier, in most states the piecemeal application to HMOs of various laws which were enacted with far different organizations in mind hardly constitutes anything as organized and unambiguous as a "policy." It was partly to correct this problem that state HMO enabling acts were advocated and passed. As reported by Holley and Walker (1974a; 1974b), by mid-1974, 17 states had such laws; seven states enacted their legislation in 1974, seven in 1973, two in 1972, and one in 1971.[9] In addition, similar legislation was pending in several other states.

While it is too early to determine the effect of these new laws on HMO development, our analysis suggests that their contribution to HMO development will be mixed. On the positive side,

[9]The states included in this list, with the year of enactment in parentheses, are: Arizona (1973), Colorado (1973), Florida (1972), Idaho (1974), Illinois (1974), Iowa (1973), Kansas (1974), Kentucky (1974), Michigan (1974), Minnesota (1973), Nevada (1973), New Jersey (1973) Pennsylvania (1972), South Carolina (1974), South Dakota (1974), Tennessee (1971), and Utah (1973).

most enabling acts require the state to monitor the quality of care the HMO delivers, require HMOs to have an established mechanism for processing enrollee grievances, and require some form of enrollee participation in the HMOs' policy-making body. All these seem to be positive provisions for protecting consumer interests. In addition, nearly all of the enabling acts also release HMOs from restrictions on advertising and the corporate practice of medicine, though these restrictions do not seem to have greatly burdened many HMOs.

However, the new enabling laws also impose new and more burdensome requirements on HMOs which probably will not advance consumer interests. For example, several states' enabling laws impose financial-reserve requirements on HMOs similar to those applied to insurance companies. While appropriate for insurers, these requirements are not appropriate for an HMO, which contracts to provide medical services and not dollar benefits. Some enabling laws also require state approval of an HMO's rates; most fail to exempt HMOs from certificate-of-need laws, which were designed for traditional hospitals (and are further discussed below). Several laws also require HMOs to have various open-enrollment provisions, which can be expected to significantly increase an HMO's costs and decrease its ability to compete, since few states impose analogous requirements on insurance companies or traditional providers. Few state enabling laws have "dual choice" [10] provisions, which would increase HMOs' access to the market, and in only one state to date (Michigan) does the dual-choice provision apply to more than state employees.

In our view, many of these regulatory requirements will do little to protect consumers and will unnecessarily limit opportunities for HMO development. For instance, in Arizona the HMO enabling act imposes new requirements of $50,000 deposits and $100,000 reserves per HMO and a 1 percent tax on net charges. These requirements hindered at least one organization in its efforts to form an HMO. Yet while imposing these financial requirements, the Arizona enabling act is silent in the areas of quality monitoring, grievance procedures, and enrollee participation in policy making.

---

[10] "Dual choice" is a provision requiring employers to offer employees an option to apply their health benefits to either an HMO or a conventional health insurance plan. As discussed later, this is a key provision of the federal HMO Act.

Nevada is another example. In the regulations evolving from the enabling act, fledgling HMOs are required to have a minimum net worth of $100,000; purchase a surety bond of not less than $250,000; maintain a blanket fidelity bond of at least $1,000,000; and establish a monthly reserve equal to 3 percent of collected enrollee payment. These new requirements appear to have driven two formational plans from the market and threaten the continued operation of a third. Thus, paradoxically, in many states an HMO "enabling act" may not increase the consumer's protection from shoddy HMOs or encourage fair competition between HMOs and other modes of health care delivery, but may instead decrease the likelihood of effective competition from HMOs.

State Certificate of Need Laws

Certificate-of-need laws require hospitals and certain health facilities to obtain approval, a certificate of need, from a regulatory authority prior to undertaking new construction or certain modifications in services.[11] These laws originated as a legislative response to the continuing increases in the cost of hospitalization. Advocates of certificate-of-need legislation saw these cost increases as a result of several factors: oversupply of hospital beds, the overutilization incentives of third-party cost reimbursement, and the excessive zeal of nonprofit hospitals in undertaking new capital expenditures for elaborate but economically inefficient facilities. Twenty-three states had certificate-of-need laws as of January 1974, and most of these were applied to HMOs. Judging by the number of certificate-of-need bills now pending, it seems very likely that more states will be adopting certificate-of-need legislation in the future. In addition, as of April 1974, 32 states had reached agreements with the federal government for implementation of Section 1122 of the 1972 Social Security Amendments (P.L. 92-603), which in effect establishes a certificate-of-need requirement under federal law for Medicare and Medicaid reimbursement of capital costs.

Although the rationale for and probable effectiveness of certificate-of-need laws in curbing hospital costs is not the subject

[11]An analysis of these laws, with particular attention to their potential impacts on HMOs, can be found in Havighurst (1973; 1974).

of this article, they have been questioned (Havighurst, 1973) by others. The applicability of such laws to HMOs rests on even weaker logical footing, since the central characteristic of the HMO is its incentive to minimize the cost of needed medical care. An HMO's viability depends on its ability to *compete* with other providers. However, it seems likely that the very forces within the traditional system whose stubborn resistance to efficient utilization and cost considerations brought on the passage of certificate-of-need laws in the first place will eventually control the control mechanism. When those controls are then applied to HMOs as well, the outcome is likely to be a reduction of effective competition from HMOs and other innovative health delivery approaches.[12] Anecdotal evidence suggests that this has already occurred in some states.

While most of the HMOs InterStudy surveyed in mid-1973 had formed before many certificate-of-need laws were in operation, many had felt the inhibitory force of these laws on their growth. In states with certificate-of-need laws in effect or pending, 48 percent of the responding HMOs cited such laws as moderate or severe barriers to their growth. Although the overall impact of certificate-of-need laws remains to be seen, it appears unlikely at this point that they will contribute to fair market competition.

Medicaid

Although Medicaid is a joint federal-state program, most of the responsibility for program operations is lodged at the state level. The 1969 Social Security Act Amendments made approving mention of prepayment plans for providing Medicaid services, but participation by HMOs in Medicaid was complicated by requirements that all Medicaid eligibles in a state were to receive the same scope of services, that those services were to be available throughout the state, and that Medicaid eligibles be allowed to choose where they would receive their medical attention. The 1972 Social Security Act Amendments (P.L. 92-603) allowed the states to waive these requirements. Unfortunately, specific regulations

---

[12]Professional Standards Review Organizations (PSROs) are another control mechanism subject to this danger, since providers from the traditional system will be able to rule on the "quality" of care provided by their competitors in HMOs and elsewhere.

for implementing the Medicaid-HMO provisions of the Amendments were not proposed until 1974 (Federal Register, 1974b), suggesting a less than maximal effort to encourage HMOs to participate in Medicaid.

In view of these facts it is not surprising that HMO participation in Medicaid is not great outside of California. According to the responses of 112 organizations to InterStudy's July 1974 enrollment survey, about 6 percent of the about 5 million HMO enrollees are Medicaid recipients. Although nearly half the HMOs in that survey had some Medicaid recipients enrolled, over half of these HMOs were in California. However, as discussed below, the attractiveness to HMOs of participation in Medicaid may increase as the result of the preference given by the federal HMO Act of 1973 to HMOs with Medicaid members.

If Medicaid participation does increase, this will not necessarily mean an improvement in fair market competition among delivery systems. The states vary considerably in the requirements they impose on both HMOs and fee-for-service providers. Oregon and Maryland illustrate (HEW, 1973) the different financial incentives states provide for HMO participation in Medicaid.

In Oregon an HMO must absorb all financial losses and can keep none of any savings it achieves, while in Maryland an HMO bears no losses and can receive half the savings. Measured against our view of fair market competition, both methods err, although in opposite directions. Oregon may be too harsh on HMOs; Maryland too lenient. To be consistent with our fair market standard, an HMO should absorb any loss it incurs in meeting its contractual obligations. By the same token, when an HMO can meet its obligations at an agreed-upon capitation rate, the HMO should be allowed to retain any savings. Unfortunately, this ideal is not yet a part of the Medicaid program.

Medicare

As noted above, historically most of the important laws affecting HMOs were at the state level; the emphasis has now shifted to the federal level. The remainder of this article focuses on the two most important recent federal actions affecting HMOs: recent Medicare modifications and the 1973 HMO Act. Our subsequent discussion draws heavily on the work of McClure (1973; 1974) and the Institute of Medicine (1974).

Medicare is presently the federal government's largest health program. As with Medicaid, HMO involvement in Medicare has not been extensive. While close to half (46 percent) of the 112 HMOs responding to InterStudy's mid-1974 survey enrolled Medicare beneficiaries, these beneficiaries accounted for less than 5 percent of all HMO members. In our view, the Medicare program fails to meet fair-market-competition criteria, but for different reasons than the laws previously discussed. This is best shown by an examination of Medicare's policies for HMO reimbursement. Although only one reimbursement method is in use now (under section 1833 of the Social Security Act), two additional alternative reimbursement methods were authorized by Section 1876 of the 1972 Social Security Amendments; but regulations for these methods were still being developed in early 1975.

The "old" cost-reimbursement method. HMOs now enrolling Medicare beneficiaries are reimbursed on a cost basis. Reimbursement must be related to the allowable costs of providing covered services. The HMO neither absorbs any losses nor obtains any surpluses and thus has no financial incentive to provide care efficiently to Medicare enrollees.

The "new" cost-reimbursement method. Under the new cost-reimbursement method provided for by the 1972 Social Security Amendments, an HMO can be paid an advance capitation payment for both parts A and B of Medicare. However, this mechanism is still essentially cost reimbursement, because the capitation payment will be *retrospectively* adjusted to reflect the HMO's Medicare-allowable expenses for providing care to beneficiaries. Again the HMO can neither keep any savings nor sustain any losses.

The risk-sharing reimbursement method. The other new reimbursement alternative is a risk-sharing plan which theoretically would bring an HMO's efficiency incentives partially into operation. Unfortunately, however, few HMOs will be able to qualify for participation under this arrangement in the near future. The proposed regulations (Federal Register, 1974c) provide that to be eligible for a risk-sharing contract an urban HMO must have a current enrollment of 25,000 members and have had an enrollment of at least 8,000 for each of the two preceding years. For rural HMOs the current enrollment must be 5,000 and for each of the preceding three years have exceeded 1,500. HMOs meeting these requirements are called "mature" HMOs. Other HMOs, denoted as "developing," are expected to use a cost-reimbursement method. Most of the 112 HMOs responding to InterStudy's mid-1974 enrollment survey were located in urban areas, only 18 reported an enrollment of over 25,000, and even some of these could not meet the requirement of at least 8,000 enrollees for each of the two preceding years.

Even if many HMOs could qualify for the risk-sharing method, they would have little financial incentive to do so. Under this reimbursement mechanism, any losses the HMO sustains must be borne by the HMO. However, any savings are split between the HMO and the Medicare Trust Funds, with the added stipulation that any savings beyond 20 percent of costs go entirely to the Medicare Trust Funds.

Thus, given the eligibility problems of the risk-sharing mechanism, and the small potential for financial reward it offers, we expect few HMOs to undertake that relationship with Medicare. This leaves cost reimbursement as the alternative. From our point of view, the problem with cost reimbursement is not that it is burdensome for an HMO, but that it is irrational, given the HMO's incentives.[13] Cost reimbursement treats an HMO like a fee-for-service provider, bypassing and possibly disabling the HMO's prepayment incentive for efficiency. In our estimation, this denies to the Medicare program the efficiency advantages of HMOs and will tend to subvert HMO efficiency incentives or even encourage cost maximization. It might even be possible for an HMO to use its "reasonable cost" Medicare reimbursement to subsidize its other non-Medicare enrollees and thereby gain an unfair competitive advantage over fee-for-service providers.

[13]Other federal policies have shown a greater awareness of HMOs' uniqueness. See the Cost of Living Council's regulations for HMOs (Federal Register, 1974a) under what was to be Phase IV of the Economic Stabilization Program. These regulations were never implemented.

The unattractiveness of risk sharing under Medicare is evident in data from InterStudy's July 1974 survey. Fifty-two HMOs then enrolled some Medicare beneficiaries, and 36 more intended to do so by July 1975. In all, however, only *two* of these 88 HMOs indicated they expected to participate in a risk-sharing contract. Forty-four expected to use one of the cost-reimbursement arrangements, and the remaining 42 were undecided or did not answer. While it is certainly desirable to extend the benefits of HMO services to Medicare beneficiaries, cost reimbursement will not further fair market competition between HMOs and the fee-for-service sector. This is especially ironic since the federal HMO strategy began with the proposal (Finch, 1970) to use the Medicare program as a catalyst for HMO development.

The Health Maintenance Organization Act of 1973 (P.L. 93-222)

The most significant new federal policy affecting HMOs is the HMO Act of 1973 (P.L. 93-222). The act establishes a precedent for governmental attempts to encourage structural change in the health care delivery system. Because this legislation had bipartisan support, it could legitimize and encourage many kinds of health-delivery innovations in addition to HMOs, and could thereby prove to be landmark legislation.

Since the act has been law only since December 29, 1973, it is too early to gauge its impact on fair market conditions for HMOs. Regulations have been developed only for portions of the act. Despite its recency, however, some indications of the act's impact can be gained from the statutory provisions and regulations (Federal Register, 1974d) and from InterStudy surveys of operational and planned HMOs conducted in May and July of 1974 to determine HMOs' reactions to the new law.

In examining the act according to fair-market-competition standards, we divided its provisions into four general topic areas: (1) funding, (2) consumer protection, (3) enabling, and (4) regulation. The HMO Act is worded so that it applies only to those HMOs which choose to become "certified" under the act. However, we believe (as discussed below) most HMOs will feel compelled to certify. Certification requires that the HMO be in compliance with the regulation and consumer-protection aspects of the act, and certification is required before an HMO can benefit from the act's funding and enabling provisions.

Funding. In our view, the funding aspects of the act will probably be of only modest significance. As first introduced by Senator Kennedy in Senate Bill 14, the act provided $5.2 billion for HMO development. By the time the HMO Act became law it had been pared to an authorization for $375 million over a five-year period, of which $50 million is specified for research and evaluation studies of quality assurance. Experience from 1971 to 1973 discussed above suggests that funding at this level will probably not have a major impact. This is, however, desirable under our fair-market-competition standard. Except in cases where more drastic action is necessary to bring health care to underserved groups, fair market competition requires that government policy aim at encouraging conditions which allow HMOs to enter and compete their way into the market, rather than having their way paid for them.

Unfortunately, however, the funding provisions also introduce certain market distortions. For instance, the act distinguishes between nonprofit and for-profit HMOs. The former are eligible for grants, contracts, and loans, but not loan guarantees, while the latter are eligible only for loan guarantees and then only when serving medically underserved areas. The loan program will make available federal money to nonprofit HMOs at the Treasury rate plus an add-on for administrative costs. For-profit HMOs will be borrowing private money under federal guarantee but at significantly higher market rates. This is discriminatory against for-profit HMOs and creates an incentive for new HMOs to adopt the organizational contortions we noted earlier that are presently used by many nonprofit HMOs to claim that status.

Consumer protection. We feel that in the long run the most effective safeguard for HMO consumers is the existence of fair market conditions which give consumers the opportunity to make a free and informed choice among HMOs and between HMOs and other providers. This freedom of choice coupled with programs aimed at measuring the quality of care received in *both* fee-for-service and HMO settings should ultimately be the most effective protection for the HMO consumer. However, long-run safeguards are not enough; short-run abuses should also be averted. Ideally, government intervention to protect consumers should insure against market-safeguard failures but, at the same time, should enable the market to deliver those safeguards ultimately. Achieving this ideal is a difficult balancing act. If too many safeguards are applied (as appears to be the case with many state HMO enabling acts), HMOs will be unnecessarily hindered in entering the market. If too few safeguards are used, allowing well-intentioned (or even ill-intentioned) but slipshod organizations to operate, the quality of care may suffer. We feel the consumer safeguards of the HMO Act effectively balance these two opposing forces.

Under the act, a certified HMO is required to make its services accessible and available to enrollees. When medically necessary, services must be available and accessible 24 hours a day, seven days a week. Certified HMOs are also required to have a fiscally sound operation, and adequate provision against insolvency satisfactory to the Secretary of HEW. In addition, certified HMOs must have grievance mechanisms for enrollees, and are not allowed to expell an enrollee for reasons of health status.

The act also specifies that certified HMOs must have a quality-assurance system and report pertinent data to the Secretary. While there has been little empirical evidence that the quality of HMO care is worse than the traditional system, and some evidence that it is better, there is the theoretical argument that HMOs may underserve their members. To guard against both the appearance and possibility of underservice, it is important to have quality safeguards and to concentrate on *outcome* rather than *process* measures of quality. However, since quality assurance and reporting entail additional expense and are not at this time required of other providers (PSROs may change this), and since the measurement of quality is still more art than science, we feel it is desirable to keep these requirements mimimal until all providers are required to meet them.

Perhaps one of the most powerful and simple safeguards in the act prohibits an HMO from enrolling more than 75 percent of its enrollees from a medically underserved population (where the underserved are defined to include Medicare and Medicaid enrollees). This provision will prevent HMOs from enrolling large numbers of the underserved unless the HMO has also been successful in attracting other enrollees. This consumer safeguard should strengthen market competition as well as protect the underserved.

Enabling. Besides funding, the act offers HMOs other benefits from certification. The most important (a) preempt various restrictive state laws, (b) require employers who offer their employees health plans to allow employees to apply their benefits to HMO membership (referred to as "dual choice"), and (c) allow advertising of the nonprofessional aspects of an HMO's services. We refer to these provisions as the "enabling" aspects of the act.

The dual-choice provision is of most importance to the HMOs, as evidenced in the responses shown in Table 4 of 97 operational HMOs to InterStudy's May 1974 survey on their reactions to the HMO Act.[14] Nearly two thirds of the responding HMOs indicated dual choice was a significant advantage to be gained from certification under the act.[15] Far fewer HMOs viewed the funding or preemption benefits as significant advantages.

Even with the potential gains from certification, only half the HMOs responding to the survey indicated they intended to apply for certification. Most of the rest were undecided. A major reason for this uncertainty becomes clear when one examines the regulatory aspects of the act and their potential for reducing HMOs' ability to compete effectively.

Regulation. The major regulatory aspects of the act are:

(1) A very rich basic benefit package. The HMO Act not only requires the generally recognized minimum essential benefits of preventive and therapeutic physician services, emergency and inpatient hospital services, diagnostic X-ray and laboratory services, and out-of-area emergency coverage, but also re-

---

[14]Organizations planning HMOs provided similar responses to a survey conducted in July 1974. For the sake of brevity, we report here only the results for the operational HMOs.

[15]This is consistent with InterStudy's 1973 survey results reported earlier, which indicated that HMOs perceived gaining access to employee groups as their greatest problem in forming and growing.

TABLE 4

Enabling Provisions of the HMO Act
(Percentage of Respondents Indicating Relative
Attractiveness of Selected Provisions)

Provision	*Significant Advantage*	*Moderate Advantage*	*No or Slight Advantage*	*No Response or Undecided*
Funding: grants, contracts, loans, loan guarantees	36	18	41	5
Preemption of restrictive state laws and practices	12	21	61	6
Dual-choice requirement for employers	62	19	13	6

quires that HMOs offer many other services such as short-term mental-health serivces and alcoholism and drug-abuse services. Seventy-one percent of the HMOs responding to our survey said they could not meet these requirements without increasing their present benefit package and, hence, their premium.[16]

(2) Permanent regulation. Section 1312 of the act gives the Secretary permanent regulatory power over any HMO which becomes certified. No time limit or escape clause is provided whereby the HMO could remove itself from such regulation For example, if a certified HMO (even one receiving no federal funds) found the minimum basic benefit package too highpriced and unmarketable in its service area, there is no way that it could seek relief. No such regulatory conditions have to date been imposed on health insurers or other providers.

(3) Open enrollment. The act requires that a certified HMO have an open-enrollment period of not less than 30 days a year during which it accepts individuals up to its capacity in the order in which they apply, without regard to health status. This provision could greatly increase HMO costs relative to other insurers with which they must compete, since open enrollment is

[16]The act does allow the use of co-payments for the provision of specific services, although only in very specific and limited ways.

not required of other insurers. One study (McClure, 1974) found that an HMO's costs for persons joining during open enrollment were 80 percent greater than for other enrollees.[17]

(4) Community-rate rating. Except for some administrative cost differences, HMOs are to charge the same premiums to all their members. Obviously, this means low users of services "subsidize" the high users. Such subsidization may be desirable from a societal viewpoint, but such requirements are usually not placed on insurers or other competitors of HMOs.

(5) Other miscellaneous requirements. The act also requires each certified HMO to have one third of its policy-making board be enrollees, requires that (after three years) group-practice-based HMOs obtain at least half their revenues from HMO activities, limits HMO purchases of reinsurance, and imposes other reporting, quality-assurance, and continuing-education requirements. Again, while many of these requirements are societally desirable they are usually not imposed on insurers and providers which compete with HMOs.

Obviously, meeting all the above requirements will not be costless for HMOs, and, in most cases, similar costs will not have to be borne by those who compete with HMOs. InterStudy's May 1974 survey shows that the HMOs recognize these potential problems, especially with the open-enrollment and community-rating requirements, as shown in Table 5.

In light of the cost increases likely to be caused by the richness of the basic benefit package, we were surprised that most HMOs did not see this as an important disadvantage, particularly since nearly three-fourths of the HMOs also said this would require changing their minimum-benefit package. Perhaps this optimism is based on a hope that potential enrollees will recognize and desire to pay for the increased services which the act will require.

---

[17]It is possible for an HMO to obtain a waiver of the open-enrollment requirement if it can show that open enrollment has or would result in the enrollment of a "disproportionate" number of high-risk persons which will "jeopardize its economic viability." This could mitigate the negative effect of the open-enrollment requirement, but is also gives more arbitrary power to government regulators and increases the complexity and uncertainty for HMOs in making cost projections and establishing premium rates.

TABLE 5

Regulatory Provisions of the HMO Act
(Percentage of Respondents Indicating Relative
Unattractiveness of Each Provision)

Provision	*Significant Disadvantage*	*Moderate Disadvantage*	*No or Slight Disadvantage*	*No Response or Undecided*
Permanent regulatory power given to HEW Secretary	23	26	33	18
Minimum basic benefits	12	28	58	2
Open-enrollment and community-rating requirement	40	21	33	6
Requirement that one-third of policy-making body be enrollees	18	16	61	5
Ongoing quality-assurance-program requirement	3	13	78	5
Requirement that medical group's principal activity be prepaid group practice	37	10	42	10

In sum, it seems likely that the ambivalence toward certification which many HMOs indicated in the survey is due to their reluctance to accept the burdens of the regulatory provisions of the act. This, however, raises a crucial dilemma. The dual-choice provision of the act may, in effect, compel HMOs to seek certification. The provision will require employers to offer their employees the option of joining an available certified HMO. Offering a non-certified HMO would not meet this requirement, and would probably create additional administrative costs for the employer. Thus, non-certified HMOs could have great difficulty gaining access to employer groups in areas with certified or potentially certified HMOs. HMOs may thus feel compelled to seek certification, even though certification is likely to increase their costs, possibly to the point that it will be extremely difficult to compete with traditional insurers and providers. Thus the HMO Act could well stifle fair market competition by forcing the majority of HMOs to become high-priced, "Cadillac" HMOs.

There are other aspects of the act which, while desirable on the surface, might have detrimental effects on competition. For example, the priority in funding given to HMOs which enroll the underserved may lead HMOs to seek increased Medicare and Medicaid enrollment. While this is laudable in many respects, we have indicated the pernicious incentives which Medicare's cost-reimbursement system for HMOs creates. Another potential danger is that the certification costs built into the act and the resulting increased competitive pressure could cause HMOs to underserve as a means of holding premium rates down to competitive levels. Ironically, this is precisely what those who advocated the costly regulatory requirements for certification.

While we have not discussed all the ramifications or details of the HMO Act, it is clear that the act escapes simple characterization. It has several very positive characteristics from a fair-market-competition viewpoint. It is a precedent for governmental encouragement of structural change in the delivery system to improve the market's operation. The funding provision of the act, while somewhat biased, should stimulate competition without overly subsidizing HMOs. The act also contains valuable protections for the consumer and an assist for certified HMOs by removing some of the more serious marketing and state legal barriers. However, in our view. the act has drawbacks which offset many of its positive features. While many of the regulatory provisions of the act would be desirable if applied to all health care providers and insurers, their unilateral imposition on HMOs could seriously weaken HMOs' ability to compete in a large segment of their potential market.[18]

Conclusions

No single delivery mode can incorporate incentives for achieving all the quality, cost, and distribution goals our society has set for health care delivery in the United States. Given this impossibility, we feel the best approach is a system which uses different delivery modes—based on different incentive structures—actively competing with one another.

[18]Rhode Island's recently enacted catastrophic health insurance plan law (HEW, 1974a) appears to adopt a more even-handed approach by requiring *all* insurers and providers to meet certain minimal conditions.

At this point, the future of HMOs and meaningful competition in the health sector is uncertain. Our evidence from the 1970-73 period suggests that HMOs can successfully compete with the fee-for-service delivery mode even when conditions are less than strictly fair. Now, however, the conditions for HMO development have changed. Ironically, many of the new federal and state laws which purportedly are designed to encourage HMOs may inhibit rather than promote competition and pluralism in health care delivery because those laws apply certain constraints only to HMOs.

Yet even this situation is subject to an even greater change in the conditions for competition in health care delivery. The most massive intervention in the health care marketplace yet attempted appears imminent in the form of national health insurance. This intervention presents tremendous potential for either improving or crippling effective competition in health care delivery. The uniform application to all health care insurers and providers of many of the provisions now applied solely th HMOs under the HMO Act would do much to promote effective and beneficial competition.

Richard McNeil, Jr.
InterStudy
123 East Grant Street
Minneapolis, Minnesota 55403

Robert E. Schlenker, PH. D.
InterStudy
123 East Grant Street
Minneapolis, Minnesota 55403

Research for this article was supported in part under a Health Services Research Center grant from the Bureau of Health Services Research, Department of Health, Education, and Welfare (Grant No. HS 00471-06). Paul M. Ellwood, Jr., M.D., made valuable comments on a previous draft, and the latter portion of this article draws heavily on the work of Walter J. McClure. Ph.D.

References

Donabedian, Avedis
1969   "An evaluation of prepaid group practice." Inquiry VI. 3.

Ellwood, Paul M., Nancy N. Anderson, James E. Billings, Rick J. Carlson, Earl J. Hoagberg, and Walter McClure.
1971 ''Health maintenance strategy.'' Medical Care 9 (May–June): 291–298.

Federal Register
1974a ''Phase IV Health Care Regulations.'' Federal Register 39 (March 27): 11378–11380, 11390–11393.

1974b ''Medical Assistance Program Proposed Contracting Requirements.'' Federal Register 39 (June 5): 20042–20044.

1974 ''Federal Health Insurance for the Aged and Disabled: Health Maintenance Organizations.'' Federal Register 39 (August 27): 30935–30941.

1974d ''Health Maintenance Organizations.'' Federal Register 39 (October 18): 37308–37323.

Finch, Robert H.
1970 ''Statement by Robert H. Finch, Secretary of Health, Education and Welfare, on Medicare and Medicaid Reforms.'' Washington, D.C.: Medicare and Medicaid Guide, Supplement No. 11, March 28, 1970, Commerce Clearing House, Inc.

Greenberg, Ira G., and Michael L. Rodburg
1971 ''The role of prepaid group practice in relieving the medical care crisis.'' Harvard Law Review 84 (February): 887–1001.

Havighurst, Clark C.
1970 ''Health Maintenance Organizations and the market for health services.'' Law and Contemporary Problems 35 (Autumn): 716–795.

1973 ''Regulation of health facilities and services by 'certificate of need'.'' Virginia Law Review 59 (October): 1143–1232.

1974 Regulating Health Facilities Construction (ed.). Washington, D.C.: American Enterprise Institute for Public Policy Research.

HEW
1971 Towards a Comprehensive Health Policy for the 1970's. A white paper (May). Washington, D.C.: U. S. Government Printing Office.

1973 ''Analysis of prepaid Medicaid contracts for comprehensive health benefits.'' HEW internal memo (August).

''Rhode Island Catastrophic Health Insurance Plan.'' Research and Statistics Note No. 33. Office of Research and Statistics, Social Security Administration (December 9).

1974b Health Maintenance Organization Program Status Report. Washington, D.C.: Health Services Administration, (March, processed).

Holley, Robert T., and Robert W. Walker

1974a   Catalog of 1973 State Health Maintenance Organization Enabling Bills. Monograph. Minneapolis, Minnesota: InterStudy (February).

1974b   Catalog of State Health Maintenance Organization Enabling Bills: January through June, 1974. Monograph. Minneapolis, Minnesota: InterStudy (August).

Institute of Medicine

1974   HMOs: Toward a Fair Market Test. A policy statement. Washington, D.C.: National Academy of Sciences (May).

InterStudy

1973–74   A Census of HMOs. Published quarterly by InterStudy.

Lavin, John H.

1970   "HEW's new drive to change health care delivery." Medical Economics, May 25.

McClure, Walter J.

1973   "Detrimental effects of applying the present Medicare amendments to Medicaid." Memo. Minneapolis, Minnesota: InterStudy (November).

1974   "A critique of the Health Maintenance Organization Act of 1973." Memo. Minneapolis, Minnesota: InterStudy (February).

Medical Care Review

1973   "California Medicaid." Medical Care Review 30 (March): 282–287.

Roemer, Milton I., and William Shonick

1973   "HMO performance: the recent evidence." Milbank Memorial Fund Quarterly, Health and Society 51 (Summer): 271–317.

Saward, Ernest W., and Merwyn R. Greenlick

1972   "Health policy and the HMO." Milbank Memorial Fund Quarterly 50 (April): 147–176.

Schlenker, Robert E., Jean N. Quale, and Richard McNeil, Jr.

1973   Socioeconomic and Legal Factors Associated with HMO Presence: An Examination of State Data. Monograph. Minneapolis, Minnesota: InterStudy (October).

Schlenker, Robert E., Jean N. Quale, Rhona L. Wetherille, and Richard McNeil, Jr.

1974   HMOs in 1973: A National Survey. Monograph. Minneapolis, Minnesota: InterStudy (February).

Schlenker, Robert E.
  1974   Why are HMOs in some urban areas and not in others? Minneapolis,
          Minnesota: InterStudy (November).

Schumpeter, Joseph A.
  1934   The Theory of Economic Development. Cambridge, Massachusetts:
          Harvard University Press.

The Federal Government as Venture Capitalist: How Does It Fare?

JOHN K. IGLEHART

Kaiser Foundation Health Plan, Inc.,
Washington, D.C.

I N THE ANNALS OF FEDERAL PROGRAM DEVELOP-
ment, the Office of Health Maintenance Organizations (OHMO)
is a unique enterprise. The office is charged with the specific
assignment of creating new private businesses that ultimately must
succeed or fail by their own capitalistic devices. The very notion
that government should so boldly challenge private medicine says a
great deal about its dissatisfaction with the status quo, but perhaps of
more importance now is a report on how this federal experiment in
venture capitalism is faring.

First of all, one must recognize the formidable obstacles that loom
before a government agency that strives to crack a private market.
These obstacles stem from the complex nature of government itself,
its role as a redistribution agent, and its political inclination to be all
things to all people (or at least as many as can be accommodated at any
one time). Congress posed additional obstacles by its complicated
design of the Health Maintenance Organization Act of 1973.

The HMO concept emerged as a government initiative during the
Republican administration of Richard M. Nixon. The concept proved
politically and ideologically attractive to Nixon's conservative administration because of its reliance upon financial incentives rather than
regulation to contain spiraling health-care costs, thus reducing gov-

Milbank Memorial Fund Quarterly/*Health and Society,* Vol. 58, No. 4, 1980
© 1980 Milbank Memorial Fund and Massachusetts Institute of Technology
0160/1997/5804/0656-12 $01.00/0

ernment's role. But the HMO act, as Birnbaum (1980) points out, became ensnared in inflexible language, delayed rule-making, and bureaucratic wrangling, thus complicating OHMO's role as administrator. Organizationally, OHMO is part of the Public Health Service and currently falls under the Office of the Assistant Secretary for Health, Department of Health and Human Services (HHS).

The challenge of creating new businesses is a tall order for any organization. For an agency like HHS, it was a totally foreign undertaking. Three broad social purposes dominate the works of the department: administering income transfer payments to eligible individuals (aid to families with dependent children and Social Security, for example), financing medical care for eligible elderly and poor people (Medicare and Medicaid), and awarding grants to nonprofit organizations that are engaged in activities deemed worthy of public support (medical schools, for example) but cannot conceivably generate enough revenue on their own to become self-sustaining. Thus the orientation and skills of most HHS employees do not lend themselves readily to venture capitalism.

Karen Davis, deputy assistant secretary for health planning and evaluation, and Howard R. Veit, director of OHMO, characterized OHMO's mandate in a June 11, 1980, memorandum to Dr. Julius B. Richmond, assistant HHS secretary for health and U.S. surgeon general:

> As we considered HMO legislative issues and general program direction, we continually encountered the conflict between the social goals the HMO program was endowed with at its inception and the difficult and complicated task of creating viable, self-sufficient businesses. This conflict is difficult, but not always impossible, to reconcile. In general, OHMO and OHPE [Office of Health Planning and Evaluation] have recommended protecting the social responsibility features of the HMO statutes. You should be aware, however, that the "pro-competition" proponents in OMB [Office of Management and Budget] and the Congress will attempt to weaken these aspects.

Venture capitalism is a form of private investment in which government usually plays no central role except, in select instances, one of oversight through the Securities and Exchange Commission. Venture capitalism involves individuals or organizations that invest their money in high-risk development opportunities, hoping for a high return on equity. OHMO's development activities characterize some, but not all, features of venture capitalism. OHMO invests public dollars in high-risk situations with a hope that the return for society will be the creation of private organizations that are capable of delivering quality health care at a reasonable price.

A fundamental difference between the federal funding of HMO development and of other HHS health service projects is the matter of self-sufficiency. From the outset, HMOs are expected to work toward the day when they do not depend on federal dollars to operate, except for those that pay for services rendered through Medicare and Medicaid. Virtually all other health service projects funded by HHS are expected to depend entirely on the federal dollar for survival. When federal support is removed, the projects are abandoned, except in those instances when state or local governments are willing to assume the costs.

The task of creating new HMOs has taxed the capabilities of OHMO's small staff. Initially, OHMO felt most comfortable awarding grants to HMO project applicants, but staff lacked the expertise to offer the kind of financial planning and marketing advice so critical to the success of a new prepaid group practice. But there has been progress on this front. OHMO staff is in a better position today to offer technical assistance and also it is using industry experts in financial matters to help new plans. Veit recognizes that the future of the HMO industry hinges in good part on its ability to attract capable managers to the field. Also, the General Accounting Office (GAO), the monitoring arm of Congress, has worked closely with OHMO to increase the management skills of the program and its grantees.

OHMO has evolved in its six years of operation—and countless reorganizations—from essentially a grant-making office to an office that has come to recognize, if not yet totally implement, its complex mandate. In talking with me on March 23, 1980, Veit said:

> OHMO is much more analytical now than before, much tougher in its review of grant applications. But it's difficult in our program to separate the bad risks. It's a painful process to get staff to look with discernment at potential grantees. But we strive to be unrelenting on that score because funding bad grantees today only leads to failures tomorrow.

The difficulties of creating a private business usually are a revelation to HMO grantees as well. Many of the grantees represent consumer-based organizations that do not have staffs with the necessary business background to successfully launch a new enterprise. One HMO official described this dilemma in a personal interview April 14, 1980, but did not want to be identified; Veit himself, however, also subscribes to these views:

> We've found that the health-care field is not a field that has attracted a lot of people with corporate skills. HMOs are businesses that generate millions in income and expenses. You can't have a nice guy who is a social worker running that kind of an organization. Most of our grant applications derive from community groups that are striving to change the delivery system a little. OHMO has tried to adjust to this problem by becoming more aggressive itself in seeking out organizations that have some of the necessary skills to create HMOs.

OHMO's mandate is further complicated by the conflicting nature of its several roles. Besides serving as a venture capitalist, OHMO also is charged by law with promoting the HMO concept in the hope of stimulating development through private capital and with regulating federally qualified HMOs. Thus, the OHMO must serve as the prime HMO booster and the major overseer of HMO performance— conflicting assignments that cause no end to strife within the program. A federally qualified plan is an HMO that abides by operational requirements set out in the HMO act, including the offering of a comprehensive package of benefits. In return, the act provides access to the market through a requirement that all employers of 25 or more individuals must offer their employees an opportunity to enroll in a qualified HMO if one is available in the area. HMOs that accept federal funds and become operational must seek federal qualification.

Veit's directorship also is hindered by other realities of the bureaucratic life. Almost one-third of OHMO's full-time employees—62 of 177—work in the ten regional offices of HHS. These staff members, however, report to the respective regional health directors, who, in turn, are responsible to the assistant secretary for health, not to Veit. OHMO, like most government programs, also operates under the vagaries of a political system that is constantly reordering its priorities

—not the kind of environment needed to bolster health maintenance organizations in an uncertain market. Veit (1980) referred to this problem in a speech:

> The impact of the federal program could have been greater if the government's commitment to HMO growth had remained consistently higher during the 1970s. In 1975, there were ample funds appropriated by Congress to start new HMOs. In 1976 and 1977, scarce dollars for new programs together with poor administration by HEW [now HHS] impeded growth. In late 1977, the department began to reorganize the federal program. This, plus increased congressional appropriations in 1978, 1979, and now in 1980, has allowed us to bring many more new HMOs into development.

The foregoing list of obstacles that stand before OHMO is by no means an apology for its performance. Any individual who spends time observing or participating in the life of a government program soon recognizes that things never run as smoothly as one would prefer, the staff is never as capable as it could be, and funds never seem to go far enough. OHMO is certainly no exception to this rule. The marvel, perhaps, is that OHMO has accomplished anything as a tiny outpost favoring marketplace solutions in a department that tilts to regulation.

Performance

One measure of OHMO's performance is the growth of new prepaid health plans in the 1970s, though a cautionary note seems appropriate. Most plans started with federal funds are small. And though they serve as symbols of one direction of reform favored by government—prepaid group and individual practices—their impact on the system thus far has not been dramatic. Zealous rhetorical overkill in the early days of the program, even while Congress was still debating the legislation that led to the 1973 HMO act, far surpassed what could realistically be expected to occur in the relatively short time that has passed since then. The overwhelming number of members enrolled in HMOs today belong to plans started long before the federal government began its romance with prepaid group practice.

Since 1970, the number of HMOs has increased from fewer than 30 to 230. This includes federally qualified plans and plans that have not sought qualification. Enrollment nationally in prepaid health plans, or HMOs as they have been called since the federal government got in the act, has increased from 2.9 million to almost 9 million, according to OHMO. Since 1974, the federal government has awarded grants of $130 million and committed $175 million in loans. Of the 230 HMOs that now are providing care, 113 are federally qualified, a regulatory stamp of approval affixed by OHMO that was defined earlier. Of the 113 qualified HMOs, 80 have received federal grant and/or loan assistance. Veit (1980) notes that federally assisted HMOs are "for the most part, still small and still striving toward self-sufficiency. Although the federal program has already had a considerable impact on the growth of the field, 85 per cent of all members are in HMOs that have developed privately. The federal government has, however, put in place a number of new programs that represent substantial capacity for future growth."

OHMO, not surprisingly, has encountered failure, too. Any time government intervenes in a private market, it assumes risks that private investors are generally thought to be unwilling to take. OHMO has revoked the qualification of 7 plans,[1] leaving 113 so designated.[2] Thus, the current failure rate is 6.0 percent. The overwhelming cause of failure was inadequate plan management, according to OHMO, but lack of capital and poor location also were factors.

Another relevant measure of OHMO's performance is the failure rate on loans advanced to qualified HMOs to subsidize their operations until they become self-sustaining (Department of Health, Education, and Welfare, 1979). As of January 1, 1980, the Department of Health, Education, and Welfare (HEW) had extended $157 million in

---

[1] Sound Health Association, Takoma, Washington; Central Essex HMO, Orange County, New Jersey; Health Alliance of Northern California, Los Gatos, California; ChoiceCare Health Services Inc., Fort Collins, Colorado; Gem Health Association, Boise, Idaho; Group Health Plan of New Jersey, Hudson County, New Jersey; and HMO Concepts, Anaheim, California. After they failed as separate entities, Sound Health Association was taken over by Group Health of Puget Sound and Group Health Plan of New Jersey by Health Insurance Plan of Greater New York.

[2] Regarding nonqualified plans, an informal list prepared by OHMO's division of development estimates that 60 plans have failed since records were first kept in 1970. Judith M. Mears, a lawyer for the Kaiser Foundation Health Plan who conducted a survey on failures, concluded, on the basis of a 1979 census, that a total of 174 nonqualified plans existed between 1970 and 1979. Thus, she estimated a failure rate of 34 percent for nonqualified HMOs in the 1970s.

loans and loan guarantees to qualified plans. Of that total, $6.9 million remains outstanding from the qualified HMOs that ceased operations in 1979. That amounts to a 4.4 percent loan default rate for qualified HMOs in 1979.[3]

While Mears found it possible to calculate a fairly accurate rate of both federally qualified and nonqualified HMOs, she concluded that the data necessary to compute a failure rate for small businesses or service businesses are not being collected by any private or governmental entity. The rate that business people and personnel in federal agencies attribute to the Small Business Administration (SBA) is that one of every two small businesses goes out of business within the first two years of operation, but the SBA does not use this statistic in any of its official material.

One question Congress undoubtedly will ponder in early 1981 when it considers extension of the Health Maintenance Organization Act is how to judge a failure. Can the termination of an operational HMO be judged a total failure, given the knowledge that it is a risky venture? Were there valuable lessons learned that justify the public investment? Should the federal government reduce its potential for loss by investing only in HMOs that look like sure winners?[4]

One thing OHMO has learned through the failures is that the demise of an HMO is accorded far more publicity than is the bankruptcy of most small businesses. In a story from Fort Collins, Col-

---

[3] Mears, in her survey, found that a loan default rate of 4.4 percent falls about in the middle of a list of default rates for selected federal loan programs: farm ownership, 0.1 percent; rural housing, 0.2 percent; farm operating loans, 1.0 percent; farm emergency loans, 1.0 percent; Hill-Burton loans, 1.7 percent; FHA hospital loans, 1.7 percent; health professions student loans, 2.0 percent; FHA Title II (group practice facilities and physicians' offices), 3.5 percent; Small Business Administration loans, 3.8 percent; all HUD loans, 5.4 percent; nursing student loans, 5.4 percent; economic development loans, 7.1 percent; Federal Housing Administration nursing home loans, 9.6 percent; guaranteed student loans, 11.5 percent; direct student loans, 17.4 percent; Federal Housing Administration Section 235 program loans, 19.5 percent.

[4] OHMO's current development strategy calls for placing first priority on cities where health care costs are considered above the national average. OHMO places in this category the following areas: Boston-Lawrence-Haverhill-Lowell, Massachusetts; New York City and environs; Buffalo, New York; Newark, New Jersey; Philadelphia and Pittsburgh, Pennsylvania; Washington, D.C.; Baltimore, Maryland; Atlanta, Georgia; Miami, Tampa, St. Petersburg, Florida; Chicago, Illinois; Detroit, Michigan; Cleveland, Ohio; Milwaukee, Wisconsin; Houston and Dallas, Texas; St. Louis, Missouri; and Denver, Colorado.

orado, headlined "Health Maintenance Organization Collapses as Its Doctors Drop Out," the *New York Times* reported on January 2, 1980:

> Insured medical care for 30,000 people in northeastern Colorado is ending today because almost all the area doctors abandoned the local health maintenance organization. The doctors' decision to withdraw from ChoiceCare Health Services, Inc., left subscribers scrambling for coverage, federal officials fuming and creditors holding a debt of more than $1 million.

In Veit's view, the program has not been operating long enough to accurately calculate what its failure rate ultimately will be:

> The ultimate success of the program depends on the number of [HMO] programs that are both financially viable and deliver high-quality care. Determining success rates requires many years given the long development period for an HMO. Our experience shows that it takes three or four years to become operational, and an additional four to five years to reach the break-even point. Thus, it takes seven to nine years of development before we can talk definitively about success. (Veit, 1980)

On a more pessimistic note, Veit told a newspaper interviewer, "It's a miracle that more haven't failed. Like any business, an HMO that isn't run effectively will fail. In the coming years, we anticipate 5–10 failures a year" (*American Medical News,* 1980).

One of the more interesting results of federal HMO development is the evolution of a particular model—the individual practice association, or IPA as it is known in industry parlance. When Congress designed the HMO act, it lumped under the HMO definition a form of practice in which member doctors remain in their individual offices but are compensated on a prepaid basis. IPAs are formed by solo fee-for-service practitioners as a defensive measure, in fear of the economic consequences of the creation of a prepaid group practice in their area. IPAs generally are closely affiliated with the local medical society. Private physicians have taken advantage of the availability of federal funds to create IPAs. Strumpf (1980) found that the growth of IPAs from fewer than 5 before enactment of the HMO law to 89 today stemmed largely from federal funds, in the case of 42 plans, and from support by the Blue Cross and Blue Shield Association, in 15 other instances. He said:

When development is viewed from this competitive perspective, we find that 55 currently operational IPAs developed after a PGP [prepaid group practice] was established [in the same service community].[5]

Fee-for-service physician response to the federal HMO initiative has led to the development of more new plans than has the response from the business community, despite the increasing expressions of concern by businessmen about the rising cost of medical care (Demkovich, 1980). Those corporations that have become involved in the HMO movement have done so not by sponsoring their own HMOs but rather by encouraging their employees to enroll in already operating plans.

InterStudy (1979) made this point in reporting to the Health Care Financing Administration its progress under a grant for "Stimulation of Alternative Health Care Delivery System Development": "One of the original intents of the project, actual corporate development of an ADS [alternative delivery system], was found to be an impractical alternative for most firms."

The National Association of Employers on Health Maintenance Organizations (Employee Benefit Plan Review, 1979) reported a similar conclusion in its Survey of National Corporations:

There appears to be little interest among respondents to develop their own HMOs—even though this group would have access to the necessary capital—and of the survey respondents only 4.6 percent have developed a company HMO, and 93.4 percent indicated no interest in developing one.

The Future

Congress enacted legislation in 1973 that sought to promote HMOs, but the act was so laden with costly requirements that new organizations developed under it found competing against traditional insurers

---

[5] IPAs require physicians conditioned to fee-for-service patterns to change their practice modes in order to live within the fixed budget that prepayment dictates. The Physicians Health Plan of Minnesota, an IPA organized by the Hennepin County Medical Society, published a fascinating account entitled, "A Case Study of Utilization Controls in an IPA," which details how one organization coped with the challenge. The study was prepared for OHMO under Contract No. 342804.

almost an impossible task. In two subsequent sets of amendments approved in 1976 and 1978, Congress removed some of these requirements and relaxed others in the hope of stimulating more HMO development. New provisions also were added, reflecting the critical need to train HMO managers and bolster OHMO's capacity to provide technical assistance to developing plans.

These amendments included minor changes in the mandated benefit package, relaxation of the open-enrollment requirement, higher ceilings for grant awards, extension of the loan eligibility period, establishment of an HMO management training program and a technical assistance authority. Other amendments included a new requirement for employers to arrange for HMO payroll deductions and authority for HMOs to seek payment from workmen's compensation and other insurance for enrolled members who had double coverage.

The HMO act expires September 30, 1981, and the administration now is preparing its recommendations for extension of the law. The Carter administration has been resolute in its commitment to HMO development and there is no reason to believe that the president will change course on this question, despite a view held by his Office of Management and Budget that the HMO concept has demonstrated its effectiveness and now it is time for the private sector to assume responsibility for further plan development.

The major legislative issues involved in the extension are similar to the kinds of questions debated in 1976 and 1978. Should more flexibility be included in the mandated benefit package so that HMOs can compete more effectively? Should the development authorities be streamlined so that financial assistance flows without major disruption to HMO projects? A new thrust also will impact on the 1981 debate. A small but growing number of members of Congress believe a medical marketplace virtually free of federal sanctions would be the most favorable environment in which competition could thrive. These members may strive to remove requirements such as community rating in the hope of making HMOs more competitive. Most of the HMO industry would resist such a move because of the importance of community rating as a major distinguishing characteristic of prepaid group practice, because of its value in helping to achieve financial stability, and because it provides high-risk groups better access to HMOs.

In sum, government must recognize that it has created a unique program. OHMO is charged with using tax dollars to develop new private businesses, a mandate that places the office in a role uncharacteristic of a government agency. But in carrying out this assignment, OHMO cannot in all instances be a hard-nosed entrepreneur looking for the best risk because another dimension of its mandate is to increase access to care to the most vulnerable segments of American society. Balancing these mandates in a responsible manner will be a demanding assignment even under the best of circumstances.

References

American Medical News. 1980. Lack of Good Managers Called Biggest Problem Facing HMO Industry. June 13.

Birnbaum, R. 1980. Health Care Regulation and Competition: Are They Compatible? Health Maintenance Organizations. Paper delivered at Project Hope Symposium, Millwood, Va , May 22–25.

Cassidy, R. 1980. The HMO Flop That Gave Fee-for-Service a Black Eye. *Medical Economics* 57:73–77.

Demkovich, L. 1980. Business, as a Health Consumer, Is Paying Heed to the Bottom Line. *National Journal* 11:851–854.

Department of Health, Education, and Welfare. 1979. *National HMO Development Strategy through 1988.* DHEW Publication No. (PHS) 79-50111. Washington, D.C.: Government Printing Office.

Employee Benefit Plan Review. 1980. NAEHMO Survey of Health Care Coverage and Industry Involvement in Cost Containment. April.

InterStudy. 1979. Grant Application 18-p-97019 prepared for the Health Care Financing Administration. Excelsior, Minn.

New York Times. 1980. Health Maintenance Organization Collapses as Its Doctors Drop Out. January 2.

Strumpf, G. 1980. The Present Status of HMOs. Paper delivered at a seminar on Challenge of the Next Ten Years for HMOs Sponsored by the Esselstyn Foundation, Claverack, N.Y., June 19–21.

Veit, H. 1980. Future Roles for the Federal Government in the Development of HMOs. Speech before the Group Health Institute. Boston, May 4.

Address correspondence to: John K. Iglehart, Kaiser Foundation Health Plan, Inc., 900 17th Street, N.W., Washington, DC 20006.

HMOs, Competition, and the Politics of Minimum Benefits

DONALD W. MORAN

Former Legislative Assistant to
Congressman David A. Stockman

O BSERVERS OF FEDERAL POLICY-MAKING HAVE
long noted the tendency of policy fads to acquire a long train
of fellow travelers and advocates of convenience as they march
eastward across the Potomac. Over the last seven years, for example,
the national goal of energy independence has been putatively pursued
by a mysterious coalition of corn farmers with alcohol stills, suppli-
cants to the Highway Trust Fund, and ailing automotive giants.
National security has always been a favorite, justifying everything
from welfare steamships to hothouse sugar mills. When added to the
drive for "free trade, but fair trade," any Washington lawyer worth
his salt can weave a patriotic bunting to clothe even the most humble
special interest appeal.

Health care policy, of course, has never been immune from this
sort of private interest masquerade. In the 1970s, the push for cost
containment was used to whitewash all manner of otherwise antisocial
behavior on the part of the government and the various provider
groups scrambling for the federal health dollar. Although the Congress
has apparently rejected expanded regulatory efforts designed to control
hospital costs, it still smiles daily on a wide range of appeals from
provider and consumer groups that are justified as cost-reducing
measures.

Milbank Memorial Fund Quarterly/*Health and Society*, Vol. 59, No. 2, 1981
© 1981 Milbank Memorial Fund and Massachusetts Institute of Technology
0160/1997/81/5902/0190-19 $01.00/0

In the last two years, a new banner has been raised on the federal health policy scene in the form of proposals to inject *competition* into the market for health care financing. Predictably, a wide range of interests have now taken to automatically incorporating an appeal to competition into their justifications for more even-handed (i.e., favored) treatment within the heavily regulated health care delivery structure. Given the novelty of the notion, such efforts have met with mixed success. To date, in fact, the only real victories won under the competition banner have been the growing list of dispensations—such as certificate-of-need (CON) exemption and favorable treatment under Medicare—awarded to health maintenance organizations (HMOs) because of their perceived accordance with the competitive model.

To most observers such legislation is not considered to be of a special interest nature; on the contrary, HMOs, because of their assumption of normal investment risk in the health care marketplace, are viewed as fundamental elements of the brave new world envisioned by competition advocates. The Carter administration, for example, in a position paper on competition and its role in health care, cited its efforts to foster the growth of HMOs as the main evidence of its commitment to the competitive ideal. Moreover, all the empirical evidence available to date in support of the viability of the competitive model is based on experience in those markets, such as Minneapolis and the West Coast, where the establishment of HMOs has generated economic competition between prepaid plans and the traditional fee-for-service (FFS) system. All in all, far from being just a special interest entree for HMOs, the competitive model appears to be inextricably linked to the fate of the HMO movement.

A Market of Competing Prepaid Plans

According to Alan Enthoven, the *doyen* of the "competition" movement, and many other proponents of the market strategy, a market composed solely of competing prepaid health care plans is the best feasible formulation of the strategy. In his view, the market must in fact be biased toward the formation of prepaid plans lest unique characteristics of the market for health care financing render the market strategy unworkable.

First, according to Enthoven, the market for health care services is fraught with consumer information deficiencies. In order to overcome the inability of consumers to choose between complex presentations of widely differing health insurance offerings, the market should be constrained so as to limit the number of choices to a set of roughly similar plans competing on the basis of price and quality for a standard set of benefits (1980a:81).

This, in turn, will cause the market to tend toward a structure of competing, vertically integrated provider groups. Because competitors will not be allowed to segment the market through product differentiation, only those who successfully control both investment and service utilization will survive. Explicit utilization controls, such as provider decisions to withhold or delay care, will in general be more successful in restraining utilization than more indirect methods, such as copayment requirements or deductibles that are small relative to the total cost of service. Thus, it is anticipated that comprehensive, prepaid plans will emerge the victor in any head-to-head battle with more loosely organized FFS providers once the allowable product offering has been suitably constrained (Enthoven, 1979:2, 1980a:5).

Nor, according to Enthoven (1979:4–6; 1980a:80), are information defects the sole justification for imposing minimum benefit constraints that ultimately lead to market dominance by prepaid plans. In the absence of fairly high minimum benefit requirements, the market would suffer from severe preferred risk selection. That is, low-risk persons would gravitate toward lower-option plans providing only bare-bones emergency coverage, while high-risk persons would gradually sift out into the high-coverage plans. The results would be that the insurance character of the market would be broken, and the cost of providing comprehensive benefits would soon be prohibitively high.

A related problem is that of "free riders," who could be expected to "game" the system if choices were wide and annual changes between plans were allowed. The notion is that those who are well would select low-cost coverages until such time as high-cost elective surgery or treatment were imminent. At that point, they would switch over to a comprehensive plan, receive the needed services at little or no additional cost, and then return to the low-option plan during the subsequent enrollment period. Hence, high-option plans would find themselves experiencing costs far in excess of collected premiums (Enthoven, 1979:2; 1980a:79).

In summary, Enthoven would hold that *only* a market where benefit choices were severely constrained—hence a market that would over time perforce evolve into a sort of "duelling HMO" model—can introduce competition into health care financing without creating a whole new raft of problems.

Another argument for the competing prepaid plan model of competition has been advanced by McClure (1979, IV:50–59). Noting the traditional tendency of physicians' groups to act in concert on economic issues, he raises the specter of pervasive provider collusion and subsequent market failure, unless steps are taken to prevent the providers in the community from unanimously resisting the efforts of financing plans to effect cost controls. To prevent such collusion, McClure argues that strict limits should be placed on the percentage of physicians that can be involved with any one plan in each HMO area. In addition to the effect of forestalling collusion, of course, such a step would provide a direct stimulus toward a market of competing closed panel health care plans.

These criticisms may be valid, but the legislative future of *competition* is not necessarily bright. It may well prove, as these analyses suggest, that a market of competing prepaid plans offering standardized benefit packages is the optimal form of competition. There is still, however, the question of how to get from here to there. For, while the models with which the competition notion is being sold are, at the least, internally consistent, the same cannot be said of the *political process* through which any solution of this sort would be implemented.

If anything, the track record of the Congress to date suggests that the key design elements of the new market system the rules by which providers compete—will be the brokered outcome of a process whereby existing market participants will attempt to give as little away as possible in exchange for the opportunities and problems of a more wide-open market for health care goods and services. In such an environment, I will argue, legislation contemplating a market solely composed of prepaid plans along the lines enunciated by Enthoven and McClure is the *least likely* outcome of congressional deliberation over injecting competition into the health care field.

The HMO Movement:
Competition with Whom?

One major reason why a market composed solely of competing HMOs is unlikely to be generated by an act of Congress lies in the fact that

HMOs will not be judged in a vacuum, solely on arguments related to the desirability of internalizing investment risk or on the incentives for HMOs to promote preventive care strategies. Rather, they will be judged on the basis of whether their track record to date offers strong and compelling evidence that what HMOs sell is itself so inherently desirable that all other types of competitors should be barred from the race. On this point, the historical record is, at best, mixed.

The HMO movement—or more generically, the development of health care financing on a prepaid capitation basis by a closed panel of health care providers—did not begin as a competitive response to the presence of FFS practitioners; instead it began for the opposite reason: a dearth of other means of providing health care to impoverished or isolated communities.

The modern precursors were born in the slums of the eastern seaboard when mutual aid societies of ghetto immigrants pooled their resources to hire physicians who otherwise would not practice in the ghetto for financial reasons. Although such plans were common in the nineteenth century, they eventually faded away as traditional physicians, in response to the alleviation of poverty in the ethnic communities after the turn of the century, moved into these areas to establish more traditional FFS practices.

The next major growth area for prepaid plans was the physician-sparse West Coast, where the huge influx of workers to man the vital defense industries during the Second World War far outstripped the ability of local physicians to provide needed health care services. Kaiser Industries, for example, faced with a lack of adequate physician man-power to provide care for its imported workforce in its steel plants and shipyards along the coast, sponsored the establishment of Kaiser Plans in Oregon and California, with enrollment at first restricted to its own employees.

After the war, these plans went public and began to effectively compete against the traditional physician community for patients. Yet, the original motive for creation of all of these plans can hardly be described as competition for patients in the health care marketplace. Instead, the plans were at first effective natural monopolies, created because markets abhor a supply vacuum.

In fact, the only prepaid plan of any size created before 1947 in direct competition to traditional practice was the Ross-Loos Plan in Los Angeles, established in 1929. Yet, this plan neither sought nor achieved a major market share among the insured population; instead, it was content to accept those families willing to eschew the free choice of a traditional physician, offered by other insurers, in favor of the prepaid plan.

The real competitive drive for patients in these markets came, not from the prepaid plans, but rather from the traditional medical community, which viewed the prepaid plans, both from an economic and professional perspective, as threats to continuation of their prevalent mode of practice. The competitive response of traditional medicine proceeded on a number of fronts.

The most common was a long string of probable antitrust violations designed to starve the prepaid plans out of the marketplace. The Oregon State Medical Society, for example, made a habit, until admonished by the Justice Department, of expelling all members of the medical society who did business with the prepaid plans. In general, the professional response, as embodied in the American Medical Association's (AMA) Code of Ethics as early as 1932, was to declare contract practice and competition for patients unethical for a member physician and to discipline transgressions through formal and informal procedures.

It is thus ironic that organized medicine *as a body* entered into a strong economic competitive effort with the prepaid plans by promoting their own prepaid plan alternatives, generally known either as individual practice associations (IPAs) or foundations for medical care (FMC)s, to draw patients interested in prepaid plans away from the HMO heretics. A classic case in point, described by Goldberg and Greenberg (1977), is the competitive response of the local medical society to the entrance of the Kaiser Plan into the Pittsburg, California, area in 1953. Citing Gabarino (1960), they note that Kaiser's decision to appeal to the giant U.S. Steel plant in the area for enrollments produced a hurried decision to form a "Doctor's Plan" to be marketed to the employees before their deciding vote on health benefits selections. The physicians sponsored full-page newspaper ads and even went so far as to park participating doctors and their wives in the company parking lot to leaflet the membership, augmented by a sound truck exhorting the employees: "retain your family doctor"; "don't be a captive patient." In the end, the fact that the "Doctor's Plan" lost the deciding vote by a 4 to 1 margin does not diminish the obvious competitive zeal of the traditional medical community.

At about the same time, the desire of the Kaiser Plan to dilute criticism from the traditional medical community induced it to undertake a number of seemingly competitive ventures. First, it instituted a requirement of "dual choice," whereby the Kaiser Plan would only be offered to employees if the employer also agreed to offer a second plan giving employees the option of selecting FFS practitioners. This backfired to a certain extent because it allowed dominant FFS insurers to effectively freeze Kaiser out by refusing to have their plans offered as a choice alongside Kaiser. For example, in Portland, Oregon, the Oregon Physician's Service, the local Blue Shield plan, simply refused to participate in dual-choice arrangements; while the competing Blue Cross plan would participate only if it was guaranteed a 75 percent enrollment share.

A second effort, generated by the active refusal of many hospitals in HMO plan areas to provide admitting privileges to HMO physicians, was the decision by Kaiser to build its own hospitals instead of relying on local facilities used by FFS practitioners. While both these actions are consistent with the notion that Kaiser was attempting to solidify its competitive position in the marketplace, the alternative hypothesis cannot be rejected: that the decision by Kaiser and other large HMOs to draw back into their own facilities and, in the Kaiser case, to eschew head-to-head competition with FFS insurers for total employee group enrollment evidenced a desire to de-emphasize *economic* competition between prepaid plans and the traditional sector in favor of an enhanced promotion of the differences between prepaid plans and the traditional sector in terms of *medical practice style*. As Goldberg and Greenberg (1977:78) note in describing the California market:

> In some respects, for instance, Blue Cross competes more vigorously with Blue Shield than it competes with Kaiser since Blue Cross and Blue Shield must compete initially for the designation of the employer's health insurance offering. It is also interesting to note, however, that Kaiser generally does not react to any competitive response Blue Cross might make because Kaiser already offers comprehensive benefits and reviews carefully hospital admissions and length of stay. Furthermore, Kaiser has a policy against advertising and charges what it believes to be the lowest premium consistent with its standard of medical care.

This approach to competition on the part of Kaiser, and to a certain extent the other large, established HMO plans, provides the key to analyzing the likely fate of HMOs under a relatively unconstrained regime. For unlike the FMCs, IPAs, and other physician-sponsored HMOs that have sprung up in response to Kaiser, Group Health, and other major prepayment plans, the traditional HMOs refuse to meet head-to-head on price with traditional insurers; rather, they effectively compete against the entire fee-for-service system via product differentiation.

The rationale for the sort of competition preferred by the traditional HMOs is captured nicely by Christianson (1978:1):

> The notion that competition among health care providers can help control costs would seem to contradict the historical evidence. In the past, competition among providers for patients has contributed to the excessive performance of surgery, the proliferation of expensive and underused equipment, and the construction of excess hospital beds [citation omitted]. Since these and other outcomes of "provider competition" have contributed to rising health care costs, why should competition between traditional providers and alternative organizations for delivering care, such as HMOs, now be encouraged?

The answer, according to Christianson, is that this second sort of competition "can restructure the incentives and influence the decisions of traditional participants in the medical care marketplace to the benefit of business and other consumers." Thus, as HMO advocates Ellwood, Malcolm, and Tillotson (1979:1) conclude:

> The competitive health system strategy requires three main elements:
> —creating forms of health delivery systems that are more efficient than the present system, and that are hence able to compete on price, benefits, access, and style of medical care;
> —such units must be installed across the country; and
> —once the majority of health care providers in any given community are involved in competing alternative delivery systems, the workability of the approach can be evaluated.

Thus, they came down squarely on the side of a finding of inherent desirability in the HMO style of practice. Moreover, they effectively concede that a wide-open market for health care financing, unless operated under the sort of constraints proposed by Enthoven and McClure, would fail to generate the desired competition model in the natural evolution of things. That is, the proposed constraints, whether or not they are sufficient conditions for the establishment of a market of competing prepaid plans, are at least necessary conditions.

In order for the Congress to accommodate this vision, then, it will be forced to rig the rules of any competitive game in order to ensure that prepaid plans win. Given the likely resistance of other groups (e.g., traditional insurers, hospitals, and physicians), it would take a strong conviction on the part of the Congress that prepaid health care delivery had intrinsic merits. To date, the history of federal involvement in the HMO movement offers little evidence that such a conviction will soon materialize.

HMOs, Competition, and the Congress

The congressional fascination with HMOs began during the Nixon administration, as the result of that administration's frantic search for a method of appearing to deal with exploding costs under Medicare and Medicaid without atypically resorting to heavy-handed, sector-specific cost control regulation.

HMOs, at least in theory, filled the bill nicely. They were private enterprises, at risk in the free marketplace, and held out the promise of keeping the politically powerful traditional medical practitioners in line with a decentralized barrage of good, clean Republican competition. Yet, because of their reformist aura, they could be sold to a Congress drifting increasingly leftward due to the political polarization attendant on the administration's other preoccupation, Vietnam. In fact, in Nixon's special health message to the Congress in February of 1971, touting HMOs as the solution to the problem of rising medical care costs, the word *competition* is conspicuously absent. Instead, Nixon extolled their potential as a "new method for delivering health services," characterized as having a "strong financial interest in preventing illness." The proposed demonstration projects designed to test their effectiveness under a dual choice model would generate a "health care supermarket" in which the notion that there were economies of scale in the group practice of medicine could be tested. By 1973, when legislation effecting Nixon's proposed demonstration program was imminent, the rhetoric grew bolder: HMOs were now a "promising innovation of group medical centers" that would ultimately "reform the health care delivery system."

Even while debating the HMO demonstration program, the Congress had already enacted legislation allowing HMOs into mainstream federal health policy by establishing a favorable arrangement for prospective payment of HMOs enrolling Medicare and Medicaid beneficiaries. The *quid pro quo* at that time, of course, was that HMOs were subjected to facilities review and approval under Section 1122 of the 1972 Social Security Act Amendments. In the same year, the Senate passed and sent to the House a bill that went far beyond the administration's original proposal, calling for $1.3 billion to launch a full-scale commercialization project for HMOs and other prepaid plans.

The House, accepting for the moment the administration's conviction that such an effort was far too costly, failed to consider the measure; and it died when the Ninety-Second Congress adjourned.

By 1973, however, the House was ready to go to work and produced a bill modeled more closely along the lines of the original administration proposal. Yet, several new wrinkles crept in, setting the stage for a debate that continues to this date. In its efforts to make the bill more flexible, the administration was pushing for the broadest possible definition of an organization eligible for assistance in order to promote diversity in plan structure (and, not incidentally, to open the door for assistance to physician-sponsored plans, lest the AMA and its legislative muscle derail the entire effort).

The Congress, however, urged on by such groups as the American Public Health Association, approached the bill like a committee bent on designing a horse and produced a far narrower definition of a "qualified HMO" than the administration had hoped for. The bill produced by the House-Senate conference committee established a definition of an eligible plan that was so restrictive only some 20 of the 133 extant HMOs would qualify. The balance were relegated to the lesser status of "health service organizations" and "supplementary HMOs," whose access to the federal funds—and to the highly important overrides of troublesome state laws—was sharply restricted compared with the benefits attendant on federally qualified HMOs.

This outcome was probably the result of the high degree of confusion then prevalent over what HMOs were, what the bill was likely to do, and what the future direction of federal efforts affecting the overall delivery system would be. For example, the Senate committee report on the bill states the objective of the legislation as an effort to "increase options available from the point of view of the consumer" but "not . . . to remake the delivery system." Yet, paradoxically, the committee believed that HMOs would in the future "largely eliminate many of the problems presented by the prevalent fragmented solo practice model."

A second seeming paradox is found in the bill's treatment of the copayments question. The HMO Act allows federally-qualified HMOs to require only nominal copayments for covered services. Copayments, of course, are instituted for the sole purpose of introducing price sensitivity—i.e., price rationing—to services that might otherwise be overutilized. Yet, the report explicitly states the intent of Congress that such copayments should be "no barrier to care"; instead, they were "solely a device to enable an HMO to market its benefit package at a competitive price." The net effect of this provision was to proscribe copayments as a means of controlling utilization but to condone them as a sort of under-the-table premium increase for qualified plans.

The Congress did, however, seem to have an inkling of the likely natural market outcome of its experimental delivery system, as demonstrated by a reference to the distinction between qualified and "supplemental" HMOs. The committee argued for its decision not to provide the latter with start-up funds on the grounds that they would occur naturally in the marketplace without help; qualified plans meeting the committee's specifications, on the other hand, were not expected to survive without significant direct federal support.

Thus, far from being interested in the potential of HMOs for generating competition, the Congress was instead attempting to outwit the normal functioning of a competitive marketplace and install in the field its own horse, which, while more reminiscent of a camel, was nevertheless expected to win the race with liberal applications of financial dope. Subsequent federal efforts in the HMO arena lend credence to the view that despite the rhetoric, federal efforts to promote HMOs have precious little effect in promoting competition in the marketplace.

In 1979, for example, the Health and Environment Subcommittee of the House Interstate and Foreign Commerce Committee produced and pushed through the House a bill reauthorizing the Health Planning Act. The most controversial feature of the bill was a section providing a sweeping exemption from certificate-of-need laws for all "providers of ambulatory and inpatient care on a prepaid basis." This broad exemption was justified by its sponsor, Congressman W. Philip Gramm (D-Texas), in the name of competition; i.e., that the degree of investment risk assumed by HMOs and other such plans was, due to the normal operation of market forces, an effective discipline against overinvestment in facilities and equipment, obviating the need for a surrogate regulatory discipline.

The broadness of the definition of an entity eligible for the Gramm Amendment exemption was not unintentional. It held out the promise that any health care financing entity which assumed risk for its own investments could effectively exit the regulatory maze of facilities franchising and compete in the open market. By further exempting from CON (certificate-of-need) requirements the activities of non-HMO hospitals that provided services primarily to such providers, the Gramm Amendment language was, in effect, a procompetitive loophole through which a truck could be driven.

While the broad language of the Gramm Amendment survived the House, it proved too much for the House-Senate Conference Committee, which severely restricted the exemption's scope by allowing the exemption only for HMOs with enrollment in excess of 50,000 persons. Only a handful of HMOs—notably such giants as Kaiser, Group Health Association of Puget Sound, the Health Insurance Plan of New York, and the other long-established traditional HMOs— were thus released from the market entry barriers of the certificate-of-need laws. The balance, including new plans that might start up to compete against the established HMOs, remained subject to the CON entry restraints.

In fact, it could be argued that, given the persistence of CON requirements for new prepaid plan entrants, the 1979 Health Planning Act exemption, far from being procompetitive, granted the traditional HMOs a major new tool to preempt the field in those areas in which they were already established, obviating the need for whatever new HMO-style entities might otherwise materialize in competition.

The Minimum Benefits Route

The contention that the Congress would willingly bequeath the entire market for health care services to competing prepaid plans is very difficult to support based on this history. While halting steps have been made in the direction of promoting HMOs that might not otherwise arise, these efforts have been justified more in terms of remedying prior discrimination against prepaid plans than because they are preferred competitors per se (see, for example, Goldberg and Greenberg, 1977).

It is possible, however, that during the course of consideration of legislation to promote competition in medical care markets, the Congress might unconsciously predispose the market toward the competing prepaid plan model by imposing either high minimum benefit requirements or outright benefit package standardization. As noted earlier, the inability of financing entities representing loosely organized FFS providers to constrain service utilization to the level achieved by prepaid plans could place them at a decided disadvantage over time.

Enthoven would argue that this would be a desirable outcome. Enthoven (1980a:45–50) distinguishes the practice styles of FFS practitioners and prepaid plans as the tendency of FFS providers to perform services that increase costs in excess of marginal benefits. Thus, unless FFS practitioners could adjust their practice styles to the utilization levels experienced by prepaid plans, he would argue that FFS plans should *not* survive in a cost-conscious competitive market.

Here, I believe, lies the crux of the problem. In essence, Enthoven argues that many of the amenities that accompany the FFS practice system today—such as short waiting times for services; free choice of physician and hospital; and the exercise of individual preferences respecting, for example, decisions of whether or not to hospitalize— bear costs far in excess of their true utility to consumers. As such, they are quirks of the current incentive structure rather than the outcome of conscious consumer choice.

An apposite view would be that this thesis should be put to the test in the marketplace. Stockman (1980) has argued that failing to allow individuals to choose among a wide range of different delivery modalities and practice styles would forestall the tremendous potential for innovative approaches to health care financing that might otherwise arise. Moreover, he argues that these amenities have, in certain instances, positive value for consumers.

The trade-off then—if there is one—is between different sorts of costs associated with different market formulations. On the one hand, a wide-open market with only minimal benefit package constraints would promote provider innovation. The standard benefits market, by contrast, would forestall many of these innovations, which would largely result from product differentiation. On the other hand, the wide-open market would induce individuals to sort themselves out to some extent on the basis of perceived risk and degree of risk aversion. In such a market, Enthoven argues, comprehensive benefit plans could not survive (1980a:79).

The question, then, is whether the costs associated with obviating product innovation are greater or less than the costs associated with creating a bias against plans that offer relatively comprehensive benefits. Interestingly, the Congress has, at least to date, tended toward the view that comprehensive benefits per se are a more desirable feature than freedom for innovation. As the record shows, however, this congressional tendency generates additional costs that must be factored into the equation.

Minimum Benefits and the Congress: Medicare and Medicaid

Posturing about comprehensive national health insurance aside, the Congress has shown a bias toward expansive definitions of allowable benefits under those programs where the federal government has control over benefit specifications.

Since at least 1950, the Congress has been hard at work adding ever wider benefits to government financed health programs. The original Aid to Families with Dependent Children (AFDC) program, enacted in 1935 under the Social Security Act, contained a simple income disregard for the amount of bona fide health care expenditures, i.e., expenditures for health care were deducted from the income of families in determining eligibility. In close cases, this practice effectively passed through, dollar-for-dollar, the health care spending of the poor. The Social Security Act Amendments of 1950 converted spending for medical care for the poor to a vendor payment system. Thus, rather than merely passing through medical care expenditures, the Social Security system made direct payments to health care providers for needed health care services for the AFDC-eligible poor. In 1960, the Kerr-Mills Act expanded both benefits and eligibility under the vendor payments program, including, for the first time, low-income aged persons without children in the home. Six years later, this program was dramatically expanded by the enactment of Medicare and Medicaid.

As originally conceived, Medicare was to be simply a program of hospital insurance for the aged. By the time it emerged from the House of Representatives, however, physicians' services were also covered. The Medicaid component, calling for a sweeping program of medical care services to low-income Americans, was also added by the House version. Since enactment Medicare has been amended seven times, and Medicaid nine times. In each instance, either eligibility has been expanded or required benefits have been substantially upgraded.

In 1968, Medicare benefits, originally covering ninety days of hospitalization annually, were upgraded by adding a *second* ninety days of coverage, called the "lifetime reserve," upon which the aged could call in any given year if the original ninety-day coverage was exhausted. At the same time, Medicaid was amended to include the "early and periodic screening, diagnosis, and treatment" (EPSDT) program, a major effort to provide a full range of comprehensive care to eligible children.

Shortly thereafter, in 1972, two large new blocks of eligibles were added to Medicare—those receiving disability insurance and those with end-stage renal disease. In addition, those receiving Supplemental Security Income, except in certain instances, were made eligible for Medicaid.

During the balance of the 1970s, virtually every Congress has added on to this growing laundry list of coverages and benefits. Chiropractors' services and the services of podiatrists are allowed in many instances. Psychiatric services have been expanded widely, particularly in Medicaid, and optometrists, skilled nursing facilities, and dentists have been able to have their services added on to the list.

Even in the budget-conscious 96th Congress, efforts were made to add to the federal programs laundry list. Legislation passed the House calling for, among other things, the expansion of both eligibility and mandatory services for children under Medicaid, the addition of the treatment of planter's warts, the provision of pneumococcal vaccine, new home health benefits, expanded dental services, ad infinitum. When budgetary considerations threatened enactment, the ingenious ploy of loading in benefit additions to the Omnibus Budget Reconciliation Act—the bill designed to reconcile spending with budget totals by *reducing* federal outlays—nearly succeeded. In the end, a number of the proposed additions survived the House-Senate conference on the budget.

The Implications for Legislation
to Promote Competition

The most direct indication of the unfortunate congressional tendency to load up the cart with new goodies is the Health Maintenance Organization Act itself. In order to qualify for federal subsidies and the boon of "dual choice" requirements for employers, "qualified HMOs" must offer an incredible array of services, including extensive mental health coverage, treatment for alcohol and drug dependency, home health services, family planning, infertility services, and optometry services for children. To the extent that few, if any, other insurers offer anywhere near this package, federally qualified HMOs often find themselves, despite cost-reducing utilization patterns, at a severe competitive disadvantage. In fact, many have held out the benefit requirements of the HMO Act as one of the major impediments to the nationwide development of health maintenance organizations. Even advocates of a market of competing prepaid plans, notably McClure (1979, IV:120–121), have commented on the disadvantages of too narrow a definition of elegible entities and benefit offerings.

Given this tendency on the part of the federal government to promise all things to all people, those who promote high minimum benefits or standardized packages must be given pause. For over and above the questions of the potential for market innovations and of whether wider choices would offer consumers greater utility (for an excellent discussion of this point, see Meyer, 1980:7–10), there is the plain political question of whether Congress, faced with the task of determining what the minimum package would be, would so load up the requirements as to make the task of financing health care fabulously expensive.

To be sure, Enthoven (1980a:143–144), among others, is not unaware of this potential problem. He notes that a means must be found to minimize the "gatekeeper" role of government in this and other respects. Yet, this problem is not merely a technical design point that can be forever resolved during consideration of enabling legislation. For, if the government is given a determining role in deciding what the market shall offer, it will retain that right in perpetuity. Moreover, as the evidence to date shows, it will not fail to exercise that right frequently in the name of equity, i.e., constituency-group appeasement.

The Stakes Are Far Too High

If anything, legislating minimum benefits in a program that covers all Americans will have a far more pervasive effect than the experience to date in Medicare, Medicaid, and the HMO Act. The great majority of competition schemes envision that whatever qualifying requirements are enacted for plans will, by virtue of leveraging the Internal Revenue Code and the Social Security Act, become a blueprint for virtually all saleable health insurance in the United States.

Faced with such a prospect, the various provider constituencies—and the victims of peculiar diagnoses known affectionately on Capitol Hill as the "Disease-of-the-Month Club"—will be motivated by more than sheer convenience or desire. They will be motivated by the impulse for survival. For to be left off the minimum benefits list will be, perforce, to shift for themselves in a world where whatever federal preferences they now have will be dissolved. To chiropractors, podiatrists, psychologists, naturopaths, faith healers, and other practitioners outside the "physician" umbrella, getting into the game via congressional mandate will make the difference between prosperity and perpetual fringe status.

It is possible that the heavy political pressure of the traditional organized groups and institutions—including, of course, the HMOs, who have not been notorious for welcoming mandates to include nontraditional providers—will keep these groups off the list for a time. Yet, sheer economic necessity will force these groups to return again and again until they are finally successful. Arm in arm with those desperately needing kidney dialysis, interferon treatments, and every other imaginable group of "outs," they will form a coalition to force reopening of the minimum benefits question. Eventually—and inevitably—the wheel will be greased.

The "Third Best" Options

Given this political reality, it may well be time to set aside the pursuit, among health care theorists, of the optimal "second best" market structure—of either the constrained market form preferred by Enthoven or the regulatory "second best" promoted by such commentators as Altman and Weiner (1978). Instead, it may be necessary to turn to a "third best," from which can be distilled a solution that provides for some constraints on adverse selection and free riders; some constraints on plan innovation and product differentiation; some bias against FFS solo practitioners; and some risk that, left to themselves in an open system, the American people may spend more, rather than less, on health care.

Unless such an accommodation is reached, the result of pushing procompetition legislation through the Congress may well be far different from what the proponents anticipate. Either the legislation will melt under the heat generated by warring factions, or else whatever market-based incentives the approach might generate will be buried under the special interest trophies won in the competition for inclusion on the minimum benefits list. It is hard to see how either outcome would be an improvement over the present morass.

References

Altman, S.H., and Weiner, S.L. 1978. Regulation as Second Best. In Greenberg, W., ed., *Competition in the Health Care Sector: Past, Present, and Future.* Washington, D.C.: Federal Trade Commission.

Christianson, J.B. 1978. *Do HMOs Stimulate Beneficial Competition?* Excelsior, Minn.: InterStudy.

Ellwood, P.M., Malcolm, J., and Tillotson, J.K. 1979. The Status of Competition in the Health Industry. Unpublished manuscript.

Enthoven, A.C. 1979. Why We Cannot Have a "Free Market" in Health Insurance. Why Some Rules Are Needed to Produce Good Results. Unpublished manuscript.

———— 1980a. *Health Plan.* Reading, Mass.: Addison-Wesley Publishing Co.

———— 1980b. Supply Side Economics of Health Care and Consumer Choice Health Plan. Unpublished manuscript: American Enterprise Institute Conference on Health Care, September 26.

Gabarino, J.W. 1960. *Health Plans and Collective Bargaining.* Berkeley: University of California Press.

Goldberg, L.G., and Greenberg, W. 1977. *The Health Maintenance Organization and Its Effects on Competition.* Washington, D.C.: The Bureau of Economics, Federal Trade Commission.

McClure, W. 1979. *Comprehensive Market and Regulatory Strategies for Medical Care.* Excelsior, Minn.: InterStudy.

Meyer, J.A. 1980. Health Care Competition: Are Tax Incentives Enough? Supply Side Economics of Health Care and Consumer Choice Health Plan. Unpublished manuscript: American Enterprise Institute Conference on Health Care, September 26.

Stockman, D.A. 1980. Can Fee-for-Service Medicine Survive Competition? *Forum on Medicine* (January), 21–25.

Address correspondence to: Donald W. Moran, 212 E. Alexandria Avenue, Alexandria, VA 22301.

II Determinants of Choice

Factors Affecting the Choice Between Prepaid Group Practice and Alternative Insurance Programs

RICHARD TESSLER
DAVID MECHANIC

This paper examines the basis for the selection of prepaid group practice in a dual-choice situation, and the social, attitudinal, and health characteristics of populations choosing prepaid programs in contrast to other plans. When asked in an open-ended way why they made the decisions they did, those selecting prepaid group practice most frequently referred to the more comprehensive coverage provided and to the fact that at the time of choice they lacked a continuing or adequate relationship with a physician. Enrollees in the prepaid program were better educated and, contrary to previous research, more likely to be unmarried. There was little evidence that enrollees in the prepaid plan brought with them distinctive kinds of attitudes and orientations toward illness and medical care. Enrollees in the prepaid program were also comparable to those retaining an alternative health insurance option on a number of indicators of health status. However, prepaid practice enrollees tended to report more chronic conditions than persons who declined to enroll in the prepaid program. Although the overrepresentation of persons with chronic illnesses is not large, data drawn from a related study suggests that persons with several chronic conditions tend to be heavy users of medical services.

In order to minimize the number of dissatisfied patients in closed medical panels, it is customary to offer eligible participants a dual choice between prepaid group practice and alternative insurance programs. When prepaid group practice is offered as a possible option, an alternative fee-for-service insurance plan, which provides less comprehensive coverage but which does not in any way restrict the patient's choice of physician or location of service, is almost always offered.

The purpose of this paper is to examine the basis for the decisions made in dual-choice situations, and the social, attitudinal, and health characteristics of populations that have made varying choices. Through such an analysis, it is possible to better understand those aspects of health plans that are viewed as attractive by particular groups in the population. Previous studies of enrollment in prepaid plans relative to alternatives indicate the importance of such features as breadth of insurance coverage, em-

M M F Q / Health and Society / *Spring 1975*

phasis on preventive medicine, and the availability of one's total pattern of medical care at a single location. Among the reasons people give for not selecting prepaid practice options are such factors as pre-existing ties with a private physician, concern about possible impersonality of care, and physical distance from the prepaid practice facility (Anderson and Sheatsley, 1959; Metzner and Bashshur, 1967; Wolfman, 1961).

It is particularly important to understand the extent and nature of selective biases in choices among alternative plans. From a practical standpoint, the relative costs and benefits of one alternative versus another depends on the health needs and characteristics of persons in various plans and how they regard and use medical services. To the extent that important differences in populations exist among plans, such information is significant in evaluating the relative performance and impact of alternative plans. Knowledge of such selectivity is also important in evaluating research findings comparing alternative health care programs. For pragmatic reasons, almost all of what we know about the performance of alternative plans comes from cross-sectional studies of enrollees in different plans who have selected their particular health care program. When we observe differences in the performance of plans, or the behavior of patients within them, it is difficult to know to what extent the results reflect real differences in performance in comparison to the special characteristics of patients choosing one or another health care program. Information on the selection process, although it does not compensate for the lack of randomized controlled trials, informs our interpretation of results from cross-sectional studies (Mechanic, 1972:102–111; 1974a). For example, in studies of mortality among patients in the Health Insurance Plan as compared with alternative populations, it is difficult to evaluate to what extent the results are a product of the special organizational characteristics of the HIP program in contrast to selective characteristics of consumers who have chosen this program relative to others (Shapiro et al., 1958; Shapiro et al., 1967).

One important type of selectivity, examined in this study, concerns individuals and families who anticipate or require, because of pre-existing conditions, higher than average needs for medical care. Commonly known as the risk-vulnerability hypothesis (Bashshur and Metzner, 1967; 1970; Metzner et al., 1972; Bice et al.;), the notion is that people who estimate the risk of illness as great, and who feel vulnerable to high costs for medical care, are predisposed to enroll in prepaid plans because of the protection against out-of-pocket costs provided. Although various studies have addressed the issue, most of them concentrate on socio-demographic characteristics as proxies for need, and do not directly examine data on health status or health consciousness. In talking with researchers who have investigated this issue, we have also come to suspect that the published literature may not be representative of research experience in this area. Investigators probably expect to find difference between prepaid and nonprepaid group practice in health status or health consciousness; when such differences are not found, such data are probably less likely to be written up or submitted for publication.

There is evidence in the literature that prepaid group enrollees are more likely to be older, married, and to have young children than people choosing alternative options (Bashshur and Metzner, 1967; Wolfman, 1961; Moustafa et al., 1971; Bice, 1973; Hetherington et al., 1975). On the other hand, Yedidia (1959) reports that the age composition of prepaid-group-practice enrollees is not distinctive, and on this basis questions the proposition that high-risk families are attracted to prepaid plans. More direct evidence concerning the relative vulnerability of enrollees in prepaid group practice comes from studies which included measures of health status and illness. Anderson and Sheatsley (1959) report no differences in the perceived health status of members of families enrolling in prepaid group practice and an alternative insurance plan. They also found that individuals selecting the prepaid option were no more likely than those in the comparison group to have experienced an expensive illness prior to enrollment. Hetherington et al. (1975) found higher proportions of families with chronic and acute illnesses in prepaid as compared with alternative plans, but it is difficult to be sure that such differences existed at the time of the choice. Bice et al. (1974), studying a lower-income area in Baltimore, found that families' previous use of health services was predictive of enrollment in a prepaid group practice for a group of people lacking an alternative option other than episodic outpatient care.

It should be appreciated, of course, that prepaid group practice, and the populations given an opportunity to enroll in them, may vary in many important dimensions, and, thus, it should not be surprising that the findings vary from one study to another. Any over-all assessment must be based on the research literature as a whole and cannot depend on any single study or study population.

Another selective bias to be examined concerns the possibility that people who enroll in prepaid plans bring with them distinctive kinds of attitudes and orientations toward illness and medical care. Anderson and Sheatsley (1959) were unable to find any consistent differences between health attitudes of individuals participating in prepaid and fee-for-service insurance plans. However, they did not probe systematically for the possibility that enrollees in prepaid group practice are more oriented toward health maintenance and preventive health utilization. A number of other studies have reported evidence of high rates of preventive health utilization in prepaid plans (see Donabedian, 1969; Roemer and Shonick, 1973; Hetherington et al., 1975), but it is not clear to what extent such differences reflect the organization of the plans or the attitudes of their enrollees.

In addition to examining each of the above issues, this study will also consider the possible effect of neuroticism (Eysenck and Eysenck, 1964) on choice behavior. We wish to examine indirectly the allegation that prepaid group practice tends to attract large numbers of "worried wells," people who are prone to present problems which physicians regard as trivial (Garfield, 1970); there is some evidence indicating that this contention may be very much exaggerated (Jackson and Greenlick, 1974). The "worried well" hypothesis, however, may be supported in part by the finding by Hetherington et al. (1975) that "hypersensitivity" to physical symptoms was higher among subscribers in a large group practice than in other insurance plans, but on more careful inspection of the data this is doubtful. Hetherington and his associates had physicians rate various symptoms in terms of the extent to which they required medical care. On the basis of these ratings, symptoms could be classified as high- and low-need symptoms. The measure of hypersensitivity took into account symptoms for which patients indicated they would seek medical care despite low-need ratings by the physicians. Inspection of the low-need symptoms indicates that they include such items as insomnia, "nerves," and general fatigue. The reader can make his own assessment as to whether seeking care for such symptoms can appropriately be regarded as the behavior of the "worried well" or as trivial.

Procedures in the Present Study

Data are reported from a telephone survey of individuals following a choice between prepaid group practice and an alternative Blue Cross – Blue Shield insurance plan. The study was designed so that interviewing took place soon after the choice situation, usually before those in the prepaid plan had any experience with the medical group. Thus we attempted to measure selectivity in terms of socio-demographic characteristics, attitudes, and illness experience prior to the time that these might be modified by the particular plan selected. The sample was drawn from public employees of a major metropolitan area including both blue- and white-collar workers.

For many years this city had offered the Blue Cross–Blue Shield plan to its employees. In June of 1973, the city gave to its employees the option of retaining the old plan or enrolling in the prepaid group practice. In order to obtain the prepaid group practice health insurance, city employees were required to pay part of the health insurance premium ($11.77 per month for a family plan and $4.03 per month for a single plan). The city, however, paid the entire Blue Cross–Blue Shield premium. Of approximately 7,000 city employees, 183 (2 percent) chose the prepaid plan, and this entire group was included in our study. A random sample of Blue Cross–Blue Shield subscribers was selected as a comparison group. Because of the requirement of an additional monthly payment, this sample is biased in favor of maximum social selection; under the risk-vulnerability hypothesis, we would expect that those willing to pay the additional cost would anticipate or have a particularly high need for medical services.

Whenever possible, women (usually wives of employees) were interviewed concerning their own health, the health of their spouse, and the health of children included within the insurance plan. If an interview could not be obtained by phone, we attempted to obtain the desired data through a household interview. Eighty-six percent of the Blue Cross sample ($N = 165$) and 93 percent of the prepaid practice sample ($N = 168$) were successfully interviewed.

Concurrent with the choice study was a second inquiry of patient satisfaction with prepaid practice and alternative insurance plans. Since we included almost all of the same questions used in the choice study in the satisfaction study, we had a particularly good opportunity to replicate the analysis with a different sample. The satisfaction study included patients from one to two years of exposure to prepaid group practice, and thus, it is not prospective in the sense of the choice study. It provides, however, an excellent opportunity to examine consistencies and inconsistencies between the various populations used in these studies.

The sample for the satisfaction study was drawn from two large industrial firms which offer a dual choice including the same prepaid group practice involved in the choice study. However, in these situations the employer assumes the full cost of insurance irrespective of the plan selected. In contrast to the choice study, the alternative plans in the satisfaction study are more generous in benefits and include more outpatient services (for further details, see Tessler and Mechanic, 1974). Employees from these two firms included semi-skilled and skilled hourly workers, and salaried personnel. Representative samples of individuals choosing each option were obtained from each firm, and data were collected through a household interview. Ninety-one percent of eligible respondents were successfully interviewed.

The Health Insurance Plans

The prepaid group practice plan is a relatively new program (two and a half years old at the time of the study). Care is provided by a multispecialty hospital-based practice staffed by full-time physicians. Enrollees in the prepaid practice obtain a fairly comprehensive benefit package on a prepayment basis including outpatient visits, specialty services, consultation services outside the group at the request of a group physician, diagnostic and laboratory procedures, physical examinations, and eye examinations by an ophthalmologist (but not lenses or frames). Among the services excluded from coverage are drugs, dental care, most cosmetic care, and sterilization services. Inpatient services are comparable to Blue Cross, and private health insurance policies generally except that hospital services, excluding emergencies, must be provided by a single hospital associated with the program.

The alternative insurance plan involved in the choice study provided emergency medical care, accident care within 72 hours, outpatient surgical procedures, X-ray and radiation thereapy, $200 diagnostic services per year, and major medical insurance. The major medical program involved a $50 deductible and 20 percent coinsurance thereafter with a $20,000 maximum per person.

Results

Data descriptive of the socio-demographic characteristics of prepaid group practice and Blue Cross respondents are presented in Table 1. A significantly larger proportion of respondents who enrolled in Blue Cross — Blue Shield in contrast to the prepaid group practice were married and selected family plans. In addition, prepaid group respondents were significantly better educated than those retaining Blue Cross — Blue Shield health insurance. There were no significant differences in the two groups in terms of the respondent's age, sex, employment status, religion, or in the terms of family income. Nor were the two groups of respondents significantly different in terms of the number and ages of their children. Comparable patterns were replicated in the satisfaction study. Although the educational difference was in the same direction as in the choice study, it was not statistically significant.[1]

Explicit Reasons for Choice

In order to assess respondents' reasons for the choices made, we asked respondents in an open-ended way why they made the decisions they did. We followed this question by suggesting various reasons for making the choice and asking respondents to indicate how important each reason was for their family. Finally, we asked respondents to select the single reason among those suggested that was of greatest importance to their families.

In the open-ended question,[2] Blue Cross–Blue Shield respondents indicated most frequently that they were satisfied with Blue Cross coverage (32 percent), that they had inadequate information about the choice (22 percent), that they were satisfied with their

[1] Also in the satisfaction study, Blue Cross respondents were more likely to be women and less likely to be employed than respondents in the prepaid practice plan.

[2] Since many respondents gave several reasons for their choice, we aggregated the data so as to indicate what proportion of the sample mentioned each reason spontaneously.

TABLE 1

Socio-demographic Characteristics of Prepaid-
Group-Practice and Blue Cross Enrollees

Socio-demographic Factors	Blue Cross (N = 165) %	Prepaid Group Practice (N = 168) %	p[a]
Respondent—Married	77	57	< .001
Family health plan	80	62	< .001
Number of children			
0	46	55	
1–2	32	23	NS
3 or more	22	22	
Number of children under 12			
0	71	76	NS
1 or more	29	24	
Age of respondent			
30 or less	24	29	
31–45	34	30	
46–55	27	30	NS
56 or more	15	11	
Sex of respondent—Female	73	73	NS
Respondent employed	72	80	NS
Education of respondent			
Some high school or less	19	14[b]	
Completed high school	52	41	< .01
Some college or more	28	46	
Religion of respondent			
Protestant	37	25	
Catholic	51	56	NS
Other	12	19	
Respondent—Black	11	6	NS
Family income			
Under $8,000	7	13	
$8,000–$11,000	39	34	NS
$11,000–$14,000	27	29	
Over $14,000	27	24	

[a]Statistical significance is computed using the X^2 distribution and the criterion used is the .05 level.

[b]Percentages may not add to 100 percent because of rounding errors.

present doctor (21 percent), that they did not wish to assume the additional cost to enroll in the prepaid plan (15 percent), and that the prepaid-practice clinic was inconveniently located for them (14 percent). Other reasons given were inertia (15 percent), preference for a wider choice of doctors or hospitals (9 percent), and concern about a clinic atmosphere at the prepaid practice (5 percent). Those selecting prepaid group practice most frequently referred to the more comprehensive coverage this program provided (30 percent) and to the fact that at the time of choice they lacked a continuing or adequate relationship with a physician (23 percent). Other reasons given included the fact that the plan covered office visits (15 percent), that it was a good deal for the money (14 percent), that physical exams were paid for (13 percent), that they knew about particular doctors at the prepaid practice clinic (13 percent), that a family member had a condition requiring a great deal of medical attention or the possibility of this occurring (9 percent), that the prepaid plan offered complete care at one location (7 percent), and that it provided preventive medicine (8 percent).

Table 2 shows the reactions of respondents choosing each option to eight possible reasons for their choice. Except for the item dealing with size of family, responses to all of the other items differed among respondents choosing each of the two options. Those retaining the Blue Cross–Blue Shield policy were more likely to rate as important the location of the prepaid-practice clinic and the fact that the family physician would be restricted to the prepaid group practice. It was clear that these were seen as disadvantages to the Blue Cross group and as advantages to those selecting the prepaid plan. For example, among the Blue Cross sample, 87 percent indicated that the location of the prepaid practice was a disadvantage, 81 percent indicated that its association with a particular hospital was disadvantage, and 90 percent indicated that the restriction of their family physician to the prepaid-practice group was a disadvantage. In contrast, among the enrollees in the prepaid plan, 76 percent said the location of the clinic was an advantage, 97 percent said its association with a local hospital was an advantage, and 93 percent indicated that it was an advantage that their family physicians would be part of the prepaid group practice. A majority of respondents choosing both options agreed that having one's medical care in one place was an advantage, although 100 percent of prepaid practice respondents gave the response in contrast to 69 percent of the Blue Cross respondents.

Table 2 also shows the proportion in the various subgroups who indicate each reason as the single most important one for them, and there is a significant difference in the pattern of response for the two subgroups. Blue Cross respondents cite as most impor-

TABLE 2

Proportion of Respondents in the Choice Study Rating Fixed
Alternative Items as Very Important in Choice

	BLUE CROSS–BLUE SHIELD (N = 165)		PREPAID GROUP PRACTICE (N = 168)		
	% Rating Item Very Important	*% Saying it Is Most Important Reason*	*% Rating Item Very Important*	*% Saying It Is Most Important Reason*	*p*[a]
Location of Northpoint Clinic	37	25	28	8	NS[b]
Northpoint's association with St. Mary's Hospital	16	2	22	3	<.05
In Compcare, all the family's medical care would be provided in one place	24	7	58	24	<.001
In Compcare, your family physician would be a member of the Northpoint group	48	34	27	12	<.001
Availability of medical care at night and on weekends at Northpoint	22	9	56	18	<.001
Knowing in advance what your medical care costs would be for the year	18	2	45	19	<.001
Importance of the size of your family in choosing health plan	19	7	24	3	NS
Chance that a member of your family might need a lot of medical care	29	14	40	14	<.05

[a]Statistical significance computed by the X^2 statistic and the criterion used is the .05 level. In Table 2 the probability figures shown refer to the ratings of importance of each item and not to the ratings of the single most important item.

[b]Probability is < .06.

tant in their choice the restriction of their family physician to the prepaid group practice and the location of the clinic. In contrast, prepaid-group-practice respondents indicate as most important the fact that all of the family's care would be provided in one place, knowing medical care costs in advance, and the availability of medical care on nights and weekends. Although more prepaid-practice respondents rate as very important the chance that a member of their family might need a lot of medical care, an identical proportion in the two groups—14 percent—rate it as most important.

Selectivity Resulting from Health Status

In order to determine whether there were any differences in health status between families enrolling in prepaid group practice and families retaining their Blue Cross–Blue Shield policies, respondents were questioned about their own medical histories and current health problems, and about those of other family members as well. As one indicator of selectivity resulting from health status, respondents were presented with a list of 34 chronic health problems and, for each problem, asked to indicate whether anyone in their family had ever had that problem. The mean number of chronic problems reported is presented in Table 3 for Blue Cross and prepaid-practice respondents, their spouses, and children. Inspection of the results shows that prepaid group-practice respondents reported significantly more chronic conditions than Blue Cross–Blue Shield respondents. As Table 4 shows, 14 percent of prepaid-practice respondents reported five or more chronic illnesses in contrast to 7 percent in the Blue Cross group.[3]

Although the chronicity differences observed for respondents are not very large in percentage terms, any addition of enrollees with a high level of chronic illness can result in considerable use of service. Analysis of the relationship between chronicity and utilization was undertaken with data from the satisfaction study. The results are presented in Table 5. Examination of the results reveals significant relationships between respondents' reports of their own chronicity and various indicators of medical-care utilization. Respondents with five or more chronic illnesses were overrepresented among those making four or more office visits in the past year, those spending six or more days in the hospital, those with the highest total cost of hospitalization, and those undergoing surgery.

[3]As Table 4 shows, when the distribution of chronic illnesses among the two groups of respondents is tested for significance using *chi* square rather than the F distribution, as was the case in the result presented in Table 3, the difference between Prepaid Practice and Blue Cross respondents does not achieve statistical significance.

TABLE 3

Health Status of Families Selecting Blue Cross
and Prepaid Practice Options

Health Status Indicator	Blue Cross $\bar{X}$	Prepaid Practice $\bar{X}$	p^a
1. Chronic problems			
a. respondents ($N = 333$)	1.67	2.12	$< .05$
b. spouses ($N = 221$)	1.24	1.33	NS
c. children ($N = 164$)[b]	.71	.84	NS
2. Perceived health			
a. respondents ($N = 333$)	1.61	1.61	NS
b. spouses ($N = 221$)	1.64	1.56	NS
c. children ($N = 164$)	1.35	1.36	NS
3. Bed-disability days			
a. respondents ($N = 333$)	.42	.44	NS
b. spouses ($N = 221$)	.36	.13	NS
c. children ($N = 164$)	.34	.43	NS
4. Major illnesses			
a. respondents ($N = 333$)	1.08	1.09	NS
b. spouses ($N = 221$)	1.07	1.02	NS
c. children ($N = 164$)	.01	.05	NS
5. Hospital days			
a. respondents ($N = 333$)	1.26	1.26	NS
b. spouses ($N = 221$)	1.17	1.00	NS
c. children ($N = 164$)	.25	.72	NS
6. Perception of family's medical problems ($N = 333$)	1.52	1.51	NS
7. Perception of family's utilization patterns ($N = 333$)	1.51	1.54	NS

[a]Statistical significance is based upon unstandardized regression coefficients, employing the F distribution. The criterion used is the .05 level.

[b]The total number of chronic illnesses among all children in the family, coded 0, 1, 2 or more, is represented here. All other figures for children included in this table are based on the average score for children in each family.

While there were no over-all differences among spouses and children of prepaid and Blue Cross respondents in number of chronic problems reported (refer to Table 3), there was a tendency for differences to emerge in a direction consistent with the risk-vulnerability hypothesis for low-income families for whom we would expect degree of chronicity to have its greatest impact on perceived vulnerability to medical-care expenditures. Tables 6 and 7 show the distribution of reports of chronic illnesses among spouses and children of Blue Cross and prepaid-practice enrollees

TABLE 4

Number of Chronic Illnesses Reported by Respondents
in Blue Cross and Prepaid Practice Plans

Reported Chronic Illness	Blue Cross ($N = 165$) %	Prepaid Practice ($N = 168$) %
No chronic illnessess	28	23
One	26	21
Two	23	25
Three	11	13
Four	5	5
Five	4	6
Six or more	3	8

$X^2 = 6.53$

$df = 6$

$p > .05$

TABLE 5

Relations Between Chronicity and Use of Services Among
Respondents in the Satisfaction Study ($N = 989$)

	NUMBER OF CHRONIC ILLNESSES					
	0	1	2	3-4	5 or more	
	($N = 272$) %	($N = 276$) %	($N = 180$) %	($N = 182$) %	($N = 79$) %	p[a]
Office visits						
0	39	32	21	24	10	
1-3	48	48	52	41	33	< .001
4 or more	13	20	28[b]	35	57	
Days in hospital						
0	89	90	90	84	75	
1-5	8	5	5	9	8	< .01
6 or more	3	6	5	7	17	
Cost of hospitalization						
0	89	90	90	84	75	
Less than $1019	10	6	8	11	14	< .01
$1019 or more	1	4	2	5	10	
Surgery						
Yes	4	4	3	9	16	< .001
No	96	96	97	91	84	

[a]Statistical significance is based on the chi square distribution.

[b]Percentages may not add up to 100 percent because of rounding errors.

TABLE 6

Number of Chronic Conditions Reported for Spouses by Insurance Plan
Among Families with Incomes of Less than $11,000

	Blue Cross (N = 44) %	Prepaid Practice (N = 25) %
Number of chronic illnesses		
0	41	32
1	36	28
2 or more	23	40

$X^2 = 2.31$
$df = 2$
$p > .05$

whose family income was less than $11,000. Forty percent of the prepaid-practice spouses were reported to have two or more chronic illnesses as compared to 23 percent of the Blue Cross spouses. Thirty-two percent of the prepaid respondents, in contrast

TABLE 7

Number of Chronic Conditions Reported for Children by Insurance Plan
Among Families with Incomes of Less than $11,000

	Blue Cross (N = 28) %	Prepaid Practice (N = 25) %
Number of chronic illnesses		
0	64	44
1	14	24
2 or more	21	32

$X^2 = 1.13$
$df = 2$
$p > .05$

to 21 percent of the Blue Cross respondents, reported two or more chronic illnesses among their children.[4]

Indicators of health status other than chronicity were all unrelated to choice of health plan (refer to Table 3). When asked to assess the health status of each member on a scale ranging from excellent to poor, prepaid and Blue Cross respondents did not differ in their ratings of their own health, their spouses' health, or the health status of each of their children. When they were questioned about the number of days spent in bed because of illness by family members within the last three months, prepaid-practice and Blue Cross respondents showed no significant differences in their responses. Similarly, no consistent differences emerged when respondents were questioned about the total number of days spent in a hospital in the preceding year, or about major illnesses in the past three months (indicated by reports of illnesses for which a physician was seen five or more times). There were also no significant differences in respondents' ratings of the seriousness of their family's medical problems as compared with other families, or the extent to which their families were prone to utilize medical services. Each of the foregoing analyses was repeated for those in the low-income groups, but no relationship worthy of note emerged.

Thus far the health status results have been presented separately for individual health-status measures, employing respondents, spouses, and children as units of analysis. Another approach was undertaken in which individual measures of health status were aggregated into a summary index with the total family employed as the unit of analysis. For respondents who had a spouse and at least one child covered by the insurance plan, an index of over-all family risk was constructed employing five pieces of information concerning the health status of family members prior to the interview. These were number of chronic illnesses, perceived health status, bed-disability days, major illnesses, and days spent in a hospital. Each of these pieces of information was available for respondents, spouses, and children. The empirical

---

[4]Because of the small sample sizes on which these differences are based the results do not achieve statistical significance even though the percentage differences are relatively large.

TABLE 8

Scores on 15-Point Family Risk Index
Based on the Choice Survey

	Blue Cross ($N = 85$) %	Prepaid Practice ($N = 65$) %
Score on risk index		
0–3	4	3
4	28	31
5	29	23
6	22	23
7 or more	16	20

$X^2 = .46$

$df = 4$

$p > .05$

[5]The reader should note that in the satisfaction study sample the information concerning the health status of family members will reflect the structure of the varying health care plans as well as patient characteristics and behavior.

distributions on each were examined, and extremes on the end of each distribution were designated as high-risk categories. One point was then assigned to a family whenever the respondent's, spouse's or children's score fell into a high-risk category. The total possible range on the risk index was 0-15.

Table 8 shows that over-all family risk was not significantly related to choice of health care plan, though the difference in the highest-risk category is in the direction predicted by the risk-vulnerability hypothesis. Twenty percent of the families enrolling in prepaid practice, in contrast to 16 percent of the families retaining Blue Cross–Blue Shield health insurance, received scores of 7 or more on the risk index. These differences are small and could represent chance variation.

A comparable analysis was carried out on the satisfaction-study sample in order to determine whether the same trend would emerge.[5] Unfortunately a measure of major illness was not included in the satisfaction study and therefore the risk index was

TABLE 9

Scores on 12-Point Family Risk Index
Based on the Satisfaction Survey

	Blue Cross $(N = 309)$ %	Prepaid Practice $(N = 301)$ %
Score on risk index		
0–1	1	1
2	27	24
3	28	29
4	22	23
5	13	13
6 or more	7	11

$X^2 = 2.48$
$df = 5$
$p > .05$

based on four rather than five types of information about respondents, spouses, and their children. Thus the index had a total possible range of 0–12. For the four pieces of information that were
available, the same cutoff points for assigning risk points which
were employed in the choice study were also used in the cross-
validation. Table 9 shows that a similar trend emerged in the cross-
validation sample, though once again it is weak and not statistically
significant. Eleven percent of the families participating in the prepaid practice, in contrast to 7 percent of the families participating
in Blue Cross, received the highest scores on the risk index.

Selectivity Resulting from Health Attitudes and Behavior

In evaluating whether there was any relationship between orientations toward preventive health practices and the choice of prepaid
group practice, we questioned respondents about their propensities
to use medical services under varying circumstances for both
themselves and their children, their perceptions of the importance
of regular checkups, when they last had a routine checkup, and
whether they owned a medical reference book. We also asked a
variety of more general questions concerning perceived control

over illness, faith in doctors, and skepticism about medical care. The results are presented in Table 10. Inspection of the results shows that no significant differences emerged. As with the health-status data, each of the analyses was repeated with the higher-income families excluded from the analysis. None of the resulting coefficients exceeded .10.

We did find, however, one exception to the general proposition that there is no selectivity resulting from preventive health attitudes and practices. Unlike the choice study, the satisfaction study included items designed to determine whether children covered by alternative insurance plans had received specific immunizations. Evidence for selectivity in immunization patterns is clearest for children, five years old and over, who had been participating in the prepaid program for one year only. These respondents were asked when, if ever, each of their children had been immunized against measles, polio, rubella, and mumps. The

TABLE 10

Reports on Use and Attitudes Toward
Preventive and Other Services

Measures of Use and Attitudes Toward Preventive and Other Services	Blue Cross ($N = 165$) $\bar{X}$	Prepaid Practice ($N = 168$) $\bar{X}$	p[a]
1. Propensity to use medical services for oneself	12.77	13.09	NS
2. Propensity to use medical services for young children[b]	13.46	12.86	NS
3. Importance of physical checkups	3.08	3.11	NS
4. Months since last checkup	48.98	38.89	NS
5. Importance of physical checkups for young children	2.64	2.58	NS
6. Perceived control over illness	8.93	9.01	NS
7. Faith in doctors	3.11	3.01	NS
8. Skepticism about medical care	8.50	8.75	NS
9. Possession of a medical reference book	1.59	1,54	NS

[a]Statistical significance is based upon unstandardized regression coefficients, employing the F distribution. The criterion used is the .05 level.

[b]Items 2 and 5 were only asked of respondents with children under 12; $N = 93$.

TABLE 11

Reports of Number of Immunizations Received One Year or More Prior to
Interview by Children Five Years of Age and Over

	Blue Cross ($N = 373$)	Prepaid Practice ($N = 445$)
	%	%
Number of immunizations received		
None	6	4
1	22	18
2	20	19
3	29	26
all 4	23	32

$X^2 = 11.47$
$df = 4$
$p < .025$

results, presented in Table 11, show that 32 percent of the children in the prepaid program, in contrast to 23 percent of those covered by Blue Cross health insurance, were reported to have received all four of the immunizations more than a year prior to the interview. It appears that children currently covered by the prepaid plan were more likely to be fully immunized prior to enrolling in prepaid practice than children of families choosing to retain Blue Cross health insurance.

A final question addressed by the present study was whether people with psychoneurotic symptoms would enroll in disproportionate numbers into a prepaid group practice plan. The results indicate that prepaid-group-practice respondents were no more neurotic ($\overline{X} = 7.86$) than Blue Cross–Blue Shield respondents ($\overline{X} = 7.88$). There were no significant differences in neuroticism in the satisfaction study, comparing prepaid-practice and Blue Cross respondents.

Discussion

Two socio-demographic factors were found to differentiate enrollees in prepaid group practice from families who chose to retain their fee-for-service insurance plan. Enrollees in the prepaid program were better educated and more likely to be unmarried. The education finding is consistent with other relevant research (Metzner et al., 1972), but the marital status result is more puzzling, since most other studies of choice report that married people are *more* likely than single people to enroll in prepaid plans. Single people were also found to be overrepresented among prepaid-group-practice participants in the satisfaction study where the employer was paying the entire health insurance premium.

The findings concerning perceptions of choice, based on the reasons people gave for their decisions, were generally consistent with previous research. Physical distance from the prepaid practice clinic and the existence of an ongoing relationship with a personal physician emerged as major deterrents to enrollment in the prepaid plan.

More than one quarter of prepaid-practice respondents reported that they had no regular doctor before joining the prepaid plan. Of those who had a regular doctor, about half indicated they were very satisfied with him when they joined the prepaid plan, and about 70 percent reported being either very or fairly satisfied. Although there was some dissatisfaction with existing medical care that led respondents to be attracted to prepaid practice, the majority were not dissatisfied, but rather were drawn to the prepaid program by positive attributes including centralization of all medical care in one place, insurance against risk, and availability of care on nights and weekends.

The risk-vulnerability hypothesis received little support in the present study. Socio-demographic indicators of risk-vulnerability (age, number of children, etc.) did not predict enrollment. Indeed, the relationship which emerged between marital status and enrollment is contrary to some of the implications of the risk-vulnerability hypothesis. Similarly, most of the data on health status does not support the risk-vulnerability formulation. There was little sign of selectivity due to perceived health status, bed disability, major illnesses, or hospitalization either when these variables were examined separately or when they were examined as part of an index of over-all family risk.

Some support for the risk-vulnerability formulation came from analyses of the distribution of chronic illnesses in the two groups.

Prepaid-practice respondents reported more chronic illnesses than Blue Cross respondents, and although the overrepresentation of respondents with chronic illnesses in the prepaid program was not large, our data suggests that persons with many chronic illnesses tend to be heavy users of medical services. From a practical point of view, therefore, any overrepresentation of persons with chronic illnesses is a significant matter. There was also a tendency for spouses and children of lower-income families enrolling in prepaid group practice to have more chronic illnesses than spouses and children of lower-income families who chose to retain the Blue Cross plan.

The evidence for selectivity resulting from preventive-health attitudes and behavior was somewhat mixed. In the choice study itself, there is no evidence of selectivity in choice resulting from health attitudes and propensities. The enrollment decision was found to be unrelated to several questions included in the interview schedule designed to tap health consciousness and readiness to use medical services. If a conclusion is to be drawn on the basis of this study alone, it would be that prepaid-group-practice and Blue Cross enrollees are basically the same in their propensities to use preventive services and in their attitudes toward care. On the other hand, retrospective data drawn from the satisfaction study concerning immunization of children participating in alternative insurance plans indicated that children of prepaid-practice respondents were more fully immunized at the point of enrollment than children of respondents who chose to retain Blue Cross–Blue Shield.

There was no evidence of selectivity due to neuroticism in the present study. Thus the results provide no support for the proposition that prepaid practices tend to attract disproportionate numbers of "worried wells" (also see Mechanic, 1973; 1974b).

In concluding, it is important to emphasize that this is basically a case study. Any conclusions about degree of selectivity into prepaid plans must be made on the basis of cumulative experience in varying social settings. The people under study here were drawn from an employed population and the Blue Cross–Blue Shield alternative was quite liberal with respect to its outpatient coverage. It is possible that selective influences on choice will prove to be greater in other populations where the savings in costs resulting from enrollment in prepaid group practice plans is more obvious and clear-cut for individuals and families at risk.

Richard Tessler, PH.D.
Department of Sociology
University of Massachusetts
Amherst, Massachusetts 01002

David Mechanic, PH.D.
Center for Advanced Study in the Behavioral Sciences
Stanford, California 94305

The study described in this paper was supported by grants from the Milbank Memorial Fund and the Robert Wood Johnson Foundation.

References

Anderson, W., and B. Sheatsley
1959   Comprehensive Medical Insurance: A Study of Costs, Use, and Attitudes Under Two Plans. Health Insurance Foundation. Research Series No. 9.

Bashshur, R. L., and C. A. Metzner
1967   "Patterns of social differentiation between Community Health Association and Blue Cross–Blue Shield." Inquiry 4: 23–44.

1970   "Vulnerability to risk and awareness of dual choice of health insurance plan." Health Services Research (Summer): 106–113.

Bice, T. W.
1973   "Enrollment in a prepaid group practice." Unpublished manuscript. Deaprtment of Medical Care and Hospitals, The Johns Hopkins University.

Bice, T. W., S. Radius, and L. Wollstadt
1974   "Risk vulnerability and enrollment in a prepaid group practice and disenrollment from a prepaid group practice." Unpublished manuscript. Center for Metropolitan Planning and Research, The Johns Hopkins University.

Donabedian, A.
1969   "An evaluation of prepaid group practice." Inquiry 6: 3–27.

Eysenck, S. F. G., and H. J. Eysenck
  1964   "An improved short questionnaire for the measurement of ex-
          troversion and neuroticism." Life Sciences 3: 1103-1109.

Garfield, S. R.
  1970   "The delivery of medical care." Scientific American 222: 15-23.

Hetherington, R., C. E. Hopkins, and M. I. Roemer
  1975   Health Insurance Plans: Promise and Performance. New York: Wiley-
          Interscience.

Jackson, J. O., and M. Greenlick
  1974   "The worried-well revisited." Medical Care 12: 659-667.

Mechanic, D.
  1972   Public Expectations and Health Care. New York: Wiley-Interscience.

  1972   "Patient behavior and the organization of medical care." Research
          and Analytic Report Series, 1-73. Center for Medical Sociology and
          Health Services Research, Madison, Wisconsin.

  1974a   "The comparative study of health care delivery systems." Research
          and Analytic Report Series, 12-74. Center for Medical Sociology and
          Health Services Research, Madison, Wisconsin.

  1974b   "The organization of medical practice and practice orientations among
          physicians in prepaid and nonprepaid primary care settings."
          Research and Analytic Report Series, 13-74. Center for Medical
          Sociology and Health Services Research, Madison, Wisconsin.

Metzner, C. A., and R. L. Bashshur
  1967   "Factors associated with choice of health care plans." Journal of
          Health and Social Behavior 8: 291-299.

Metzner, C. A., R. L. Bashshur, and G. Shannon
  1972   "Differential public acceptance of group medical practice." Medical
          Care 10: 279-287.

Moustafa, A. T., C. E. Hopkins, and B. Klein
  1971   "Determinants of choice and change of health insurance plan."
          Medical Care 9: 32-41.

Roemer, M. I., and W. Shonick
  1973   "HMO performance: the recent evidence." Milbank Memorial Fund
          Quarterly: Health and Society (Summer): 271-317.

Shapiro. S., S. L. Weiner, and P. M. Densen
  1958   "Comparison of prematurity and perinatal mortality in a general

population and in the population of a prepaid group practice medical care plan.'' American Journal of Public Health 48: 170–187.

Shapiro, S., J. J. Williams, A. S. Yerby, P. M. Densen, and H. Rosner
1967   ''Patterns of medical use by the indigent aged under two systems of medical care.'' American Journal of Public Health 57: 784–790.

Tessler, R., and D. Mechanic
1974   ''Consumer satisfaction with prepaid group practice: a comparative study.'' Journal of Health and Social Behavior, forthcoming.

Wolfman, B.
1961   ''Medical expenses and choice of plan: a case study.'' Monthly Labor Review 84: 1186–1190.

Yedidia, A.
1959   ''Dual choice programs.'' American Journal of Public Health 49: 1475–1480.

HMO Enrollment: Who Joins What and Why: A Review of the Literature

S.E. BERKI and MARIE L.F. ASHCRAFT

Department of Medical Care Organization,
School of Public Health,
University of Michigan;
Health Services Research and Development Program,
Ann Arbor Veterans Administration Medical Center,
Ann Arbor

I F HEALTH MAINTENANCE ORGANIZATIONS (HMOS) are to be economically viable alternatives in the medical care market they must be able to attract providers and consumers. The quantity and quality of their enrollee base is a principal determinant of their ability to provide services at competitive prices. Hence the question of who enrolls and why is basic.

Enrollment may occur on an individual or a group basis. Individual enrollment, during open enrollment periods, is a voluntary exercise of choice. Group enrollment is also the result of choice by individual members. Although the decision to offer an HMO option may frequently be subject to collective bargaining or some other type of joint decision-making, once such a choice is offered, it must be one alternative between two or more plans from which consumers are individually free to choose.

Milbank Memorial Fund Quarterly/*Health and Society,* Vol. 58, No. 4, 1980
© 1980 Milbank Memorial Fund and Massachusetts Institute of Technology
0160/1997/5804/0588-46 $01.00/0

The requirement of free choice among alternative plans, with different benefit packages, costs, and provider systems, indicates that the decision to enroll in a given plan can best be considered in the framework of choice behavior. Models of choice behavior generally assume that the individual decision maker will select the alternative that, given his level of information, is expected to maximize his satisfaction or utility. This assumes that the individual, informed about the characteristics of available alternatives, is the best judge of which particular combination of such characteristics, as represented by a given plan, is the most suitable for him, or in other words, is likely to yield the highest level of satisfaction. This does not imply that individual decisions are not influenced by the choices of others or by group values and decisions.

The assumption of individual choice is an important one. The approach here presented is not applicable to situations where group members do not exercise individual choices, a long-standing objective of unions (Munts, 1967). Further, although in dual- and multiple-choice situations group members must *de jure* be free to exercise individual decisions, *de facto* they may not always be so where collective choice by a group, such as a union, is paramount. That possibility is also not encompassed here. Both of these situations would require a different framework for their understanding.

In the past, the choice, if any, was between a service benefit or indemnity health insurance plan, and a closed-panel, prepaid group practice—hence the studies of dual choice. Current alternatives often include a third model, the individual practice association with its open panel of physicians. The question of "Who joins HMOs?" is now, therefore, *"Who* joins *what* kind of HMO and *why?"*

Whatever framework is employed to analyze enrollment, the enrollment decision is clearly related to expected service use. Hence the issue should be viewed as a set of iterative, interrelated decisions, specifically, 1) the decision to enroll; 2) the decision to remain enrolled; and 3) the decision to utilize services. The development of a complete model of enrollment, retention, and utilization, each of crucial significance to HMO performance, is beyond the scope of this paper, and beyond the current state of the literature.

This paper sets out a framework for analyzing the enrollment decision and then summarizes the literature on it.

Enrollment Choice: An Analytic Framework

Choice among alternative plans with different benefit packages, costs, and provider systems results in the observable decision to enroll in a given health insurance plan. Concepts of risk, of expected costs and benefits, are applicable directly to situations involving service benefit or indemnity plans only. In such situations the purchase of health insurance is a transfer of the risk of financial losses incurred by the use of medical services. Selection of providers of services is a separate decision, subsequent in time to the choice of insurance coverage. Since the decision is between insurance plans only, and is independent of the choice of providers, it can be considered strictly in terms of *insurance characteristics:* 1) the benefit package covered; 2) premium cost to the enrollee; and 3) cost-sharing provisions such as deductibles, copayment, coinsurance, and benefit ceilings.

Enrollment in an HMO is a simultaneous choice of both insurance coverage of the cost of medical services and their system of delivery. Decision variables relating to aspects of the delivery system, the *delivery characteristics,* must also be considered. Principal dimensions that consumers may consider include 1) spatial, psychosocial, and temporal dimensions of access; 2) continuity of care; 3) comprehensiveness; 4) clinical quality, and 5) social quality. Individuals are likely to evaluate the importance of these delivery characteristics in terms of their relative attractiveness, relative among alternatives and relative to the system or plan in which they receive services at the time the decision is made.

The framework for the analysis of enrollment decisions is summarized in schematic form in Figure 1, with direct relationships shown in solid lines. The economic characteristics and risk factors of the decision unit (family or individual), modified by its beliefs about medicine, determine its expected volume and type of health services use, its utilization pattern.

The expected utilization patterns and their associated costs are the principal factors influencing choice among the insurance characteristics of alternative plans. Financial aspects of that choice are analyzed in terms of the financial vulnerability hypothesis. The effect of expected utilization patterns resulting from family risk factors is analyzed in terms of the risk perception hypothesis.

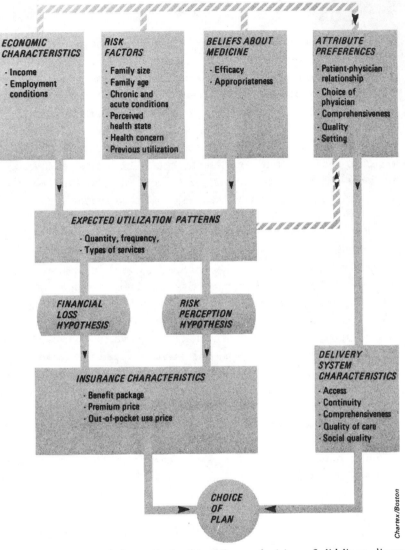

FIG. 1. Framework for analysis of enrollment decisions. Solid lines, direct relationships. Barred lines, indirect relationships.

Expected utilization patterns and the desirability of the delivery characteristics of alternative plans are the decision variables in the choice of delivery system. The decision unit's socioeconomic characteristics and its health risk factors influence its preferences over delivery characteristics, indicated in dotted lines.

The economic characteristics, risk factors, beliefs, and preferences for plan attributes are the variables describing potential enrollees. The insurance and delivery characteristics of the alternative plans are evaluated by the potential enrollees in terms of these variables. Given expected utilization patterns and attribute preferences on the one hand, and, on the other, the insurance and delivery characteristic bundles available, enrollment will represent the choice of plan whose dimensions are thought to best fit the potential enrollee's utilization and system preferences. The nature and extent of the trade-offs between insurance and delivery system characteristics, and their relation to such characteristics of alternate plans, are the basic issues to be considered in delivery system design, siting, and pricing.

Plan Characteristics, Perceived Characteristics, and Plan Valuation

Specific alternatives have objectively existing insurance and delivery characteristics. Each plan offers a defined set of covered services, specifying exclusions and/or the conditions under which the services are available, such as out-of-area coverage; indemnity plans similarly specify types of services and situations that will result in the payment of predetermined amounts. Among the attributes that define the plan are premium and cost-sharing provisions and rates, as well as delivery characteristics, such as the ability to choose a physician either from a specified and limited group or from a large number of individually located physicians, or, alternatively, the ability of a potential enrollee to retain an existing relationship with a physician. In their totality, these attributes comprise the plan. Hence they can be said to exist objectively. The extent to which they exist equally for all enrollees, and hence enrollees' experience with them, is principally related to the decision to remain enrolled and, to some extent, to the plan's "reputation" and its potential effect on enrollment decisions.

The enrollment decision, however, is based on information about these objectively existing characteristics. To the extent that plan characteristics are considered in the decision to enroll, it is the decision makers' beliefs about them that become the deciding factors. It is the perceived attributes of plans, what potential enrollees believe them to be, and not necessarily what they actually are, upon which decisions are likely to be made. The degree of conformance between actual and perceived attributes and the role of information are principal marketing issues and will not be developed here. What is important to note, however, is that preferences are translated into choice based on attributes that decision makers believe to exist. The match between the state of the world that can be said to exist objectively, and what decision makers believe it to be, is not necessarily exact.

How objective attributes are perceived, their salience, is likely to be dependent on their relative valuations by decision makers. The principal issues in assessing the roles of perceived attributes in the enrollment decision are how these perceptions came about and how the attributes are valued.

The roles of insurance characteristics are best understood in terms of risk perception and financial vulnerability hypotheses.

Insurance Characteristics

The *risk perception* hypothesis states that the higher an individual's perceived likelihood of the occurrence of future events that will require the use of medical services, the more likely that individual is, other things being equal, to choose a more comprehensive benefit package and to pay the higher premium.

The *financial vulnerability* hypothesis argues that the larger the expected utility loss associated with a given level of expected financial loss, the more likely that the individual will purchase a plan that reduces the cost of utilization of medical services.

The risk perception hypothesis is derived from a formulation in which medical care services are single-purpose goods and yield satisfaction only when the consumer considers them to be needed for therapeutic, maintenance, or preventive purposes. They are not considered to be substitutes for other goods and services and hence do not yield satisfaction except in the case of perceived present or future need. Hence it is the individual's subjective probability estimate of future events, illness, maintenance, or prevention—that is, his perception of risk—that assigns a value to medical services, the benefit package.

The level of perceived health risk is likely to be a function of the individual's health history, present state of perceived health, age, and experience in health services utilization. The magnitude of subjective risk is also likely to be influenced by attitudes toward risk, that is, risk avoidance or preference, as well as future orientation and perceptions of locus of control. Thus individuals who are not future-oriented and operate within relatively short time horizons, in the belief that they themselves are not in control of future events, are less likely to have high risk perceptions or assign high values to risk avoidance.

The health risk hypothesis is consistent with the concepts of adverse self-selection and moral hazard. Those who believe themselves, for whatever reason, more likely to be in need of future services are more likely to choose the more extensive coverage at the same price or even at a higher price. Further, once individuals with higher risk perceptions are able to utilize services at lower out-of-pocket prices, their use of services is likely to be highly price-elastic, resulting in large increases in utilization.

To the extent, therefore, that HMOs offer extended benefit packages at zero or nominal out-of-pocket prices, they are likely to be attractive to individuals whose level of perceived health risk is higher, and who then will use excessive services. From the perspective of the HMO, the self-selection, if it occurs, is adverse.

The role of insurance characteristics is complicated by the fact that coverage is traditionally available to dependents; hence the risk perception hypothesis, while applicable to individuals, may be even more so to families. When the decision maker considers not only his own health status but also the health status and welfare of eligible family members, it is the subjective health risk of the family unit that is the appropriate unit of analysis.

In economic models of insurance (Grossman, 1972), the demand for coverage originates in a perceived need to reduce losses from present or expected future health status, by the purchase of health care services. The economic models assume that the effects of such purchased health care services on health status are determined by some externally given production function. The effectiveness of health care services, in other words, is given by the state of the medical arts. Although that may be the case objectively, individual attitudes, however acquired, toward the efficacy of medicine, and types of health care, are likely to vary. It would be expected that higher levels of belief in the efficacy of modern scientific medicine, for example, would lead to a higher valuation of the restorative function and hence, for a given level of subjective perception of health risk, to a higher demand for more extensive benefit packages. This concept is distinct from beliefs about the efficacy of the individual providers and the clinical quality dimensions of alternative plans. In fact, a certain degree of belief in the efficacy of medicine must exist for beliefs about the clinical quality of individual providers to be relevant. Clearly, at the extreme, disbelief in medicine renders moot the issue of the efficacy of its individual providers.

The health risk hypothesis, then, is the principal means of incorporating those individual, familial, experiential, and attitudinal factors that are likely to affect the decision-making unit's assessment of its subjective risk status and its evaluation of the appropriateness of the benefit packages available.

The financial vulnerability hypothesis, on the other hand, incorporates those financial aspects of the alternatives that are attendant on the use of services and the purchase of insurance. In this formulation there is no distinction between service benefit and capitated plans. From the perspective of the potential enrollee, they are both prepaid; what differ are the benefit packages and the rates and mechanisms of cost sharing. Particularly with the increasing availability of "riders" and "add-ons," from dental coverage to prescription drugs, and in the presence of comprehensive inpatient coverage in the service benefit plans, the major factor is likely to be cost-sharing rates. In this perspective, noncovered ambulatory services in service plans are seen as fully self-insured, with full cost-sharing. The extent to which financial factors are likely to play a role in the decision will depend on the expected level of total health care costs, premium and out-of-pocket, and its associated utility loss.

Utility loss arises from economic loss, reduction either of wealth or of consumption. The expected level of total health care costs, and thus its utility loss equivalent, is a function of expected service use. At one end of the spectrum, as Bice et al. (1974; 1975) have indicated, when the connection between expected utilization and financial cost is broken, as in the case of those eligible for Title XIX, the financial vulnerability hypothesis is irrelevant. It may also be that at the other end of the spectrum, at high income levels, where even relatively large potential financial losses are associated with relatively low utility losses, the purchase of the insurance characteristics of the plan may not be attractive. The extent to which this is likely to be the case, or, alternatively, the extent to which large losses even with very small subjective probabilities lead to risk aversion, the fear of a "wipe-out," is debatable. The implications of the financial vulnerability hypothesis, however, are that lower-income decision units, for whom a given economic loss is a relatively larger utility loss, and relatively higher-income decision units (but still within the middle-income range), for whom large financial losses may represent an economic wipe-out, are more likely to choose the option with the better potential for reduction of economic loss, and at a higher premium price. The stress must be on premium price, since the *total* price of any given pattern of service use is the sum of premium payments and out-of-pocket costs. Out-of-pocket costs of service use are determined by the benefit package and the cost-sharing provisions. Inclusion of fully prepaid ambulatory service benefits, that is to say, zero cost-sharing, in a benefit package (x), offered at the same premium price as another benefit package (y) with identical coverage but with 50 percent cost-sharing, represents a lower *total* price. The lower total price (of x) may reflect that the actuarial value of the premium is greater than its price, or that service use will somehow be controlled. It may also be that the premium of the cost-sharing plan (y) is predicated on the existence of moral hazard, excessive use induced by the reduction of out-of-pocket price.

Choice of Delivery Characteristics

The delivery characteristics of health care plans are their organizational, locational, and social attributes. It is useful to consider them as 1) access; 2) continuity; 3) comprehensiveness; 4) quality; and 5) social quality or social organization.

Access. Access may be considered to have three dimensions: spatial, temporal, and psychosocial. *Spatial* access refers to the location of delivery sites in relation to the potential user's domicile or, where appropriate, domicile and workplace. It is assumed that potential enrollees, other things being held constant, prefer health care plans whose delivery sites, in terms of distance or travel time, provide for greater ease of physical contact. The extent to which perceptions of spatial or physical access by potential enrollees might vary, based on their accustomed travel patterns, is not clear.

Spatial accessibility is important in both single site and multidelivery site systems. Furthermore, in multidelivery site systems offering a comprehensive set of services, the spatial distribution of specialized services, e.g., inpatient and therapeutic radiology, will necessarily differ from the spatial distribution of services used more often, e.g., primary adult and pediatric care. In such choice situations, the potential enrollee is likely to consider the spatial distribution of the totality of services, so that the formulation of hypotheses about its effect on the enrollment decision becomes more difficult.

How strongly consumers feel about spatial access is likely to be affected by their expected use patterns. In this instance the health risk hypothesis reinforces the potential significance of spatial accessibility. Those whose perceived health risk is higher and who, therefore, expect to be higher utilizers, are more likely to consider spatial access to be important than are those who expect to use few services, or specific services relatively infrequently.

The *temporal* dimension of access refers to the time lag between the patient's first attempt at establishing contact with a provider and its actualization. Under nonemergent conditions, waiting time required to get an appointment and waiting time in the office comprise the basic elements of temporal access.

The time required to contact a provider out of office hours and the time required to make physical contact during emergencies may also be considered relevant decision factors.

The relative importance of the temporal dimensions of access in the decision process is likely to be influenced by the potential enrollee's perceived health risk. As in the case of physical access, temporal access is likely to be considered more important to consumers whose perceived health risk is higher than for decision units who expect lower use rates.

An important element of both spatial and temporal dimensions of access is the enrollees' perception of whether contact with a physician can be readily obtained or not. Health care plans that deliver medical services on single or multispecialty group bases, with or without special emergency clinics, but with mechanisms that allow assured contact with a provider with a short time lag in spatially easily accessible locations, can be said to provide "assured access." Although this feature is theoretically attainable by individual solo practice settings, through the establishment of emergency coverage during off-hours and formal patient-sharing and referral mechanisms in case of overload, in practice that is not likely to be the case. Assured access may be a particularly important decision variable for individuals new to the community or who do not perceive its existence within their former delivery setting.

One of the dimensions of temporal access has been considered by economists as the "time price" of services. To the extent that time prices vary by occupational and income levels, it is expected that those whose opportunity cost of time is higher will prefer delivery systems in which time price is minimized. Whether the time price concept fully captures time preference is unclear. Time preferences may be influenced by attitudinal and ecological factors, independent of the money price of time. Thus future-oriented "time-conscious" individuals for whom longer office waiting times involve social disruptions—the socially active homemaker, the proverbial "dependent"—may well prefer shorter waiting times, more than the higher-income wage earner paid on a yearly basis.

The temporal dimensions of access, then, may be considered more important by individuals with higher perceived health risk and, other things being equal, shorter temporal access may be considered better.

Psychosocial access refers to the potential enrollee's perceived social distance to providers. The ability to communicate freely and openly with providers, an assumed preference of patients, is influenced by patient-provider social class, ethnic, racial, and cultural differences. Particularly in multiethnic and multiracial settings, it is likely that health care plans, or their delivery sites that employ providers closely identified with a particular racial or ethnic group, are going to be a less favorable option to other, different, ethnic or racial groups. The obverse, however, may also be true.

Although the relative importance of the spatial, temporal, and psychosocial dimensions of access to the enrollment decision may not be the same, it is likely that all are important decision variables to the choice of plan.

Continuity. Continuity of care refers to the ability of the patient to establish or to maintain a patient-physician relationship with a physician of choice, and having a given physician as the principal health care coordinator.

The essential elements are the ability to have a patient-physician relationship, the ability to choose that physician, and the definition of the set of physicians from which that choice may be made. This is the principal issue in the choice of closed-panel and op´ .-panel HMOs. Closed-panel HMOs offer a choice of physician, always in theory and often in practice. But that choice is necessarily limited to a group whose size and composition are defined by the plan. Open-panel HMOs, on the other hand, generally include large proportions of the practicing physician population in their community, hence the choice of a physician, if one needs to be made, is less constrained.

Individuals, and/or decision units where that is the family, who have an established patient-physician relationship of some duration are more likely to want to maintain it. The choice of HMOs in which enrollment necessitates the severing of an existing satisfactory patient-physician relationship, other things being constant, is not likely. On the other hand, if enrollment in a health care plan provides for the maintenance of an already existing relationship, the usual feature of foundation or IPA models, enrollment (other things being the same) is more likely.

For decision units without such a relationship, or with a relationship that is unsatisfactory, the choice situation is different. For them, enrollment in a closed-panel HMO does not imply severing the familiarity of an established relationship. Here the reasons for the absence of such a relationship must be considered, however. If such a relationship does not exist because the decision maker is new to the community, or because attempts to establish such a relationship were made unsuccessfully in the past, choice of a plan that offers assured access and a choice of a physician, even if from a limited group, is more likely. If, however, the decision maker has no patient-physician relationship because there was no felt need for it, enrollment (other things being equal) is problematic. Hence it is not simply whether a patient-physician relationship exists but also, if it does not, why.

Patient-physician ratios, practice loads and practice patterns, all supply side factors, as well as community net migration patterns, are important determinants of the prevalence of the patient-physician relationship and of perceived access to care. Where relationships are less prevalent, the likelihood of the choice of closed-panel HMOs is apt to be increased.

Professionals maintain the desirability of having one provider to orchestrate the provision of health care services, and some HMOs in fact attempt to provide for this, but the extent to which consumers prefer this is unclear. Thus even though such a system may be advantageous from the clinical, administrative, and economic perspectives, its role in the enrollment choice decision is unclear.

For enrollment choice analysis, therefore, the essential elements of continuity relate to the existence of the patient-physician relationship and the degree of physician choice.

Comprehensiveness. Comprehensiveness refers to the breadth of services that the patient may receive from the same set of providers or within the same physical setting. It is to be distinguished from the comprehensiveness of the benefit package, in that it refers not to the spectrum of services covered but to the system by which that spectrum of services is rendered.

Evolution of general consumption patterns, both facilitated by and encouraging "supermarket" retailing in a wide variety of fields, is thought to imply consumer preference for "one-door shopping." Physical aggregation of generalists, specialists, and ancillary services in health care may, therefore, be considered attractive in terms of service pattern preferences. It can also reduce service-connected travel time and facilitate more appropriate referral patterns, particularly intra-group referrals.

The extent to which these features are perceived and valued by decision makers in the enrollment choice situation is problematic.

Quality of care. The clinical quality of delivery characteristics encompasses the clinical appropriateness and effectiveness of the care pattern. The clinical competence of individual providers is a necessary but not a sufficient condition for the maximization of the clinical quality of the care pattern. The care pattern attains high levels of clinical quality when its individual elements, rendered by different providers, are most appropriately coordinated and are suited to the complex of clinical and psychosocial pathologies represented by the whole patient. It is a characteristic of the system, and not only of its individual elements. Even supposing that differences in these aspects of clinical quality are in fact systematically associated with types of practice settings, whether patients perceive it that way is open to question.

A subset of clinical quality, however, the competence of the providers, is more likely to be a decision variable in enrollment choices. Few if any patients have sufficient experience and clinical information to assess for themselves the competence levels of various providers. They may therefore be influenced in their enrollment .ecisions by the reputation of provider plans and beliefs about the appropriate" organization and management of medical practice. These are then used to derive associated beliefs about the competence of providers. Hence, if decision makers believe, whether based on their own experience or not, that physicians practicing in clinics do not have the same level of competence as those practicing in private settings, the HMO that offers a clinic-type delivery system may not be viewed with favor. An appropriately managed clinic-type setting may have high levels of temporal access, continuity, and comprehensiveness, yet, because of the nature of its organization, may be assumed to provide lower quality. Yet the lower levels of performance on these delivery aspects that might be found in solo settings may be associated with higher quality. Hence the role of perceived quality, not to mention its relation to actual quality, in the enrollment decision is unclear.

Another subset of clinical quality, and one that may be interdependent with psychosocial access, comprises the humaneness of providers and the dignity afforded patients, the "care" component of "cure and care." Enrollees can be assumed to prefer delivery settings in which the providers are expected to care more, to be more solicitous of patient complaints, to treat them more as individuals. It may well be that potential enrollees associate these characteristics more with individual office-based physicians than with larger-scale clinic-type settings. This may also be an important motive for the desire to establish a patient-physician relationship; hence it is unclear whether it is more appropriately considered as a dimension of that relationship or as a dimension of the quality of care. In either case, it is probably an important decision factor.

Social Quality. The concept of the social quality captures the elements of the delivery system that, although not objectively related to other delivery characteristics, are perceived by potential enrollees as relevant. The physical attractiveness and social location of delivery sites, the prestige and reputation of the plan in terms of "modernity," "innovativeness," and humane concerns, are elements of an HMO's perceived social quality or social attractiveness. For example, HMOs originating in inner cities, which then attempt to expand to middle-class suburban areas, sometimes may find it advantageous to change their names, to live down, as it were, their reputation. Alternatively, where competing HMOs exist, competitors may repeatedly refer to such plans by names designed to stigmatize them as socially less desirable, as in Rochester, where the Rochester Health Network is often referred to as the "Neighborhood Health Center Plan."

Further, social quality may include perceptions of the clientele the HMO serves. Whom the patient shares the waiting room and clinical facilities with may be considered as a factor in the decision to select one plan over another, particularly in geographically and socially heterogeneous settings. Where the delivery site is located and who the site serves, and whether the HMO is identified with a given population subset may be important variables to some potential enrollees.

The effects of these aspects of social quality are important in enrollment decisions and their implications for the economic viability of HMOs. HMOs identified by potential enrollees with an ethnic or racial group may attract only members of that group, and particularly its members from the lower-income strata. If such enrollment "success" reduces the HMO's chances of enrolling the higher-income members of other ethnic or racial groups, the economic composition of the enrollees may not ensure economic viability without subsidies. Increased reliance on subsidies directly, or indirectly by enrolling subsidized individuals, such as Title XIX beneficiaries, may further reduce the HMO's relative attractiveness to other potential enrollees, particularly in dual or multichoice options offered to employed groups. Needless to say, this is likely to have an effect on the medical staff composition, thus starting a downward spiral whose termination is the "Medicaid mill," an unattractive alternative, regardless of its geographic setting.

Social quality may be seen as an aspect of product differentiation, sometimes merely packaging. Its effect in the enrollment decision may be to segment enrollment by social class or along ethnic and racial lines. Its corollary is the drawing power of HMOs whose reputation and prestige are high.

When one of the options is a standard service benefit plan, such as Blue Cross/Blue Shield (BC-BS), that plan may enjoy several advantages in terms of social quality. First of all, it has no delivery system; hence none of the location- and facility-related aspects of social quality apply to it. Second, it will usually be the plan used by the largest proportion of potential enrollees in other plans—the incumbent plan—and its present users are socially, demographically, and economically heterogeneous. It might also be associated in the minds of potential enrollees as the "mainstream," "the American way." The extent to which these potential advantages of plans such as BC-BS can be transferred to HMOs sponsored by them is unclear.

On balance, and other things being equal, it is likely that the social quality dimensions of HMOs play an important part in enrollment decisions, with higher perceived social quality an enrollment advantage.

State of the Art

Studies of enrollment choice attempt to determine individual and family characteristics that differentiate those who select an HMO from those who do not, and to differentiate between those who select a staff model HMO and those who choose an individual practice association (IPA). By determining the relative roles of these characteristics in the enrollment decision, one should be able to predict its outcome: who enrolls, in what, and why. The design and analytic plan of most studies, however, while responding to the first and occasionally the second question, have rarely provided answers to the third. Even when only the first question is asked, differences in the methodologies render the results essentially incomparable. It is not clear whether the differing results of various studies are due to differences in population characteristics, sample sizes, instrumentation, analytic design, and study timing, or whether the enrollment groups actually differ. Nor is it clear whether lack of significant differences between enrollment groups within any study is a generalizable finding, or the result of limited variation that occurs naturally in the sample. In addition, since bivariate analyses are used almost exclusively, determining the independent or relative effects of the more important factors, such as health risk and financial vulnerability, is virtually impossible. Those are the principal reasons why answers to the questions of who enrolls, in what, and why are at best tentative.

Tables 1 and 2, respectively, show the variation among empirical studies, in terms of design and methodology, and in setting and population characteristics, all of which affect the comparability and generalizability of their results. In the sections that follow the results of those studies are discussed.

Insurance Characteristics

As stated previously, the role of the insurance factors can best be understood in terms of characteristics that define individuals' level of risk, which derive primarily from two sources: individuals' perceived or actual health state and their perceived financial vulnerability.

Risk Perception Factors. Although the risk perception hypothesis has not been tested in the precise terms stated earlier, it has been closely approximated. On the reasonable assumption that future need for medical care is related to present need, although probably not linearly, studies have focused on those direct and indirect indicators of health risk that might be predictive of future use of services. The issue is one of adverse self-selection: Do "sicker" people join an HMO?

Health risk has variously been measured by previous utilization experience, both ambulatory and inpatient, by the number and kinds of acute and chronic illnesses, by the presence of disability and its duration, by attitudinal measures such as perceived health status and health concern, and by demographic characteristics as proxy indicators, used either independently or in combination. The evidence on adverse self-selection is mixed.

Demographic characteristics of individuals and families, such as age, marital status, family size, age of children, procreative age, and retirement status, may indicate a potential need for medical care as clearly as reports of present health or perceived health status (Andersen, 1968). These measures have been used singly as well as combined in a family life stage construct to test the risk perception hypothesis. In general, the results have supported it.

In studies of choice between an HMO and either a service benefit (such as BC-BS) or an indemnity health insurance plan, HMO enrollees are more likely to be married than single (Bashshur and Metzner, 1967; Jurgovan and Carpenter, 1974; Moustafa et al., 1971), with larger and younger families (Berki et al., 1977a; Juba et al., 1980; Roghmann et al., 1975; Wolfman, 1961), than those choosing less

TABLE 1
Methodological Characteristics of Selected Studies of Enrollment Choice

Study	Study Date	Sample Characteristics	Months between Enrollment and Study	Method of Data Collection*	Number in Study Response Rate**	Respondents	Principal Type of Data Analysis
Bashshur and Metzner, 1967	1964	Stratified Random	36	S	1,201F 90%	Subscribers	Bivariate
Berki et al., 1977a	1974	Stratified Random	1–2	S	626F 83%	Employees	Bivariate
Berki et al., 1978	1974	Stratified Random	1–2	S	626F 83%	Employees	Multivariate
Bice, 1973	1971	Area Probability	Prospective	S (plus records)	826I 92%	All adults	Bivariate
Juba et al., 1980	1976	Stratified Random	‡	M	332F 46%	Employees	Multivariate
Jurgovan and Carpenter, 1974	1974	100%	1–2	M (plus records)	3,365F 57%	Employees	Bivariate
Moustafa et al., 1972	1967	100%	‡	M	271F 58%	Employees	Bivariate
Richardson et al., 1976	1976	100%	< 1	S	6,860F 90%	Adults	Bivariate
Roghmann et al., 1975	1973	Stratified Random	1–5	M	373F 30%	Subscribers	Bivariate
Scitovsky et al., 1978	1973	100%	> 6	S	1,816F 59%	Subscribers	Multivariate
Tessler and Mechanic, 1975	1975	Stratified Random	‡	T	333F 89%	Female adults	Bivariate

*S, Personal interview; T, Telephone survey; M, Mail survey

**F, Families; I, Individuals
‡No information available

TABLE 2

Site and Plan Characteristics of Selected Studies of Enrollment Choice

Study	Age of HMO (Years)	Premium Cost to Enrollee for HMO?	Hospital Control by HMO?	Comparative Plans	Characteristics of Eligible Study Population
Bashshur and Metzner, 1967	4	Yes	Yes	PGP/BC-BS*	UAW members in automotive plants
Berki et al., 1977a	< 2	No	No	IPA/2 PGPs/BC-BS*	Employees of single manufacturing plant
Bice, 1973	< 1	**	No	PGP	Residents of low-income inner city area
Juba et al., 1980	"new"	Yes	No	PGP/BC-BS*	University employees
Jurgovan and Carpenter, 1974	1	Yes	No	IPA/PGP/Indemnity*	Employees of single company
Moustafa et al., 1972	> 10	Yes	Yes	2 PGPs/BC-BS/Indemnity*	New university employees
Richardson et al., 1976	> 10	**	Yes	PGP/BC-BS	Residents of low-income target area
Roghmann et al., 1975	< 1	Yes	No	IPA/2 PGPs/BC-BS*	Employees of single company
	< 3	Yes	No	IPA/2 PGPs/BC-BS*	Employees of several companies
Scitovsky et al., 1978‡	> 10	Yes	Yes	2 PGPs	University employees
Tessler and Mechanic, 1975	< 3	Yes	No	PG/BC-BS*	Municipal employees

*Incumbent plan.
**Not applicable.
‡This study focused on choice between two HMOs (Kaiser and Stanford Clinic Plan). For purposes of display on this table, Kaiser was arbitrarily selected as the HMO.

comprehensive (and less expensive) service benefit plans, usually favored by young, single individuals (Berki et al., 1977a; Roemer et al., 1972).

Although these results generally have prevailed, contrary findings have also been reported. In one study, married families selected BC-BS more often than an available HMO (Tessler and Mechanic, 1975); in two other studies, HMO enrollee families were somewhat older than families opting for BC-BS, although all were still within the middle-age range (Bashshur and Metzner, 1967; Moustafa et al., 1971); and no statistically significant differences in age and family size between the two enrollment groups were found in another (Tessler and Mechanic, 1975).

On balance, however, the evidence seems convincing that when employee groups are offered a choice between plans differing in their insurance characteristics, single individuals and families with few or older members seem to prefer the limited coverage of the insurance plan (with its usually lower premium cost), while HMOs attract families expected to exhibit the greater demand for care that is associated with a younger and expanding life stage. It is this evidence, in fact, that indicates that HMO enrollment is a function of a perceived future health need for care among younger families. It speaks also to the nature of the services the enrolled population may demand, particularly maternity (Hudes et al., 1979; Wersinger et al., 1976) and preventive health care benefits (Dutton, 1979; Luft, 1978; Perkoff et al., 1974; Tessler and Mechanic, 1975), and to the possible duration of their membership should their expectations be met.

It should be noted, however, that this evidence derives from studies of employed populations and does not hold for populations that are not employed, among whom, if covered by Title XIX, financial risk for the cost of medical care does not exist. In the few studies of enrollment decisions where enrollment neither entailed financial obligation nor protected against future financial loss (because of Medicaid eligibility or special study circumstances), the delivery characteristics (where and how services would be obtained) seemed to assume greater importance. This was evident among low-income participants in a demonstration project, who were offered the choice between an open-panel health plan, where an ongoing patient-physician relationship could be maintained, and a closed-panel plan that required a new provider relationship to be established. Families and individuals with characteristics assumed to represent higher risk levels (e.g., larger families, older individuals, and females) preferred the open-panel arrangement over the group practice plan (Richardson et al., 1976). In another study of enrollment among low-income persons, Medicaid families exhibited similar behavior. Families who were higher utilizers of medical services, and whose family age and characteristics could be interpreted as representing higher levels of risk (e.g., presence of younger children), enrolled in the HMO less frequently than Medicaid families with lower levels of risk (Bice, 1975). Although there are important differences in these studies (see Tables 1 and 2), they support Bice's contention that where no financial vulnerability for care exists, the health risk factors that are usually predictive of enrollment become less salient to the enrollment decision than the characteristics of the delivery setting.

Further support for this proposition is found in two studies of employed populations whose enrollment choice included an IPA. Both sets of studies took place in Rochester, New York, where employee groups were given a choice between a long-standing, relatively comprehensive BC-BS plan, an IPA, and two group-practice HMOs. The insurance characteristics of the IPA and the closed-panel HMOs were essentially identical—they had similar benefit packages, copayment provisions, and service limitations and constraints but both differed from BC-BS coverage, which did not provide for ambulatory care. The delivery characteristics of the alternative plans, however, were such that the IPA and BC-BS were identical—care provided in private practitioners' offices—with both differing from the group-practice HMOs. Berki et al. (1977a; 1978) studied enrollment choice in one large employment group; Roghmann et al. (1975) reported on two surveys, one of a single employment group and the other a sample of members in each of the four plans.

Berki et al. found that the IPA attracted significantly fewer single individuals than either BC-BS or the group practice HMOs and that IPA families were the youngest and largest. They demonstrated the role of family life stage in the decision between an open and a closed-panel HMO: "As the health risks inherent in family life stage and composition increase, the probability of joining the open-panel plan also increases" (Berki et al., 1978:693). On the other hand, the analysis of Roghmann et al. (1975), which excluded individuals, found that group practice plans appealed to young families and that those who selected the IPA were more likely to be older couples. Although differences in their methods and measures prevent the direct comparison of these studies, both concluded that the delivery characteristics distinguishing the IPA from the group practice plans were as important as, if not more important than, the insurance characteristics of the HMOs.

Although not studies of enrollment choice directly, two studies have compared population demographic characteristics in defined areas with the characteristics of individuals from those populations who enrolled in HMOs. Hence they can be considered to address the enrollment predictive power of demographic characteristics. Gaus (1971), in his study of Columbia, Maryland, found HMO enrollees to have larger families and older heads of households than nonenrollees, although the mean age for both groups was under 40 years, but Nycz et al. (1976) found no significant differences in the Greater Marshfield, Wisconsin, area. The results are inconclusive, essentially because no information on the choice situation is available.

While the relatively standardized nature of demographic indicators makes it easier to interpret the results of studies in which they have been used, *health status measures* have no similar comparability. Attitudinal constructs and single items, number of chronic diseases or symptoms, disability days, and self-reported utilization measures have all been used to test the risk perception hypothesis. The results have been neither clear nor consistent.

When self-reports of utilization, occurring before the enrollment decision, have been used to examine the adverse selection issue, higher preenrollment hospitalization rates for HMO enrollees have been reported (Gaus, 1971; Roghmann et al., 1975), as well as rates that do not differ between the two groups (Berki et al., 1977a; Tessler and Mechanic, 1975). The same kind of varying findings have been reported for ambulatory utilization: more frequent among HMO enrollees (Roghmann et al., 1975); less frequent among enrollees in group practice plans, although IPA enrollees and BC-BS subscribers reported similar rates (Berki et al., 1977a); and similar rates for BC-BS subscribers and HMO enrollees (Tessler and Mechanic, 1975). In general, prior utilization of health services as a measure of health risk in dual-choice studies has not been predictive of HMO enrollment.

However, one study of a low-income population (Bice et al., 1974) found that experiential measures, as indicators of health risk, as well as attitudinal and perceptual measures of health status, were positively associated with selection of the HMO for those who were also at financial risk. It should be noted that this was not a dual-choice situation, nor was the study population the employed middle-income population that is the object of most enrollment choice research. Rather, the population was composed predominantly of Medicaid recipients who had no out-of-pocket costs, no matter which alternative was chosen, and a small number of poor but not Medicaid-eligible families who were financially vulnerable for all medical costs unless the HMO was selected; and there was only one alternative health plan available—a hospital-based group practice HMO for which there was a complete premium subsidy for all eligible residents choosing to enroll, regardless of their Medicaid status. The alternative was to continue with existing resources of care and methods of payment. For Medicaid recipients, no relation between health risk and choice was found; rather, Bice et al. found that the choice was made on the relative attractiveness of the service attributes of the two alternative delivery systems. But for low-income families not eligible for Medicaid, with high levels of health risk, that is, previously high users of medical services, the attractiveness of no-cost medical care as an HMO enrollee was considerable. Although the generalizability of these findings, based on a very small sample, is limited, they suggest that there is a trade-off between the insurance and delivery characteristics of the alternative plans, and that the trade-off assumes a more or less salient position in an individual's decision as a function of his/her financial and health vulnerability.

When Bice et al.'s findings on low-income people not eligible for Medicaid are combined with the findings from Rochester studies (Berki et al., 1977a; 1978; Roghmann et al., 1975), they seem to confirm the hypothesis that within the middle-income range there is a trade-off between the insurance and delivery characteristics of plans or, more precisely, between expenditures and access to a familiar provider. Roghmann et al. found that IPA enrollees had preenrollment ambulatory utilization rates higher than enrollees in either the group practice HMOs or the BC-BS subscribers. If previous utilization is a good indicator of health risk and the expected future demand for health care, as has been suggested (Bice et al., 1974), IPA enrollees were in the highest health-risk group. It was further found by

Berki et al. that the IPA enrollees were at lower financial risk than the other enrollment groups, by virtue of their significantly higher per capita incomes. In other words, Bice's low-income noneligibles were at one end of the income spectrum and the IPA enrollees were approaching the other. At a subsequent enrollment period, the premium cost of the IPA was significantly increased (from zero out-of-pocket to $25 per month), with the enrollee's contribution to the premium costs of the group practice HMOs and to BC-BS remaining at zero. The health risk hypothesis, since it stresses the importance of insurance characteristics, would predict that former IPA enrollees would switch to either of the group practice HMOs. But rather than enrolling in either of them, the majority of former IPA enrollees opted for BC-BS, with its much more limited ambulatory benefit packages (Ashcraft et al., 1978). Although this decision was likely to result in an increase in their out-of-pocket costs, given that their ambulatory use rates remained the same, the decision allowed them to retain the delivery characteristics that they found attractive (maintenance of a relationship with a private provider). Even though these results are not conclusive, they suggest that because of their lower financial vulnerability, these families opted for the delivery characteristic they preferred (particularly access to a known provider), regardless of the potential financial advantages of switching their enrollment to a group practice.

In addition to previous utilization rates, attitudinal measures of perceived health risk have been used in an attempt to differentiate HMO enrollees from BC-BS subscribers. Perceived health status of individuals and families has variously been measured by a single health-assessment questionnaire item (Anderson and Sheatsley, 1959; Bice, 1973; Juba et al., 1980; Richardson et al., 1976; Roghmann et al., 1975; Scitovsky et al., 1978; Tessler and Mechanic, 1975), a relative health rating item (Bice, 1973; Tessler and Mechanic, 1975), a constructed scale of several items (Berki et al., 1977a; 1977b; Gaus et al., 1976), and previously validated and tested indices of health and emotional status (Bice, 1973). Moreover, these measures, ascertained for individuals, are sometimes combined for all family members and either averaged (Juba et al., 1980), or formed into an index for the family unit (Scitovsky et al., 1978; Tessler and Mechanic, 1975), in order to obtain a family health-risk measure. Because of this diversity among research studies and the variations in instruments, there should be very little comparability among the findings. But such is not the case. With only one exception, where lower family health status was associated with a lower probability of enrollment (Juba et al., 1980), no significant difference in perceived health status has been reported when enrollees in either type of HMO and nonenrollees are compared.

This obviously raises some questions. Are these attitudinal measures so nondiscriminatory that they don't elicit any variation in the response? Is the lack of variation due to methodology, some of which seems questionable, or is there really no difference in perceived health state between HMO enrollees and nonenrollees? Is it a "true" finding or does it only appear that there is no adverse self-selection into HMOs, at least in terms of reported health status? The answers are not obvious.

This is not to suggest that no attitudinal measures related to health discriminate between those who choose to enroll and those who do not. Health concern, measured by a multi-item construct intended to ascertain individuals' present and future concern for their health, was found to be a significant predictor of enrollment in a group practice HMO, but not of enrollment in an IPA (Berki et al., 1977b; 1978). This finding was in contrast to the lack of association in the same study between perceived health status measures and enrollment in any HMO. Berki et al. concluded that although enrollees in group practice HMOs do not consider themselves to be less healthy than others, they are more concerned about, or conscious of, their health, and thus are more likely to select the plans in which such concern can be translated into increased demand for preventive care. However, in order to be confident that these results were not idiosyncratic to the study site and population, other studies of the choice between IPA and staff model HMOs are needed.

The findings of studies using reported illnesses as indicators of health risk are ambiguous. Bice et al. (1974) found a greater number of reported symptoms of ill health among low-income enrollees in a group practice HMO but found no similar relation for Medicaid recipients. Gaus et al. (1976) also found no difference in number of illnesses between HMO enrollees and a control sample of Medicaid recipients. Richardson et al. (1976) found the "sickest" families (number of bed-disability days, chronic conditions, and signs/symptoms) more likely to choose an individual provider system.

Roemer et al. (1972), on the other hand, found more chronic illness among group practice HMO members than among subscribers to any other type of health insurance plan. Gaus (1971) also found that HMO enrollees reported greater frequency of medical conditions requiring follow-up care, when compared with nonenrollees in the same community. Taken together, the findings from these latter two studies might suggest that HMO enrollees were "sicker." However, in both instances the data were gathered in a postenrollment period. Hence it is not clear whether the illnesses were in existence before enrollment, and thus possibly predictors of it, or whether the illnesses and the need for follow-up care were identifiable because of HMO experience. Tessler and Mechanic (1975) also noted that HMO enrollees had more chronic illness than BC-BS subscribers, although neither that measure nor the number of bed-disability days and the presence of a major illness were found to differ significantly between the two enrollment groups. Juba et al.'s (1980) findings that the number of family members reporting a chronic illness increased the probability of HMO enrollment, while a lower family health status decreased it, is inconsistent and neither supports nor rejects the hypothesis that HMOs tend to attract sicker families.

On the other hand, when an IPA is included in the choice situation, and multivariate analysis permits the identification of the relative importance of illness history in the enrollment decision, the role of chronic illness becomes clearer. Berki et al. (1978) found that more chronic illness in a family (the number of chronic illnesses per family member) increased the likelihood of enrollment in an IPA but not in a group practice HMO. This finding was unambiguous, but illness histories were less powerful predictors of IPA enrollment than the pre-enrollment existence of a relationship with a physician. Thus, it was concluded that although the IPA may enroll "sicker" families, the reason was the families' attachment to a physician, rather than the health risk factors per se.

In summary, past research on the relation between risk perception and enrollment in an HMO indicates that, within employed populations, HMO enrollees are at somewhat higher risk levels for future services than nonenrollees, with IPA enrollees at greater risk than group practice HMO members. The higher risk level, however, cannot be inferred from earlier utilization of medical services, which has not been found to be consistently different in the two groups, nor can it be derived from reports of lower perceived health status. Rather, HMO enrollees' higher risk levels are seen in their younger and larger families, which are in a procreative stage. The role of previous illness histories is ambiguous. Research results are sketchy, but there is reason to believe that if illness histories have led to the development of a satisfactory relationship with a physician, enrollment in an HMO may take place only if that physician is a member of the plan.

The literature based on empirical evidence provides scant support for the existence of adverse self-selection into HMOs, based on health risk. Although in its totality the evidence appears to indicate that those who enroll in HMOs are not sicker (nor do they report themselves to be so) than those who opt for the fee-for-service sector, there is no reason to believe that in fact they are healthier. The recently advanced "favorable" self-selection hypothesis suggests that relative HMO utilization performance can be read to indicate that those who select an HMO are likely to be at lower health risk (Luft, 1978). Blumberg (1980), in the only study that specifically discusses this issue, reports that there are no significant differences between HMO enrollees and others on a variety of health status measures. Although this study is based on individuals who have been HMO members for some (undefined) period, and hence the observed health risk levels may be the result of membership rather than a reason for joining, there is no direct evidence for "favorable" self-selection, or skimming. Direct studies of enrollment in well-established HMOs rather than developing ones, and of larger and more varied populations, must be undertaken before either the adverse or the favorable self-selection hypothesis can be validated.

Financial Vulnerability Factors. The financial vulnerability hypothesis posits a relation between expected financial loss due to future use of service and the propensity to enroll in an HMO. This is related to the risk perception hypothesis, since without perceived health risk and the expected future need for medical care, the financial vulnerability hypothesis may not hold. However, even in the absence of present health risk, fear of future economic jeopardy may exist. Thus, the insurance characteristics of the alternative plans may become salient in the enrollment decision.

It has long been held that the choice of an HMO is an economic decision, that "economic vulnerability is a primary basis for the choice of prepaid group practice" (Bashshur and Metzner, 1967:44). While strictly health insurance plans generally cost less in terms of premium, total price to consumers may be greater than to those selecting HMO coverage (Roemer et al., 1972). HMO enrollment transfers most of the financial risk for the costs of a wide range of services to the provider, an attribute particularly attractive to those who are financially vulnerable.

Although there is general agreement that financial vulnerability may play an important role in the enrollment decision, the findings have not been consistent. Further, how vulnerability should be measured is unclear. Risk vulnerability, an aggregation of measures of income, age, and family size (Bashshur and Metzner, 1970), which occasionally includes indices of health status and previous utilization (Roghmann et al., 1975; Tessler and Mechanic, 1975), has been used in most studies to test the financial vulnerability hypothesis. The inconclusive results led to the suggestion that the concepts of health risk and economic vulnerability should be distinguished from each other: "Risk vulnerability refers to expectations about *needs* for services, economic vulnerability, to expectations about effects of *costs* of services" (Bice, 1975:698–699).

However, even when the two concepts are disaggregated, there has been no agreement on how financial vulnerability should be measured: family income, or per capita income. Studies employing family income as the measure of financial vulnerability have produced inconsistent results: higher-income families elect the HMO (Bashshur and Metzner, 1967; Gaus, 1971; Roemer et al., 1972); no statistically significant relation between family income and choice of plan could be elicited (Moustafa et al., 1971; Roghmann et al., 1975; Tessler and Mechanic, 1975); or that HMO enrollees had lower family income than BC-BS subscribers (Juba et al., 1980; Roghmann et al., 1975). However, in all these studies in which family size was also reported, HMO enrollees were found to have larger families than those selecting the less comprehensive insurance plan.

When per capita income was used to test the financial vulnerability hypothesis, lower per capita income was associated with HMO selection (Berki et al., 1977b). This result is compatible with studies employing family income uncorrected for family size, given that those studies found that HMO enrollees had larger families.

Although HMO enrollees may be at greater financial risk than others, there is evidence that IPA enrollees are less financially vulnerable than enrollees in group practice HMOs: lower per capita income was associated with an increased probability of enrollment in a closed-panel plan, and higher per capita incomes increased the likelihood of enrollment in an IPA (Berki et al., 1978).

Financial vulnerability may also be indicated by expected future expenditures for medical care. If enrollment in an HMO is an action taken to protect against those expenditures, one would expect that higher pre-enrollment medical expenses would lead to selection of the HMO. In the few studies testing this hypothesis, however, the findings are either inconclusive, that is, no difference between enrollees and nonenrollees in previous out-of-pocket expenditures (Anderson and Sheatsley, 1959; Berki et al., 1977a; Roghmann et al., 1975), or suggest that an alternative hypothesis may be in order, one that relates to the relative importance of potential savings weighed against the maintenance of an existing provider relationship. Support for the notion of a trade-off between financial considerations and an ongoing physician-patient relationship is found in two studies, one in which BC-BS members reported higher expenditures but retained their coverage in preference to HMO enrollment (Juba et al., 1980), and the other in which IPA enrollment was preferred over the group practice HMO, although potential savings were possible through lower or no copayment provisions in the plans rejected (Berki et al., 1977a; Roghmann et al., 1975).

Although the magnitude of the potential savings that were exchanged for maintaining a physician relationship was estimated to be less than $120 annually, and was possibly not obvious to the enrollees, there is evidence that consumers are aware of their share of the premium price associated with HMO enrollment. When the premium differential was in favor of BC-BS membership, as was the case in most of the studies reviewed, the expense associated with HMO enrollment, although not very large, was frequently cited as an important reason for rejecting it (Moustafa et al., 1971; Roghmann et al., 1975). On the other hand, in a more recent study in which the increasing costs of BC-BS premiums exceeded the premiums of the HMO alternative, Piontkowski and Butler (1980) found a dramatic and increasing trend toward selection of the group practice plan. They also suggest that, in addition to premium differentials, enrollees in the HMO were sensitive to the substantial BC-BS copayment provisions for services whose prices rose rapidly during the study period (1969–1978).

This latter study lends support to the argument that it is total price (premium plus cost of utilization, whether through copayment or exclusions) that consumers consider in making their choice between HMO and plans offering less comprehensive coverage. When the total out-of-pocket price was likely to be lower with HMO enrollment, although many of the details of the benefit package were not fully understood, consumers consistently named one of these insurance characteristics as the HMO's most attractive feature. However, since each study asked the question and codifed the answers somewhat differently, the results can be considered descriptive only. The comprehensiveness of the coverage (Gaus, 1971; Juba et al., 1980, Jurgovan and Carpenter, 1974; Moustafa et al., 1971; Roghmann et al., 1975; Tessler and Mechanic, 1975), combined with prepayment, "knowing medical costs in advance" (Tessler and Mechanic, 1975), as well as particular aspects of the benefit package such as immediate maternity coverage (Roghmann et al., 1975), preventive care (Juba et al., 1980; Roghmann et al., 1975; Tessler and Mechanic, 1975), and office visits (Tessler and Mechanic, 1975), were specifically named.

IPA enrollees view their plan's insurance attributes somewhat differently from group-practice HMO enrollees. Expected savings on medical costs and undefined financial reasons were named most frequently by IPA enrollees, and particular service attributes and the comprehensiveness of the benefits predominated in the choice of a group-practice HMO when the two types of plans were offered together (Ashcraft et al., 1978; Roghmann et al., 1975).

On the other hand, BC-BS subscribers were more inclined to name delivery aspects, rather than the plan's insurance characteristics, as the basis for their choice. With one exception, where enrollees in both BC-BS and alternative HMOs gave economic reasoning as decisive in their choice (Roghmann et al., 1975), selection of BC-BS was influenced both by the existence of patient-physician relationships that could be maintained (Juba et al., 1980) and by satisfaction and experience with BC-BS (Tessler and Mechanic, 1975).

Potential enrollees may ascribe more comprehensive coverage to one alternative plan and cite it as a salient reason in their enrollment decision, but it is not clear that other characteristics of the plans are sufficiently understood. Benefit ceilings, exclusions, deductibles, and copayment provisions are complex matters to the ordinary consumer; yet it is precisely these details, plus the more obvious delivery dimensions, that distinguish the HMO from the alternative service or indemnity health insurance plans. Although some enrollees may report that they understand the choice and that the details about the plans are clear (Roghmann et al., 1975), there is contrary evidence that plan members are not aware of the services their plan offers even though they selected it over another alternative (Moustafa et al., 1971). Although an appreciation of the broad characteristics of an innovative plan may be sufficient to attract some enrollees, others prefer the status quo to making an uninformed choice. This reluctance to reject a familiar health insurance scheme for an innovation with unclear dimensions, the "incumbency effect" (Yedidia, 1959), is evident in the reports of lack of information about the alternatives (Tessler and Mechanic, 1975), failure to rank in importance the reasons for retaining BC-BS (Juba et al., 1980), and simply no consideration of unchosen alternatives (Ashcraft, 1978), which have all been given as reasons in making the choice. Although the complexity of some enrollment situations may lead to perceptions that insufficient information had been provided (Ashcraft, 1978), it is also likely that a search for alternatives is related to the perceived level of risk (Bashshur and Metzner, 1970): those who perceive themselves at risk may pay greater attention to the characteristics of the new plan, seriously considering whether it or the existing coverage offers the desired level of protection.

Delivery Characteristics

Unlike the choice between two health insurance plans that may vary in some of their insurance characteristics, such as their benefit packages or copayment provisions, the inclusion of a group-practice (staff) model HMO in the choice situation introduces variation in the delivery characteristics of the alternatives: 1) access; 2) continuity; 3) comprehensiveness; 4) clinical quality; and 5) social quality dimensions.

The effects of varying insurance characteristics fit within the concepts of risk perception and financial vulnerability, but there is no analogous scheme for determining the effects of delivery characteristics on enrollment behavior. Further, unlike demographic indicators and reported utilization and costs, all of which are reasonably straightforward and require little interpretation, preferences for delivery characteristics frequently must be inferred from expressions of satisfaction or dissatisfaction with existing arrangements, or from those sociocultural characteristics that are assumed to affect such preferences (Metzner and Bashshur, 1967).

Sociocultural Characteristics Related to Perceptions. Sociocultural characteristics that have been investigated are education, race and/or ethnic group, religion, political party affiliation, union involvement, and various measures indicating formal and informal group involvement as well as general values.

On the assumption that the likelihood of adoption of an innovation, such as an HMO, would be positively related to educational attainment, several studies have pursued this issue. The results, however, while generally supporting the notion, should be carefully interpreted since they may only reflect the uniqueness of each study population (see Table 2). Significantly higher educational attainment among HMO enrollees has been noted (Berki et al., 1977a; Gaus et al., 1976; Juba et al., 1980; Roemer et al., 1972), with a greater percentage of heads of families with "some college" selecting the HMO over BC-BS (Tessler and Mechanic, 1975). Although no statistically significant differences in educational level between HMO enrollees and nonenrollees have also been found (Bashshur and Metzner, 1967; Moustafa et al., 1971), no studies reported that BC-BS subscribers had more education than HMO enrollees.

Although the results of these studies refute Wolfman's (1961) earlier suggestion that the "free choice" of physicians inherent in BC-BS membership may be more appealing to the more educated families in spite of the HMO's economic merits, the inconsistency may be due to the nature and size of the samples used. When insufficient variation in educational level is a natural characteristic of the employment group studied, as with the auto workers studied by Bashshur and Metzner, detection of differences between enrollment groups is not likely. When, however, the employment groups contain a range of occupations, such as the municipal workers included in Tessler and Mechanic's study, the chance of finding differences in education is increased. Moreover, when statistically significant differences are found, the substantive differences have no unambiguous meaning. For instance, Berki et al.'s (1977a) finding of a higher education level among HMO enrollees passed the test of statistical significance, but the actual difference in years of education was less than one.

Investigations of other sociocultural characteristics have also produced mixed results. For instance, studies of racial and ethnic differences between enrollment groups have had contrary results. In some study sites, higher proportions of foreign-born whites and nonwhites selected HMO coverage over a service-benefit plan (Roemer et al., 1972), particularly when the HMO location was readily accessible to their residences (Bashshur and Metzner, 1967), but no racial or ethnic differences between enrollees and nonenrollees have also been noted (Moustafa et al., 1971; Tessler and Mechanic, 1975).

Neither religion (Bashshur and Metzner, 1967; Tessler and Mechanic, 1975), political party affiliation, formal organization attendance, nor other indicators of informal social organization distinguished between HMO enrollees and nonenrollees, although more active union members joined an HMO whose membership was composed predominately of union workers (Bashshur and Metzner, 1967).

Access. Access attributes generally associated with HMOs, both service and provider accessibility 24 hours a day, which are frequently ranked high as decision factors (Roghmann et al., 1975; Tessler and Mechanic, 1975), consistently ranked below expected lower costs and comprehensive benefits as the most important reasons for selecting an HMO. Other access issues have also been investigated and, as expected, easier physical access or convenience (Bashshur and Metzner, 1967; Gaus, 1971; Richardson et al., 1976; Scitovsky et al., 1978), and dissatisfaction with the convenience of previous sources of care (Bashshur and Metzner, 1967) were all associated with HMO enrollment; time-cost of travel to care was related to HMO enrollment in the expected negative direction, although the coefficient was not statistically significant (Juba et al., 1980). When the location of the HMO was viewed as a disadvantage (Tessler and Mechanic, 1975), or seen as inconvenient (Roghmann et al., 1975), the alternative plan was selected.

Temporal factors, such as waiting time for an appointment and in the office, and dissatisfaction with them (Ashcraft et al., 1978; Roghmann et al., 1975) have been named so often by HMO enrollees as influencing their choice that they must also be considered as decision variables.

Psychosocial factors, as a dimension of access, and their relation to the enrollment decision have received less systematic attention than distance, convenience, or temporal factors. Yet, when they have been investigated, it was found that an unsatisfactory interpersonal relationship with a previous physician led to increased probabilities that an HMO would be selected (Ashcraft et al., 1978; Bice, 1973).

In summary, empirical results suggest that access factors, especially those of time and distance, seem to affect an individual's choice of plan. Thus, the intuitive relation between access and enrollment seems to be confirmed.

Continuity. Almost every study of enrollment choice has investigated the desirability of the continuity dimension as a predictor of HMO enrollment. The considerable interest in the effect of having or not having an ongoing patient-physician relationship is understandable (Donabedian, 1965), since it is a critical factor especially for the development of closed-panel HMOs. Unlike developing IPAs, many of whose member physicians provide medical care to enrollees both before and after the enrollment decision, group practice HMOs must depend, for the most part, on consumer willingness to leave former arrangements and establish a relationship with a physician whom they frequently do not know. Although there are other routes for consumers to enter an HMO, most studies of enrollment choice have focused on whether an earlier patient-physician relationship existed and the nature of that relationship. Further, since the choice of an HMO physician is not as broad as it is, theoretically at least, in the fee-for-service sector, the studies have investigated consumers' attitudes toward accepting the limited choice of physician in a closed-panel HMO.

Free choice of physician has not always been mentioned spontaneously as a deciding enrollment factor, but it was named frequently enough to support the conclusion that many potential enrollees consider it a significant deterrent to HMO selection. It was given as the most important reason for selecting an open-panel plan (Anderson and Sheatsley, 1959), for choosing BC-BS (Bashshur and Metzner, 1967; Juba et al., 1980; Roghmann et al., 1975; Wolfman, 1961), and for selecting one HMO over another (Scitovsky et al., 1978), although in the latter instance it was actually possible in both.

Just as lack of free choice of physician seems to deter HMO enrollment, so also does the existence of a pre-enrollment relationship with a physician (Anderson and Sheatsley, 1959; Berki et al., 1978; Jurgovan and Carpenter, 1974), except when that provider becomes part of the HMO's staff (Jurgovan and Carpenter, 1974), or when the HMO is an IPA (Berki et al., 1977a; Roghmann et al., 1975). Moreover, when that relationship is a satisfactory one, the likelihood of terminating it by HMO enrollment is further decreased (Juba et al., 1980; Tessler and Mechanic, 1975), even when the HMO is geographically more convenient (Gaus, 1971; Scitovsky et al., 1978). Conversely, it has consistently been found that the absence of a provider relationship increases the likelihood of selecting a plan that offers the opportunity for one to be established (Berki et al., 1977a, 1978; Juba et al., 1980; Richardson et al., 1976; Tessler and Mechanic, 1975). Having a regular source of care where an enduring relationship with a single physician was unlikely to be established, such as an outpatient department, clinic, or emergency room, also raised the probability of selecting an HMO (Anderson and Sheatsley, 1959; Ashcraft, 1978; Berki et al., 1977a; Roghmann et al., 1975).

Support of the continuity hypothesis seems clear. Other factors have also been identified, however, which, while not direct evidence, may be indicative of an attachment to the traditional form of private solo practice. Length of residence in the community (Bashshur and Metzner, 1967; Juba et al., 1980; Tessler and Mechanic, 1975) and duration of employment (Bashshur and Metzner, 1970; Scitovsky et al., 1978), have been inversely related to HMO enrollment. These factors may indicate a greater likelihood that a provider relationship exists.

Comprehensiveness. This delivery attribute refers to the scope of services available in one location, the spectrum of specialty and ancillary providers within the same physical settings, and the integration among those services and providers in rendering comprehensive care to the patient.

Since preference for group practice, where family doctors and specialists work together in the same place as a group (Metzner et al., 1972), was found in cities where HMOs did not exist, it has been hypothesized that such an arrangement would be a preferred attribute by those actually offered the choice. In general, the findings confirm it.

The desirability of an indentifiable integrated organization (Richardson et al., 1976), the ability to obtain all necessary care in one place (Tessler and Mechanic, 1975), the availability of specialists in the same place as family doctors (Anderson and Sheatsley, 1959), the "group" arrangement of closed-panel plans where family doctors and specialists work together (Metzner and Bashshur, 1967), and having physicians and records all in one place (Scitovsky et al., 1978), were frequently named by HMO enrollees as reasons for their decision. Not surprisingly, both BC-BS and IPA enrollees value this attribute less highly than those choosing a staff model HMO (Roghmann et al., 1975).

Quality of Care. It was long ago suggested that consumers view the technical quality of care in a formalized group practice to be higher than in individual practice settings (Freidson, 1961). However, since there has been little systematic investigation of whether quality of care perceptions affect enrollment decision, it is difficult to know whether variations in quality are perceived. When respondents were asked to give explicit reasons for choosing one plan over another, costs, comprehensiveness of benefits, and expected and existing physician relationships predominated, but there is some indication that differences in quality have been perceived. A prospective study of enrollment in a poverty population (designed to elicit perceptions of expected quality before actual utilization) found that potential enrollees expected the HMO to have "higher-quality care" than the "poor or fair" quality associated with present, pre-enrollment medical care experience (Bice, 1973). Previous experience was undoubtedly also the basis for evaluations of quality in another enrollment study using fixed-choice alternatives. The reputation of physicians in a long-standing and familiar plan, in terms of their competency and training, was the most frequently given reason for selecting that plan over the newer alternative (Scitovsky et al., 1978). In another study, quality of care was found to be a much preferred item, achieving, along with low costs, a consensus among all respondents, with no difference between enrollees and nonenrollees (Roghmann et al., 1975).

Clearly, this limited evidence is insufficient to decide whether quality plays a substantial part in the enrollment decision. Impressions of clinical quality may be imbedded in some other reasons given for selection of a health insurance plan, but they remain to be made explicit in a systematic fashion.

Social Quality. The social quality dimensions of the HMO's delivery characteristics have been captured variously by negative statements about the clinic atmosphere (Anderson and Sheatsley, 1959;

Tessler and Mechanic, 1975; Wolfman, 1961), type of patient seen there (Roghmann et al., 1975), the plan's perceived instability or inexperience (Jurgovan and Carpenter, 1974), and its reputation in general (Scitovsky et al., 1978). However, when asked to rank these impressions relative to other features of the HMOs (specific services and benefits), consumers have rated them as relatively unimportant (Metzner and Bashshur, 1967). It is not clear whether perceptions of these social-quality dimensions of the HMO's delivery characteristics derive from marketing techniques, particularly in employed groups where the marketing staff is not independent of the alternative plans, or whether they are ranked as unimportant only when judged relative to some of the financial considerations.

Positive perceptions of the plans' social quality can also be found in reports of friends' recommendations (Richardson et al., 1976; Scitovsky et al., 1978), or recommendations about the plans provided by physicians. Enrollees have also named as salient to their enrollment decision the relation of the HMOs to hospitals or institutions that are regarded favorably in the community (Gaus, 1971; Tessler and Mechanic, 1975).

While there is a generally accepted axiom among HMO developers that the difficulties encountered in enrollment and the slow growth of certain plans result from the plan's social quality dimensions, its location, clientele, and image, the literature on enrollment does not provide any definitive answers.

Conclusions

Current understanding of who enrolls in what kind of HMO is based on an extensive series of studies, characterized by lack of comparability, ad hoc theorizing, inconsistent and often poorly designed measures and methodologies. To the extent that their internal validity is accepted, their generalizable findings appear to indicate that an HMO's ability to attract enrollees depends on its ability to offer insurance and delivery system characteristics that consumers find desirable. Broad coverage, lower expected costs of utilization, and assured access are the principal features that individuals consider to be the advantages of HMOs. Limitations on the choice of provider, absence of information, uncertainty about new, unfamiliar, perhaps innovative health care arrangements, as well as the spatial disadvantages of a centralized delivery organization, are the major factors that militate against enrollment. Of the negative factors, the most important is the cessation of an ongoing relationship with a provider, except in those instances where the provider is part of the plan—IPAs. When an IPA is not available and there seem to be potential cost advantages to HMO enrollment, preference for a continuous provider relationship is frequently expressed by retention of BC-BS membership. There is no strong evidence that potential enrollees prefer financial savings over existing health care arrangements, but the consistent finding in regard to enrollees' income level is supportive. As a measure of disposable income available for medical expenses, the family's per capita income indicates its financial vulnerability. That HMO enrollees have lower per capita income indicates either that they are willing to give up previous relationships for the protection against costs that the HMO will provide, or that they are less likely to have established a previous relationship. Further research is needed to determine the interrelations among these insurance and delivery characteristics.

The evidence so far appears to indicate that closed-panel HMOs are most likely to attract enrollees who do not have established patient-physician relationships, and who tend to be members of younger families with a larger number of smaller children. These characteristics are often found in areas with high population mobility. Individuals and families new to a community have not had the opportunity to establish a private patient-physician relationship and they also tend to be younger. The closed-panel HMO offers them assured access without their having to search for sources of routine care in a new and unfamiliar community. Having the option available through the workplace, and having the ability to gain at least some information about the delivery characteristics of the HMO, reduce the burden of searching for sources of care. The open-panel HMO, on the other hand, appears to be most appealing to those who already know the physicians within it and who can enroll and simultaneously maintain an already existing patient-physician relationship.

The concern about the quality of enrollees (their levels of risk and propensity to use services) and its cost implications is most often expressed in the concept of adverse self-selection. This issue is not clearly resolved in the literature. Although there seems to be ample evidence that families with higher risk levels, by virtue of their age and life stages, choose HMOs for their comprehensive benefit packages and their guaranteed access to certain services and providers, there is little evidence that HMO enrollees are sicker than those choosing BC-BS. However, it should be remembered that most studies have focused on dual choice, involving employed workers and their families, which, by definition, excludes potentially higher users of services—the aged and the unemployed. Enrollment open to the general population may produce different results, but there is no unambiguous evidence that HMOs are chosen more frequently by those with high expected demand than plans where existing patient-physician relationships can be maintained. Nor is there convincing evidence that those who choose HMOs are healthier or potentially lower users of services. The current evidence is not sufficient to make definitive predictions of enrollment rates or enrollee quality.

The inability to make such predictions is particularly troublesome from a policy perspective. To design an effective HMO policy, one would like to be able to predict enrollment rates and patterns over time, on the basis of the attractiveness of different types of HMOs, the available alternatives, population characteristics, and relative costs. To develop valid HMO evaluation methodologies, to be able to assess HMO performance and potential cost savings attributable to lower utilization rates, it is necessary to separate population effects from HMO effects. Thus, whether those who enroll in HMOs are sicker, healthier, or about the same as the population in the fee-for-service sector, the base line, becomes a crucial evaluation parameter. The evidence so far is substantial that there is no adverse selection in terms of health risk, yet it is equally substantial that enrollees are likely to be higher users of ambulatory and maternity-related services by virtue of their life cycle stage. For the design and evaluation of policy, current knowledge based on past enrollment behavior offers, at best, only tentative indications as to what kinds of HMOs in what circumstances are likely to become economically viable.

Our ability to predict future performance in the longer term is also inhibited by the potential roles of several factors on which there is no information at all. The effects of improving coverage offered by service benefit and indemnity plans, and increasing copayment rates in HMOs, are predictable, from our understanding of the financial loss and health risk hypotheses. The effects of other factors are not. The principal issues that might well affect future enrollment experience, and on which no information is available, are 1) HMO maturation and multi-HMO competition; 2) multiple, differentially priced benefit packages within an HMO; 3) increasing physician-population ratios; and 4) national health insurance.

Within the rubric of HMO maturation there are two separate issues: the effect of an HMO's length of experience on its enrollment, and the effect on enrollment of the diffusion of HMOs, their increasing image as part of the "mainstream." What little is known about HMO aging does not appear in the research literature, but seems to indicate that as an HMO ages, its enrollee profile begins to approach that of the population in its service area, with greater representation of the aged among its members. Open enrollment, continuation of employment-based health benefits into the retirement period, usually as supplements to Title XVIII, and the increasing numbers of aged in the population may well mean that the relatively high utilizing portion of HMOs' enrolled population will increase.

The second aspect of maturation becomes relevant when the HMO is no longer seen as "the new boy on the block." The assumed attractiveness of the "innovative" plan, as well as its opposite, the "let's wait and see if it works" attitude, will become irrelevant when HMOs have sufficiently diffused so that they no longer will be considered as either new or major departures from the dominant system of providing care. Whether, when they lose their innovative image, they will be selected by persons at greater risk than those selecting them now, remains to be seen. Should that happen, however, issues of service utilization and service capacity planning and, ultimately, costs are involved. We can speculate about the premium and copayment implications and their effects on marketing and marketing costs for the future, but little is known about them now.

Equally little is known about the enrollment effects of multi-HMO competition. The handful of studies on enrollment in multi-HMO settings, while interesting, may not have much predictive value. The methods of intra-HMO competition, whether by access, premium, copayment prices, benefit package, or some combination of these factors, are important for their enrollment effects and, of course, go to the heart of marketing strategies. Marketing strategies will also be affected by limitations on employer health-benefit contributions resulting, for example, from proposals to alter the advantageous tax treatment such contributions currently receive, but their long-run effect on subsequent enrollment is not now known.

A related issue is found in the development of variously priced benefit packages within the same HMO, or across HMOs. Increased flexibility in coverage would imply potentially increased attractiveness to larger population slices, but if the "high-priced package" means increased out-of-pocket premium payments, the beneficial effects of the coverage spread may be negated. Some plans have long offered multiple benefit packages, but little is known about their enrollment effects.

Increases in the supply of physicians and of physician services, and the expected increase in the proportion of physicians providing primary care, do not augur well for HMOs. Increases in the number and capacity of medical schools, as well as federal manpower policies, indicate that the supply of physicians will continue to increase. As the number of physicians increases, more of them, even though trained in the specialties, are likely to be shifted into rendering primary care services, as at least part of their practice. The chances, therefore, of establishing contact by would-be patients should improve. Once access in the solo office sector is improved, the assured access offered by HMOs will have less attraction. Further, areas with current physician shortage, rural and inner city, are likely to remain so in the future, since they offer the least attractive location alternatives to entering physicians. These are also the areas with the least potential for the development of economically viable HMOs, since they provide neither the manageable service area nor the economic base for maintaining self-sustaining HMO operations. Hence HMOs are most likely to develop precisely in areas where future increases in private physician supply are also most likely to take place. While one can speculate about the dynamics and effects of such a development, their effects on HMO enrollment cannot be predicted since no systematic studies exist of the effects of physician supply on HMO enrollment.

Perhaps the most important issue for future HMO enrollment and development is related to national health insurance, NHI. If NHI essentially removes the link between utilization and out-of-pocket costs, the distinguishing insurance characteristics of HMOs will become irrelevant and delivery characteristics will become the dominant decision variables. If, as currently proposed, NHI is implemented with substantial first-dollar exclusions, copayment and coinsurance provisions, and provided that the private insurance industry does not develop supplemental coverage for such provisions, HMOs may experience a beneficial enrollment effect. Should HMOs receive favorable treatment in payment schemes, groups of physicians may form HMOs and develop them on the basis of their current patient loads. Since those who are at higher risk and who are older and sicker are more likely to have established a patient-physician relationship, the initial membership of such an HMO is likely to be composed of high utilizers, high-cost members. What this implies for the viability of the organization and its attractiveness to other segments of the population is unclear.

The establishment of an enrollee base of a size required to attain economies in the provision of services is the fundamental requirement of HMO survival. The quality of that enrollee base and the time required to attain it are the two basic building blocks of HMO planning. Hence, who enrolls and why are the first questions the future research agenda should be designed to answer.

References

Andersen, R. 1968. *A Behavioral Model of Families' Use of Health Services.* Research Series No. 25. Chicago: University of Chicago: Center for Health Administration Studies.

Anderson, O.E., and Sheatsley, P.B. 1959. *Comprehensive Medical Insurance: A Study of Costs, Use, and Attitudes Under Two Plans.* Research Series No. 9. Chicago: Health Information Foundation.

Ashcraft, M.L.F. 1978. *The Impact of Previous Medical Care Experiences on Enrollment in Prepaid Group Health Plans.* Washington, D.C.: Department of Commerce, NTIS PB-281, 859.

———, Penchansky, R., Berki, S.E., Fortus, R.S., and Gray, J. 1978. Expectations and Experience of HMO Enrollees after One Year: An Analysis of Satisfaction, Utilization and Costs. *Medical Care* 16:14–32.

Bashshur, R.L., and Metzner, C.A. 1967. Patterns of Social Differentiation between Community Health Association and Blue Cross-Blue Shield. *Inquiry* 4:23–44.

———, and Metzner, C.A. 1970. Vulnerability to Risk and Awareness of Dual Choice of Health Insurance Plan. *Health Services Research* 5:106–113.

Berki, S.E., Ashcraft, M.L.F., Penchansky, R., and Fortus, R.S. 1977a.

Enrollment Choice in a Multi-HMO Setting: The Roles of Health Risk, Financial Vulnerability and Access to Care. *Medical Care* 15:95–114.

———, Ashcraft, M.L.F., Penchansky, R., and Fortus, R.S. 1977b. Health Concern, HMO Enrollment, and Preventive Care Use. *Journal of Community Health* 3:3–31.

———, Penchansky, R., Fortus, R.S., and Ashcraft, M.L.F. 1978. Enrollment Choices in Different Types of HMOs: A Multivariate Analysis. *Medical Care* 16:682–697.

Bice, T.W. 1973. *Enrollment in a Prepaid Group Practice.* Baltimore: The Johns Hopkins University, Department of Medical Care and Hospitals.

——— 1975. Risk Vulnerability and Enrollment in a Prepaid Group Practice. *Medical Care* 13:698–703.

———, Radius, S., and Wollstadt, L. 1974. *Risk Vulnerability and Enrollment in a Prepaid Group Practice and Disenrollment from a Prepaid Group Practice.* The Johns Hopkins University, Center for Metropolitan Planning and Research.

Blumberg, M.S. 1980. *Health Status and Health Care Use by Type of Private Health Care Coverage.* Oakland, Calif.: Kaiser-Permanente Medical Care Programs, Working Paper.

Donabedian, A. 1965. *A Review of Some Experiences with Prepaid Group Practice.* Bureau of Public Health Economics Research Series No. 11. Ann Arbor: University of Michigan, School of Public Health.

Dutton, D.B. 1979. Patterns of Ambulatory Health Care in Five Different Delivery Systems. *Medical Care* 17:221–241.

Freidson, E. 1961. *Patients' Views of Medical Practice.* New York: Russell Sage Foundation.

Gaus, C.R. 1971. Who Enrolls in a Prepaid Group Practice: The Columbia Experience. *Johns Hopkins Medical Journal* 128:9–14.

———, Cooper, B.S., and Hirschman, C.G. 1976. Contrasts in HMO and Fee-for-Service Performances. *Social Security Bulletin* 39(May):3–14.

Grossman, M. 1972. *The Demand for Health: A Theoretical and Empirical Investigation.* Occasional Paper No. 119. New York: National Bureau of Economic Research.

Hudes, J., Young, C., Sohrub, L., and Trinh, C. 1979. *Are HMO Enrollees Being Attracted by a Liberal Maternity Benefit?* Los Angeles: Kaiser Permanente Medical Care Program, Southern California Region. Presented at the Joint National Meeting of the Institute of Management Sciences/Operations Research Society of America (May).

Juba, D., Lave, J.R., and Shaddy, J. 1980. An Analysis of the Choice of Health Benefits Plans. *Inquiry* 17 (Spring):62–71.

Jurgovan, R.J., and Carpenter, B. 1974. *The Sandia Event: Choice and Change among One Indemnity and Two Prepaid Health Care Plans.* Final Report, Contract HSM-110-72-171. Rockville, Md.: Litton Bionetics, Inc.

Luft, H.S. 1978. Why do HMOs Seem to Provide More Health Maintenance Services? *Milbank Memorial Fund Quarterly/Health and Society* 56(Spring):140–168.

Metzner, C.A., and Bashshur, R.L. 1967. Factors Associated with Choice of Health Care Plans. *Journal of Health and Social Behavior* 8:291–299.

———, Bashshur, R.L., and Shannon, G.W. 1972. Differential Public Acceptance of Group Medical Practice. *Medical Care* 10:279–287.

Moustafa, A.T., Hopkins, C.E., and Klein, B. 1971. Determinants of Choice and Change of Health Insurance Plans. *Medical Care* 9:32–41.

Munts, R. 1967. *Bargaining for Health: Labor Unions, Health Insurance, in Medical Care.* Madison: University of Wisconsin Press.

Nycz, G.R., Wenzel, F.J., Lohrenz, F.N., and Mitchell, J.H. 1976. Composition of the Subscribers in a Rural Prepaid Group Practice Plan. *Public Health Reports* 91:504–507.

Perkoff, G.T., Kahn, L., and Mackie, A. 1974. Medical Care Utilization in an Experimental Practice in a University Medical Center. *Medical Care* 12:471–485.

Phelps, C.E. 1972. *Demand for Health Insurance: A Theoretical and Empirical Investigation.* R-1054-OEO. Santa Monica: Rand Corporation.

Piontkowski, D., and Butler, L.H. 1980. Selection of Health Insurance by an Employee Group in Northern California. *American Journal of Public Health* 70:274–276.

Richardson, W.C., Boscha, M.V., Weaver, B.L., Drucker, W.L., and Diehr, F.K. 1976. *The Seattle Prepaid Health Care Project: Comparison of Health Services Delivery. Chapter 1: Introduction to the Project, the Study and the Enrollees.* Washington, D.C.: Department of Commerce, NTIS PB-267 489.

Roemer, M.I., Hetherington, R.W., Hopkins, C.E., Gerst, A.E., Parsons, E., and Long, D.M. 1972. *Health Insurance Effects: Services, Expenditures, and Attitudes under Three Types of Plans.* Bureau of Public Health Economics Research Series No. 16. Ann Arbor: University of Michigan, School of Public Health.

Roghmann, K.J., Gavett, J.W., Sorenson, A.E., Wells, S., and Wersinger, R.P. 1975. Who Chooses Prepaid Medical Care: Survey Results from Two Marketings of Three New Prepayment Plans. *Public Health Reports* 90:516–527.

Scitovsky, A.A., McCall, N., and Benham, L. 1978. Factors Affecting the Choice between Two Prepaid Plans. *Medical Care* 16:660–681.

Tessler, R., and Mechanic, D. 1975. Factors Affecting the Choice between Prepaid Group Practice and Alternative Insurance Programs. *Milbank Memorial Fund Quarterly/Health and Society* (Spring) 54:149–172.

Wersinger, R., Roghmann, K.J., Gavett, J.W., and Wells, S.M. 1976. Inpatient Hospital Utilization in Three Prepaid Comprehensive Health Care Plans Compared with a Regular Blue Cross Plan. *Medical Care* 14:721–732.

Wolfman, B.I. 1961. Medical Expenses and Choice of Plan: A Case Study. *Monthly Labor Review* 84:1186–1190.

Yedidia, A. 1959. Dual Choice Programs. *American Journal of Public Health* 49:1475–1479.

A version of this paper was presented at the Conference on the Performance of Prepaid Health Care in the United States, Boston, Massachusetts, November 1, 1979.

Address correspondence to: Prof. S.E. Berki, Chairman, Department of Medical Care Organization, School of Public Health, The University of Michigan, 109 Observatory Street, Ann Arbor, MI 48109.

III Aspects of Performance

HMO Performance:
The Recent Evidence

MILTON I. ROEMER

WILLIAM SHONICK

Health maintenance organizations (HMOs) are being promoted as a strategy to modify the U.S. health care delivery system toward more economical patterns, encouraging preventive and ambulatory rather than costly hospital services. Evidence of HMO performance has accumulated over the years, much of it reviewed in 1969. Since then, additional evidence suggests that the "prepaid group practice" (PGP) model of HMO continues to yield lower hospital use, relatively more ambulatory and preventive service, and lower overall costs (counting both premiums and out-of-pocket expenditures) than conventional open-market fee-for-service patterns. Economies of scale in group practice per se are still not proved, but some evidence supports this theoretical hypothesis. New data point to reduced disability from the PGP model of HMO, as well as to more favorable consumer attitudes (based mainly on the economic advantages, in spite of certain impersonalities of clinics) than exist toward conventionally insured private solo practice. The medical care foundation (free choice of private practitioners with fee payments) model of HMO has yielded some evidence of economies in physician's care, but none in hospital use. HMOs entail hazards of underservicing and distorted risk-selection, but with appropriate public monitoring they constitute an approach to health planning, stressing local initiative, competition, and incentives to self-regulation.

Introduction

In a "health strategy" message of February, 1971, the President gave new prominence to an idea which had been evolving in the United States for half a century or more. Basically, the idea involves the assumption of responsibility for the health of a population by an organized entity, in consideration of a fixed, prepaid amount of money. Incentives to increase medical earnings through maximizing services are theoretically replaced by incentives to maximize earnings by prudent use of costly services. Initially a contentious deviance from the conventional open-market, fee-for-service concept of medical care, the idea gradually gained social acceptance in the 1950s and 1960s, as experience demonstrated that it could yield medical care of good quality at lower than prevailing average costs. By the 1970s, the spiraling of medical costs had become so alarming that a conservative federal administration decided to push the idea and to give it a glamorous new label: the "Health Maintenance Organization," or HMO.

Clearcut evidence of the effects of HMOs has not been abundant but it has gradually mounted. Avedis Donabedian (1969) published a comprehensive evaluation of the principal model of HMO—that based on group practice organization—and since that time additional evaluative evidence has accumulated. Most of this evidence compares the prepaid group practice (PGP) model with other patterns of health care delivery, but some of it concerns the model of the "medical care foundations," in which the key principles of HMOs are implemented under a pattern of physician's service offered through individual rather than group practices. This paper will review this recent evidence and offer interpretations of its meaning, with respect to social policy decisions on HMO strategy.

The definition of HMO applied here is an organization which:

(a) makes a contract with consumers (or employers on their behalf) to assure the delivery of stated health services of measurable quality;

(b) has an enrolled population;

(c) offers a stated broad range of personal health service benefits, including at least physician services and hospital care;

(d) is paid on an advance capitation basis.

Regarding element (c) in this definition, the investigations reviewed here have been applied to HMOs with rather widely varying scopes of benefits, not all of which offer protection for *all* physician and hospital services used or needed by a population. At this point, however, we believe there are lessons to be learned from study of some HMOs which may not fit perfectly under an ideal definition.

Since 1969, there have been published a number of other general review papers which examine the whole question of HMOs and their consequences: for health, economy, and other values. In offering this review we have naturally made use of these papers, in particular those by Herbert Klarman (1971), John Glasgow (1972),

Merwyn Greenlick (1972), and Ira Greenberg and Michael Rodburg (1971) in the *Harvard Law Review*. We shall, of course, in addition review the main findings of several other studies reported separately.

The recent material has not only provided additional empirical evidence but has also extended and deepened our understanding of the various dimensions along which analysis must proceed if we are to infer, from the accumulated evidence, generalizations useful for social policy decisions.

Previous studies

Research on comparative performance under alternative forms of organization of medical care delivery had been going on with ever increasing frequency since the issuance of the final report of the Committee on the Costs of Medical Care (1932). Particular interest centered around the performance of prepaid group practice (PGP) as compared with other modalities for delivery of care. In attempting to design research which would provide information about these effects, the investigators were faced with evaluating a phenomenon whose input consisted of a number of different and perhaps separable factors and whose output similarly consisted of a number of separately identifiable elements.

On the *input side* have been included the factors of (a) prepayment by the subscriber, (b) practice in a group setting, (c) paying the physician by salary, and, in some cases, (d) owning or at least controlling the operation of the associated hospitals. Although each of these components was often present in the operation of a PGP, not all of them existed in "pure" form in every PGP studied. The degree to which each of these factors was present varied among the PGPs studied; attributing an appropriate aliquot part of the observed effect to these several input factors was often the aim of later research, using ever more refined designs.

Similarly, on the *output side,* the criteria to be applied in judging the effects produced by the PGP, as compared with alternative practice modalities, were increasingly broken down by researchers into more particular elements, such as patient satisfaction, effects on hospital use, and the like.

As the number of such studies proliferated, publications reporting their results began to be interspersed periodically with review articles summarizing and analyzing the current state of the findings on various facets of the question. In attempting to draw generalization about the performance of PGP from the published results, the several reviewers formulated various typologies for analysis.

The earlier reviews did not discuss in great detail the various components of PGP (noted above), in general considering all such organizations to be members of one generic group. These earlier evaluation articles each focused on some particular aspect of the performance results of PGP, as compared with alternative forms of organization of practice. Klarman's initial review (1963) addressed itself to the effects of the PGP and other practice modalities upon hospital utilization; Weinerman (1964) dealt mainly with patients' perception of the medical care provided in prepaid group practice.

Donabedian's 1969 review constituted a landmark in its attempt to analyze the research results according to a broad series of criteria, considering the entire spectrum as the necessary basis for evaluating medical care system performance. He grouped these criteria, and the parameters for measuring them, as follows:

1. Patient satisfaction:
   frequency with which consumers choose PGP, when this choice is available
   expressed opinions of subscribers
   frequency of out-of-plan use by PGP members

2. Opinions of participating physicians:
   concerning conditions of medical practice
   concerning the nature and behavior of subscribers

3. Health service utilization rates:
   from hospital and insurance records
   from survey questionnaires to subscribers

4. Costs to patients:
   premiums paid (from insurance records and surveys)
   out-of-plan expenditures from surveys

5. Economic productivity:
   theoretical analysis of expectations
   economic analysis of empirical data

6. Quality of medical care:

   influence of pattern on ways of using medical services (through survey questionnaires)

   qualifications of physicians and hospitals used (from records and surveys)

   physician performance (from direct observation and "audits" of medical records)

7. Ultimate health outcomes:

   mortality rates on matched samples

Format of the present study

While this Donabedian analysis, in its multifaceted approach to PGP performance, was the most comprehensive up to 1969, it was based entirely on the author's study of previous individual investigations which he had identified and considered relevant. Indeed, Donabedian specifically states that his "review was made without reference to Klarman's 1963 and Weinerman's 1964 reviews . . ." referred to earlier in this paper.

The present review will consider the evidence on HMO performance that has been newly accumulated since the Donabedian paper, along with material that he did not include, especially from the Klarman (1963) and the Weinerman (1964) papers. In the light of present-day perspectives on HMOs, our analysis will be classified along somewhat different evaluative categories, as follows:

1. Subscriber composition
2. Participation of physicians
3. Utilization rates
4. Quality assessments
5. Costs and productivity
6. Health status outcomes
7. Patient attitudes

With respect to each of these features, we will attempt to report empirical findings under both the PGP and the "medical care foundation" (MCF) models of HMO. Finally, we will offer a few interpretive comments about the apparent need for surveillance of HMOs, the implications for comprehensive health planning, and the indications for further required research.

Subscriber Composition

The performance of HMOs will naturally be influenced by the composition of their memberships. Rates of utilization, costs, health status outcomes, and other measures for evaluation are inevitably influenced by the demographic composition of HMO members, their pre-existing medical conditions, and related factors.

A. T. Moustafa et al. (1971) reported on the characteristics of persons choosing among a series of five health insurance plans, two of which represented the PGP model (Kaiser-Permanente Health Plan or Ross-Loos Medical Group Plan). They found that married persons with children, in contrast to single persons, were more likely to choose the more comprehensive HMO-type plans, but that, otherwise, educational or income levels showed no significant relationship to plan choice. When, for some reason, persons changed their plan affiliation (at an annual open-enrollment period), those in comprehensive benefit plans—whether HMO-type or commercial insurance with wide benefits—were most likely to shift to another plan of comprehensive benefit scope.

The social acceptance of the idea of group medical practice, in contrast to the traditional pattern of individual practice, was investigated over several years in three cities (Detroit, Cleveland, and Cincinnati) by C. A. Metzner et al. (1972). A substantial majority of persons surveyed expressed preference for the idea of getting their care through group practice arrangements, even though many had no actual experience with such arrangements. The preference tended to prevail for all demographic breakdowns but was somewhat stronger in persons of higher educational and middle income levels. While this study did not explore *prepaid* group practice, the findings would seem to have implications for the HMO model as well.

Virtually all the investigations cited in the review by E. R. Weinerman (1964) were included by Donabedian (1969), and we shall not repeat them here. However, Weinerman's own analytic contribution is worth noting. He drew these inferences on the initial choices, among different patterns of delivery, made by subscribers to health insurance plans (Weinerman, 1964: 882):

> The fee-for-service plans still attract a majority of workers in a dual choice situation, especially when their benefits are broad in scope. The advantages of initial enrollment have been indicated. Certainly, the organizational effort preceding the election date is of enormous impact. . . . The group practice method is still new and unfamiliar to most patients and to most doctors. . . . The comparative advantages of group practice health plan benefits are often complex and difficult for the average worker to decipher. Most significant is the repeated observation that enrollees respond primarily to the prospect of comprehensive benefits, and seem less concerned with the alternative of group versus solo practice.

It would seem to follow that greater familiarity with the PGP pattern is likely to increase the tendency of persons to like it, in spite of some of the impersonal "public clinic" connotations of *large* group practices.

In 1973, there were reported, for the first time, the actual characteristics of random samples of *total memberships* enrolled in various types of insurance organization, including HMO models. Studying health insurance plans in southern California in 1968, Roemer et al. (1973) found that significantly higher proportions of persons with generally greater risk of sickness were members of PGP organizations than were in commercial insurance or provider-sponsored (Blue Cross and Blue Shield) plans. This was reflected by slightly higher proportions of plan members aged 41 years and over, substantially higher proportions of families with a history of one or more chronic illnesses (60.6 percent in PGP plans, in contrast to 46.6 percent and 37.4 percent in the two open-market plan-types), and somewhat greater proportions of persons scoring high on a "symptom sensitivity" test. They also found a slightly greater proportion of foreign-born and nonwhite persons in the HMO-type plans, although the average family incomes in those plans, paradoxically, was slightly higher ($11,309 compared with $10,987 and $10,398 in the other two plan-types).

These studies suggest that any advantages that may be found for HMO-type plans, in terms of lower costs or better health status outcomes (as reflected in the pre-1969 research reports), cannot be attributed to their containing a smaller membership of high-risk persons, but would seem to be associated with the opposite.

With respect to the medical care foundation model of HMO, we have found, unfortunately, no documentation on the nature of its subscriber composition. We can only point out that the MCFs operate predominantly in relatively small counties of low urbanization. Moreover, as Richard H. Egdahl (1973) notes, a major share of member composition in many foundations has been derived from Medicare and Medicaid beneficiaries in recent years.

Participation of Physicians

The performance of HMOs is bound to be influenced by the qualifications of physicians as well as of other personnel entering this pattern of health service. It is also likely to be influenced by the satisfaction of professional personnel with their general conditions of work (including earnings) in this setting.

Prepaid group practice

Careful investigation of the qualifications of doctors in PGP (compared with others) has not been made, except for what may be inferred from the espoused policies of PGP organizations. The policies of large HMO models, like the Health Insurance Plan of Greater New York (HIP) and the Kaiser-Permanente Plan, are believed to result in careful selection of properly qualified specialists for all positions requiring specialty status (Greenberg and Rodburg, 1971). Insofar as general practitioners are selected for primary care, qualifications under the new specialty board in family medicine are encouraged. Similarly rigorous criteria for appointment, however, evidently do not apply to all HMOs, such as some of the new ones with small group practice units organized mainly to serve Medicaid beneficiaries in California (Nelson, 1973).

Empirical studies have recently been made regarding the satisfaction of physicians with the conditions of work in PGP. The earlier literature on group medical practice gave the impression that, with or without prepayment, difficulties and dissatisfactions were rampant (Dickinson and Bradley, 1952). D. M. Du Bois (1970) studied in 1966 a small series of private group practices that failed and disintegrated, comparing them with a series of private group practices that grew and prospered; he concluded that organizational failure was mainly associated with "policies in conflict with the professional role"—in a word, commercialization. Other relevant factors were a hostile professional environment and poor administrative management.

Based on a national survey in 1970 of private multispecialty medical group practices, Laurence D. Prybil (1971) found that the annual turnover rate—a long-used index of job dissatisfaction—was less than 5 percent. The respondents were from institutional members of the American Association of Medical Clinics *(N —* 237), a series that might admittedly be expected to have especially high stability. Even this low rate of turnover, however, seemed to be declining; it involved physicians mainly under 45 years of age, and most of those who left went to other positions in organized settings rather than into solo practice. Low turnover was also confirmed by the study of Austin Ross (1969), who found problems of remuneration in group practices to be the major cause of departure. David Mechanic (1972) in a recent national survey also found high rates of satisfaction in group practice—95 percent were either "very" or "fairly" satisfied (over 50 percent were "very satisfied") —with no differences evident in comparison to satisfaction with solo practice. Of course, one may infer that only those physicians who like the concept enter group practice in the first place.

Focusing more specifically on *prepaid* group practice, Mechanic found these doctors most satisfied of all subgroups with opportunities for professional contacts, total time of work required, and leisure opportunities; they were least satisfied with respect to time available per patient, income level, office facilities, and community status. Nevertheless, in aggregate "general satisfaction with one's practice," the PGP physicians reported "very satisfied" in 52 percent of the cases, which was precisely the same percentage as reported by fee-for-service solo practitioners. A turnover study in the Northern California Kaiser-Permanente PGP over the period 1966–1970 by Wallace H. Cook (1971), reported under 10 percent departures per year for employed doctors and less than 2 percent for Permanente Group partners.

Considering the socially marginal character of prepaid group practice in American medical culture, the remarkable point would seem to be how little dissatisfaction is evident among physicians who have "bucked the tide" and engaged in this pattern of work.

One can readily speculate that, with the steady growth of open-market private group practice (now up to about 20 percent of clinical physicians, according to the AMA Survey reported in 1972) and the general national promotion of the HMO idea, participation in PGP will become regarded as less and less "deviant," will attract more doctors, and will become associated with greater stability.

Medical care foundations

In regard to the medical care foundation HMO pattern, participation of physicians is, of course, open to all members of local medical societies. Except for young physicians-in-training, doctors in full-time research, education, or administration, and some physicians in full-time salaried hospital employment, one may assume that local medical societies (not necessarily the American Medical Association or the black physicians' National Medical Association) contain in their memberships virtually all private clinical practitioners in their areas. In the Physicians' Association of Clackamas County, Oregon, for example, it is reported (Bechtol, 1972) that all but two members of the County Medical Association participate in the foundation. Such widespread participation, of course, implies wide free choice for patients, but says nothing about the specialty or other technical qualifications of the physicians, beyond the licensure and "ethical" requirements for medical society membership.

Studies of the San Joaquin County Foundation for Medical Care by the UCLA School of Public Health cast some light on the participation of these physicians in the care of Medicaid beneficiaries. One study (Gartside and Proctor, 1970) found a higher proportion (85 percent versus 78 percent) of all physicians and particularly of certain qualified specialists (strikingly so in pediatrics and obstetrics) from the foundation area to be serving Medicaid patients than in a closely matched comparison county (Ventura) without a medical foundation. Another UCLA study (Roemer and Gartside, 1973) found that, in the performance of surgical operations, the work was more often done by properly qualified surgeons in the San Joaquin Foundation area than in the comparison county. These findings would suggest that, in the nonmetropolitan type of county where medical foundations have tended to develop, they exert a positive influence on the qualifications of doctors serving the poor; similar disciplinary influence might possibly apply to the care of all patients in foundation-type HMOs.

Utilization Rates

The data on differential utilization rates for health services under HMOs, compared with other medical care arrangements, have continued to accumulate. One of the principal advantages long claimed for the HMO model, of course, has been its association with relatively lower use of expensive hospital days, resulting in substantial cost savings. Before reviewing the recently produced data on this (and other) utilization features, we should consider some of the earlier interpretations of them not included in the benchmark Donabedian paper of 1969.

Hospital utilization

The Klarman review (1963) was one of the earlier assessments of the general influence of health insurance on hospital utilization. Some of his interpretations, not reported in the Donabedian review (1969), should be cited. Drawing upon the studies of Osler Peterson in the United States and of G. Forsythe and R. Logan in Great Britain, Klarman noted that the concern of the 1930s about underutilization of hospitals shifted, in the 1960s, to concern about overutilization. Which concern is "correct," he notes, cannot be determined, since no objective standards for "proper" utilization exist. This implies that lower hospital utilization rates cannot appropriately be used as evidence of good performance without reference to what type of utilization is being reduced—"necessary" or "excess." Donabedian (1969) attempted to address this question by pointing to studies which analyzed certain aspects of hospital utilization between different practice modalities, in particular the diagnostic composition of this differential. Although the final verdict is far from being rendered, the prevailing pattern in the various studies of admission rates for the Health Insurance Plan of New York (HIP), as compared with other types of practice organization in New York City, was substantially lower in precisely those diagnostic categories most often suspected to comprise unnecessary admissions—tonsillectomies and upper respiratory infections.

There are two additional analytic points covered by Klarman (1963) which were either omitted or skimmed over by Donabedian. One concerns the early findings of 1940–1946 that Blue Cross–insured persons had higher hospital admission rates and lower average lengths of stay than did the general United States population. The other was the finding that, although HIP subscribers experienced lower hospitalization rates than persons under Blue Shield–Blue Cross, they showed the same rates as persons who used a union self-insured plan for ambulatory care. In the latter comparison, both the HIP subscribers and the self-insured union members used a self-insured hospital plan, leading to a hypothesis that control, specifically, of hospital use is a deciding factor. This is an important point, since it represents an attempt at identifying which structural variables in PGP affected which output results.

M. I. Roemer and M. Shain (1959) had reviewed the available evidence up to that time on hospital utilization under insurance. They conceptualized the determinants both of rates of hospital admission and hospital days in an area as derived from three sets of influences operative under conditions of economic support through insurance:

1. Patient determinants:
   incidence and prevalence of illness
   attitudes towards illness
   cost of medical care to the patient
   marital status
   housing and social level

2. Hospital determinants:
   supply of beds
   efficiency of bed utilization
   mechanisms of hospital remuneration
   availability of alternative bed facilities
   outpatient services

3. Physician determinants:
   supply of physicians
   method of medical remuneration
   nature of community medical practice
   medical policies in the hospital
   level of medical alertness
   medical teaching needs

Roemer and Shain speculated that, while all these factors must theoretically exert an influence under the cost-easing operation of insurance (and there was support from empirical data for the influence of most of these factors), the most pragmatically effective mechanism of *control* was probably through constraints on the supply of hospital beds, that is, the bed-population ratio in an area. As we shall see, the subsequent findings on hospital utilization under the HMO models have continued to point to the bed supply as an important explanatory variable. The enactment of "certificate of need" laws on hospital construction in some 20 states, moreover, seems to reflect a growing consensus on the importance of the influence of bed supply on bed demand, with obvious implications for community costs (American Hospital Association, 1972).

Subsequent to the Donabedian review, additional publications dealing with hospital utilization levels of HMOs continued to accumulate. These consisted both of additional reports of empirical results and newer evaluative and analytic works.

Another Klarman paper (1970) concentrates its analysis upon "expected savings in health services expenditures" from the PGP pattern, thus again exploring the general criterion of his 1963 paper. Reviewing again the HIP studies summarized in the Donabedian review, Klarman clarifies certain aspects of the unavoidable confounding of the many causative (independent or input) variables in those studies that resulted from the special circumstances of the HIP structure and the New York City location. Included in these variables are group practice organization; prepayment by the subscriber; capitation payments to the 30-odd medical groups, accompanied by the diverse methods of payment by the groups to the physicians; the use of part-time as well as full-time physicians; the unique nature of the New York municipal hospital system; and the limited access which HIP physicians had to community hospital beds. From these studies, as well as others involving Kaiser-Permanente, Klarman concludes that the evidence indicates that limiting physicians' access to hospital beds has been an important factor in keeping the utilization of hospitals low under the PGP pattern.

Hill and Veney (1970) offer new empirical evidence from a Kansas Blue Cross–Blue Shield experiment on insured outpatient benefits. This experiment confirmed earlier evidence supporting the proposition that increased ambulatory insurance benefits per se for patients lead to no reduction in hospital use and, in fact, result in at least a temporary increase of such use. These findings, Klarman argues, effectively rule out the availability of ambulatory care benefits as an explanatory cause for the reduced hospital utilization generally experienced by PGP organizations.

Besides limiting access to beds, Klarman notes that the salary or capitation forms of paying the physician may reasonably be expected to contribute to decreased hospital utilization on theoretical economic grounds. He cites the work of Monsma (1970), who showed that fee-for-service physicians derive a marginal increment in earnings for the performance of additional service (surgery, for example) while capitation payments (and salary) do not offer such an increment. This theory fits the findings noted in Donabedian's review that the excess hospitalization of the fee-for-service arrangement over that of PGP care modalities is centered in surgical diagnoses, particularly in tonsillectomies, cholecystectomies, "female surgery," and appendectomies. It is also supported by Bunker's findings (1970) that surgery rates are much lower in England (where there are relatively fewer surgeons, most of whom are on salary) than in the United States.

Klarman's most recent review (1971) broadened the field surveyed from PGP to the generalized HMO concept. Thus, besides reporting on some additional research and giving further analysis of PGP experience, he considered the data on medical care foundations reported in the literature and analyzed the factors in the MCF form of organization which might affect performance. Dealing with savings on hospital utilization under PGP, Klarman has summarized some of these results in the following generalizations: (1) It has been widely held, based on the implications of two HIP studies conducted in the 1950s, that there is a saving of about 20 percent in patient days and admission rates under PGP plans, compared to other health insurance plans; and (2) These results have been "subsequently reinforced in several ways."

Most of the "reinforcing" studies discussed by Klarman were cited and described by Donabedian in 1969, but there have since been additional ones. Moreover, Shapiro (1971) estimated a 25 percent lower rate of hospital utilization for HIP compared with other matched subscribers.

The Social Security Administration (1971) reported that per capita medical *expenditures* for hospital use were, respectively, 18 percent and 11 percent lower in northern and in southern California for Kaiser-Permanente, compared with care under other aus-

Table 4-5-4. New Offense in First Year After Release After Conviction for Willful Homicide, by Sex and Year, 1971–75

Year of release		Total	No offense	New offense						
				Willful homicide	Negligent manslaughter	Armed robbery	Unarmed robbery	Aggravated assault	Forcible rape	Other
1975[a]		2,897	2,824	8	3	18	6	6	1	31
1974	M	1,601	1,549	5	0	8	3	6	0	30
	F	184	182	0	0	0	0	1	0	1
1973	M	1,786	1,753	2	0	8	2	4	2	15
	F	212	210	0	0	1	0	0	0	1
1972	M	2,165	2,117	5	0	10	0	6	1	26
	F	275	271	1	0	0	0	0	0	3
1971	M	2,143	2,105	5	0	7	1	7	1	17
	F	269	268	0	0	1	0	0	0	0
Total		11,532	11,279	26	3	53	12	30	5	124

[a] Breakdown by sex not available

Source: Sourcebook of Criminal Justice Statistics 1978, p. 667; 1977, pp. 686, 688; 1976, pp. 745, 746; 1975, pp. 673, 680; 1974, pp. 489, 491.

cian under the MCF type of HMO is fee-for-service, there remains the incentive for the physician of higher income for additional services, according to Monsma's type of analysis. While the MCF type of HMO does not alter the method of paying the physician, it does broaden the ambulatory service benefits available to the subscriber. Empirical results have failed to indicate that such a broadening lowers hospital utilization rates. In addition to the Kansas findings of the Hill and Veney study (1970), Klarman also reminds us of the Avnet study (1967) for Group Health Insurance (GHI) in New York and of the reported results from extended out-of-hospital Blue Shield benefits offered in Maryland and described by Kelly (1965). All of these substantiated the theoretical expectations of no decrease (and, indeed, an increase) in hospital utilization when "physician services are broadened in a solo practice fee-for-service setting." In the Saskatchewan setting, Roemer (1958) had reported the same finding—increased hospital use associated with prepaid comprehensive doctor's care, compared with no insurance for ambulatory care—as far back as the late 1950s.

In recent years, further data on hospital utilization continued to be reported. Another study of government employees (state, rather than federal) insured under different types of health plan was reported from California (Medical Advisory Council to the California Public Employees Retirement System, 1971). Hospital utilization findings in this PERS (Public Employees Retirement System) study corresponded generally with those found for federal employees, with aggregate days per 1,000 per year being much lower than PGP plans. Unlike the federal study, the California one also reported utilization under the medical care foundation plans, which are relatively numerous in this state. Interestingly, the utilization rates for both hospital days and ambulatory doctor visits were *higher* under the foundation-type plans than for any of the other plan-types. The experience applied to a 12-month period in 1962–1963.

Still another comparison of hospital utilization under the PGP type of HMO with other types of health insurance plan in California is given by Roemer et al. (1973). This study examined the experience of random samples of the total memberships of the three main types of plan, selecting two examples of each type. In contrast to some others, this study found the differential for hospital admission rates to be relatively small, but, because of a very short length of hospital stay under the PGP plans, the differential in aggregate hospital days was great—526 days per 1,000 per year in the PGP plans, compared to 864 and 1,109 days in the commercial and provider-sponsored plans, respectively. In this investigation, out-of-plan hospital use (determined through study of a subsample) was found to involve 7.2 percent of the admissions, many of them for maternity care (short-stay cases). These cases, unlike those in the earlier Densen studies of HIP experience, however, are included within the group practice hospitalization rates reported above.

Roemer et al. (1973) also analyzed hospital utilization according to several demographic breakdowns. It became evident that the low use rate (in days per 1,000 per year) of the group practice or HMO-type plans was largely referable to the experience of families with dependents and families of other than Protestant faith. With respect to social class (as measured by educational attainment and occupation), hospital day rates in all plan-types were consistently higher in the lower-class group, but the markedly lower rate under the HMO-type plans prevailed for both social classes. The same was true of families with and without a history of chronic illness—much greater hospital use in the "chronically ill" families, but markedly fewer days in the HMO-type plans for both types of families.

Interpretations of hospital experience

The total complex of causes contributing to the lower use rates of hospital days in the PGP type of HMO remains a matter for discussion and research. As noted earlier, the absence of fee incentives, especially for elective surgical operations, has been credited by much of the data (and theoretically justified by Monsma). Easier financial (if not geographic) accessibility to ambulatory care under these plans has also been considered causative, but both the findings of the California PERS study (Medical Advisory Council, 1971) and the numerous studies of ambulatory care insurance for private doctor's care in Kansas, Saskatchewan, Maryland, and elsewhere, reported above, would not seem to support this contention. The constraint exercised by a limited hospital bed–population ratio, however, in the PGP plans would seem to be clear. The less-than-average supply of hospital beds in the Kaiser-Permanente Health Plan (below 2.0 per 1,000 members) obviously places an upper limit on the number of hospital days of care that can be provided. Striking evidence of this influence of bed supply is furnished by the differentials noted earlier in this paper on hospital expenditures for Medicare beneficiaries in the Kaiser-Permanente Health Plan in 1971, compared with other California Medicare beneficiaries; on the other hand, in HIP of New York, where the Medicare members use ordinary community hospitals, their hospital use expenditures were just the same as those of non-HIP Medicare beneficiaries (Social Security Administration, 1971). The degree to which this latter finding is due to the "opening up" of HIP physician accessibility to community hospital beds in New York, or to the other factors which Klarman postulates, cannot be determined on the basis of available data.

The point is that PGP doctors can evidently "live with" a constrained bed supply; they adjust by being prudent on hospital admissions, doing the maximum diagnostic workups on an outpatient basis, and keeping patients hospitalized for relatively short stays. Whether this results in better or poorer health for the patient is a serious question yet to be answered (refer to the section on Health Outcomes). That it results in cost savings (refer to the section on Costs and Productivity) is beyond doubt.

Aside from the PERS study reviewed above, meaningful data on hospitalization under the medical care foundation model of HMO are sparse. The Physicians' Association of Clackamas County, Oregon (Haley, 1971), reported that for 1969–1970 the average length of stay of Clackamas County patients at one Portland hospital was 5.18 days, compared to 6.82 days for patients from metropolitan Portland. No other data about the characteristics of these patients or the rate of admissions are given; since Clackamas County is essentially suburban to Portland and since its population characteristics doubtless differ from those of the central city, it is difficult to interpret these figures.

A still unpublished study of the Clackamas County Foundation by the UCLA Survey Research Center (Berkanovic, 1973) gives other data on hospital utilization under this pattern. Based on 1971 experience of Medicaid beneficiaries enrolled in the Clackamas County foundation, the preliminary findings suggest a *higher* hospital utilization rate (by a factor of 1.5 to 2.0), in days per 1,000 persons covered per year compared with a Medicaid population in a neighboring county using open-market patterns without a foundation.

Ambulatory care utilization

Donabedian (1969) noted that the sparsely reported data on ambulatory care utilization tended to indicate that, in general, such utilization increased under plans which insured for out-of-hospital benefits. The increase, however, was no different under PGP than under fee-for-service private practice. Also, there seemed to be no evidence of flagrant or obvious overutilization of ambulatory services.

Klarman (1971) attempted to assess the import of various published reports on physician-population ratios, in an effort to arrive at generalizations about respective ambulatory care utilization rates in PGP and in other delivery forms. Physician-population ratios presumably give indirect evidence of patient-doctor contact rates—if productivity levels are assumed constant. Based on the reported evidence of physician-population ratios, Klarman noted the often contradictory results of published studies, beginning as far back as 1940. In some cases the savings, in terms of per capita expenditures for physician care, were found to be greater than the proportionately lower physician-population ratio, presumably because of lower rates of reimbursement of physicians in PGP plans.

The actual rate of physician visits per capita is estimated by Klarman to be 4.50 per year for Kaiser-Permanente, compared to 4.42 for the general California population, after adjustment for out-of-plan utilization as well as for telephone and other nonphysician contacts reported as visits in the California-wide data. These estimates are based on the report of the National Advisory Commission on Health Manpower (1967) and on the Columbia University survey of three plan-types in 1962. The greater number of visits and the generally lower physician-population ratio in Kaiser-Permanente implies a higher level of production for the latter's physicians, but Klarman believes the Manpower Commission's report overstates the general California physician-population ratio. Data (Social Security Administration, 1971) on ambulatory care from the Medicare program could be used without the dubious intervention of "adjustments," except that only expenditures, not medical visits, are reported. Per capita expenditures for physician's care were 7 percent less for Kaiser-Permanente, Northern California, the same as other sources for Southern California, and 35 percent higher for HIP, as reported by SSA in 1971. Expenditures may, indeed, reflect utilization differences, but the relationship can be confounded by different levels of earnings and different productivity rates of physicians. Thus, the picture presented by Klarman (1971) provides very little information on differentials in utilization rates for ambulatory services between PGP and other forms of medical care delivery.

The Roemer et al. study (1973) does provide some comparative data on ambulatory services. Basically, the findings showed much lesser differentials among the plan-types than for hospital days; the PGP-type plans had doctor-contacts at the rate of 3,324 per 1,000 persons per year, compared with 3,108 in the commercial and 3,984 in the "Blue" plans. A revealing categorization in which these relationships, however, did not prevail was by educational level of the family head. Among persons with college education, ambulatory care use was higher under the PGP plans than under either of the other two plan-types. It would appear that better educated and probably more sophisticated persons are able to make greater use of ambulatory care in the relatively complex framework of the large prepaid group practice plans found in California; this is less true under conventional conditions of private medical practice.

Another study in California (Kovner et al., 1969) examined the effect of family income on ambulatory care utilization under two HMO patterns: both the prepaid group practice (the Ross-Loos Medical Clinic Plan) and the medical care foundation (San Joaquin County) patterns. The study found that, in both these HMO patterns, the effect of income was virtually nil—eliminating the usual correlation between poverty and low utilization of outpatient services.

It has been shown both theoretically and empirically that merely extending insured ambulatory service benefits will not reduce hospital utilization under fee-for-service practice; the same economic theory indicates that there is reason to believe that paying the physician either by capitation or salary should lead to decreased hospital utilization. If one adds to this the influence of substantial ambulatory diagnostic and treatment facilities found in a group practice setting, as well as a restriction on available beds, one may expect a *relatively* higher level of ambulatory, compared with hospital, utilization under the PGP type of HMO.

A revealing demonstration of these dynamics is given in the ratios between doctor visits and hospital days reported by Roemer et al. (1973) in the three plan-types. These were as follows:

Plan-type	Doctor visits per 1000/year (a)	Hospital days per 1000/year (b)	Ratio (a):(b)
Commercial	3,104	864	3.6
"Blues"	3,984	1,109	3.6
Group practice	3,324	526	6.3

It is apparent that the PGP-type plan gives almost double the *relative* emphasis on ambulatory, compared with hospital bed service, as does either of the open-market plan-types.

Further evidence of the influence of the PGP model of HMO on the ratio between ambulatory and hospital services came from the Columbia (Maryland) Plan in 1969–1970. Malcolm Peterson(1971) reported that physicians' office visits were occurring at a rate of about 8.0 per person per year (of which 40 percent were for well-person care), compared with 4.6 nationally; hospital days, by contrast, were at a rate of 335 per 1,000 per year, compared with about 1,100 days nationally. Although these rough figures were not adjusted for age, socioeconomic status, etc., they are still striking.

Quality Assessments

Regarding the persistently difficult question of quality evaluations, an excellent review of all the methodologies was produced by Robert H. Brook (1972) as a doctoral dissertation at the Johns Hopkins School of Hygiene. Although the evaluation of HMOs, in comparison with other patterns of medical care, figures only tangentially in this work, Brook concludes that both "process" and "outcome" measures should ideally be used in combination. Among outcome measures, he advocates greater application of the so-called "tracer" technique, in which the incidence of morbid sequelae of specified pathological conditions (e.g., middle ear infection leading to deafness or hypertension leading to stroke) is traced under varying subsystems of medical care.

In the last several years, investigators do not seem to have devoted much effort to quality assessments of HMOs based simply on "structure" or the input of resources (personnel, equipment, etc.). The unitary medical record and the greater convenience of interspecialty consultations were emphasized as structural avenues to quality care in the *Harvard Law Review* paper by Greenberg and Rodburg (1971), but these factors in the PGP model have not been subjected to quantified comparisons with ordinary medical practice. Williamson (1971) has demonstrated the discrepancies between "input" measures of the qualifications of doctors, and "output" measures of the quality of their work, pointing further to the importance of using process and outcome measures in combination as a basis for quality evaluation.

With regard to "process" evaluations, the recent years also do not seem to have produced medical audit studies comparing HMO services with traditional patterns of medical care delivery. The belief continues to be widely held, nevertheless, that peer review—whether on a day-to-day basis or on the post-hoc basis of claims surveillance in medical foundation plans—helps to assure the quality of the doctor's work. Yet Weinerman (1969), commenting on group practice (whether prepaid or not) noted: "Group conferences, medical audits, and informal office consultations . . . are common in the descriptive literature but infrequent in daily practice."

The Roemer et al. study in California (1973), from its examination of samples of actual medical records in doctors' offices or clinics, developed a "rationality index" as an approach to quality evaluation. This index was based on such documentable criteria as completeness of the medical history, extent of physical examination, frequency of consultations, and other elements of service. With the use of "factor analysis" technique, the value of this index for the HMO model plans turned out to be 0.527, compared with 0.515 in the "Blue" plans and 0.503 in the commercial plans. The fallacies of medical record analysis as a reflection of the actual medical care process have long been recognized, yet there is no reason to expect less complete records in private medical offices than in prepaid group clinics, and it is the comparative values that the above indices reflect. In fact, one might suspect that in private offices, where fees are paid for each unit of service, records would be more nearly complete than in prepaid clinics where the doctors are on salary; if so, the differentials on "rationality" indicated above may understate the relative performance level under the HMO pattern.

Another dimension of the quality of medical care is often considered to be the degree to which preventive services are provided and used. Under HMOs, there has long been discussion of the effect of incentives to preventive service, aside from the influence of early, rather than late, attention to overt symptoms. Roemer et al. (1973) have produced some of the first hard data on this question through the examination of medical records (and hospital records) under the PGP versus open-market patterns. Indicators of prevention, identifiable in patient charts, were such items as "checkup" examinations of adults, well-child examinations, vaginal cytology tests, routine rectal examinations, chest x-rays, serological tests for syphilis, and immunizations. Summating these, by "factor analysis," a "preventive service index" was derived for the three types of health plan. It was computed as 0.452 in the HMO-type plan, compared to 0.404 in the "Blue" and 0.384 in the commercial insurance plans.

Another reflection of prevention in HMOs is given in data reported by Lester Breslow (1972), derived from 1965 studies in Alameda County, California. In the sample of the "Human Population Laboratory" in that county, those persons who were insured under the Kaiser-Permanente Health Plan had a "health maintenance examination" within the past year more frequently than those covered by open-market plans; the comparisons were, respectively, 58 percent versus 43–46 percent for men and 63 percent versus 49–57 percent for women.

A study of schoolchildren in whom physical defects had been detected was reported by Cauffman and Roemer (1967), with information on utilization under the different types of health insurance plans that covered the various children's families. They found that any type of health insurance coverage, compared with noninsurance, was more likely to be associated with treatment of the child's defect, but that children in families covered by PGP health insurance plans were more likely to have received a general "checkup" examination than children in families covered by open-market plans.

Costs and Productivity

The economic dimension of HMOs, compared with other modes of medical care delivery, must distinguish between the overall expenditures by the patient or the community, on the one hand, and the "costs of production" or the productivity of the subsystem, on the other, whether or not any productive efficiencies are "passed along" to the consumer in the form of lower prices. Each of these questions will be considered separately.

Expenditures by the consumer

With regard to expenditures by consumers or costs to patients, the Roemer et al. California study (1973) produced data on the PGP model of HMO, as compared with conventional patterns. It analyzed annual expenditures by family units for physician and hospital services in terms of (a) insurance premiums (whether or not paid partly or wholly by employers) and (b) out-of-pocket expenditures. The basic findings for families of all sizes in the three plan-types were as follows:

Plan-type	Average premium	Out-of-pocket expenditures	Total costs
Commercial	$208	$156	$364
"Blues"	257	190	447
Group practice	271	52	323

Thus, it is evident that the average family premiums of the PGP-type plans are higher, but that the out-of-pocket expenditures for medical and hospital services are so much lower than in the other two plan-types that the aggregate costs are the lowest among the three types of plan. When family size is held constant, the same general findings prevail. There are, however, different relationships by other demographic breakdowns. In families of three to four members defined as "lower income" (under $11,000 per year), the lowest aggregate expenditures occur in the commercial plans; they are $391 in the latter plans, compared with $417 in the PGP-type plans. These findings may reflect the lower illness risk composition in the enrollment of commercial plans (reported earlier) as well as the lower available family incomes (even in the "under $11,000" category), also reported earlier.

For the medical care foundation model of HMO, the available data are, again, confined largely to the experience of Medicaid beneficiaries on the California scene. In a comparison (Gartside,

1971) of the four-county area covered by the San Joaquin County foundation with a similar county lacking a foundation, the monthly costs per eligible person averaged $5.81 for physician services in the MCF area and $6.66 in the comparison traditional area; the state-wide average, adjusted for the mix of Medicaid categories, was $7.33. The overall average costs for all types of health service were actually higher in the MCF than in the comparison area ($10.43 versus $10.13), although this was due almost entirely to a higher expenditure for nursing-home services in the San Joaquin area.

The MCF of Clackamas County, Oregon (Haley, 1971), reported that "generally costs in Clackamas County are 23 percent under the cost of service outside the county," but clear data in support of this statement have not been issued.

Production efficiencies

In considering the crucial question of production efficiencies under the HMO model, studies on economics of scale within prepaid group practice have figured prominently. Herbert Klarman, (1970; 1971) goes into this subject at some length. He notes at the outset that empirical results represent experience drawn entirely from fee-for-service practice since "little, if anything, has been published on variation in productivity among medical groups in the same prepayment plan" (Klarman, 1971:30). By implication at least, he minimizes the dangers of extrapolating conclusions, reached on the basis of findings from the fee-for-service group practice milieu, to the PGP model, asserting that the caveats of Roemer and Du Bois (1969) about the noncomparabilities of the two practice media "pertain to who gets the benefits of any savings, but do not appear to bear on the issue of variation in physician productivity by the size of the medical firm" (Klarman, 1971:30). Although this particular point is well taken, it would still seem that such extrapolation should be made with extreme caution.

First, much of the fee-for-service practice data have been obtained in single-specialty settings, and PGP is typically carried on in a multi-specialty setting. Second, in view of the important influence on other performance criteria believed to be associated with different methods of paying physicians, one would hesitate to assume that there is no impact on productivity just because one cannot at present make a clearcut case for it. After all, until Monsma's work (1970) articulated the issue, there was no commonly accepted theoretical explanation for the method of physician payment influencing HIP versus non-HIP hospitalization differentials in New York City. It may very well be, for example, that the management option of "pacing" physician visits, by control over the appointment system when the physician is on salary, can be more strongly asserted in large PGPs than in smaller ones. It may also be that substitution of lower-paid personnel for part of the physician's time is more feasible in the PGP model.

Many of the research findings cited by Klarman appeared in Donabedian (1969), but Klarman noted some additional works and further refined the economic analysis. The major studies again concern the work of Boan (1966), Bailey (1968), and Yett (1967). The study by Yankauer et al. (1970) is new. Klarman notes that theoretical considerations have led economists to expect returns to scale in medical care output on a priori grounds, and that Boan's and Yett's work seems to support this hypothesis. Bailey (1968), however, draws opposite conclusions. His findings (focused on specialists in internal medicine) lead him to infer that physicians in larger group practices earn more because of the profits earned on a proportionately higher rate of ancillary services performed in their establishments. The output, in terms of clinical visits per physician per unit time, was found to hold constant with increasing size of medical group. Bailey interpreted this to mean that the proportionately greater use of ancillary services by the larger groups of internists apparently did not represent a substitution of the time of allied health personnel for that of physicians, but could be viewed as merely incremental services delivered by larger groups.

Yankauer et al. (1970) reported a similar finding based on a nationwide survey of pediatric practices. This study also found the number of physician visits per unit time to be virtually constant with increase of size of the group practice. Delegation of tasks by the physician was generally in the administrative, technical, and clerical functions, but not in patient care functions. Where the latter type of delegation was found to occur, it was in response to relative local shortages of pediatricians, rather than in relation to the size of the medical group.

Klarman notes that the conflicting interpretations placed on these findings cannot be resolved by further analysis of existing data, but require additional research on medical care production, designed to answer the open questions. For the present, he concludes (1971:31) that "economies of scale have not yet been demonstrated empirically."

It should be noted that arguments which postulate a possibly greater willingness to delegate patient care tasks to ancillary personnel are related to the circumstances found more widely under large PGP conditions. These include the feasibility of close supervision of such tasks by the physician, a relative lack of concern by him that his income position may be eroded, and, in the case of large, self-sufficient PGPs, lessened fear of retaliation by competitors. Moreover, it is difficult to see why one could expect any increase in productivity, as measured solely by physician visits, under conditions which closely prescribe the tasks reserved for physician performance. In particular, in a PGP situation the number of visits to be handled by a physician per hour would largely be determined by the scheduling mechanism, and could resemble the moving assembly line in industry.

It is also necessary to note that defining physician productivity solely in terms of office visits, in fee-for-service private practice, can be illusory. Since, in the American scheme of things, physicians typically prescribe treatment for the same patient in the office and in the hospital, it is not unreasonable to postulate that solo practitioners and small private groups run up physician visit "scores" by hospitalizing freely. In that case, as Roemer and Shain (1959) have pointed out, the private physician can ostensibly increase his efficiency of practice by hospitalizing patients, passing along the heavy diagnostic work to the hospital and the expense to insurance plans. The larger, better equipped group practices may reasonably be expected to handle more of these cases in the office—spending more time with the patients, doing more tests, and hospitalizing less. Bailey's (1968) data tends to support this hypothesis, at least for solo as compared with group practice.

The important missing data in Bailey's study are the total utilization by and cost to the patients per year, per illness, etc. Lacking a defined subscriber population, these data are virtually impossible of meaningful interpretation. (If one wished to dramatize the deficiencies of these data, one could argue that all the data on visits to a particular physician might pertain to two or three patients with chronic illness making repeated visits, with astronomical cost to themselves or their insurance carriers.)

Boan (1966) stated the conclusions from his research in Canada straightforwardly. He found that physicians in group practice, compared to solo practice, had higher ratios of allied health personnel per physician, lower costs per physician for such personnel, and lower costs of investment per physician. However, these results are not strictly proof of economies of scale, since only the dichotomy between solo and group practice is examined. Furthermore, the applicability of nationwide Canadian results to the United States scene remains open to question. Direct inferences on returns to scale can be made only if one assumes that Boan's conclusions follow from observation on two discrete points along the size-of-firm scale— solo and larger than solo—and if one is further willing to assume that his upward slope of the returns-to-scale line would hold if the group practices were categorized along an increasing size scale.

Yett (1967) measured total tax-deductible expenses per physician as related to output (of computed patient visits) per physician, and found definite economies of scale. The result would suggest that practices in which the physicians were more productive, in terms of visits produced, exhibited a smaller overhead cost per physician visit. It would seem that a cost function analysis of this type does not directly address the question of economies of scale in terms of larger versus smaller group practices, and, a fortiori, does not shed light on what one might expect in an HMO situation. Furthermore, it does not directly address the problem of physician output as a function of size of practice (measured by number of physicians involved), which was Bailey's concern.

However, subsequent work by Reinhardt and Yett (1972), at the University of Southern California has produced insight on this crucial subject. The published work concentrates on fitting production functions to national data reported to the magazine *Medical Economics* (MEDEC). These investigators are now tackling the question of the output of physicians (measured in patient visits per physician per week and, separately, by annual gross patient billings per physician) as a function of inputs. The latter consist of the services of medical auxiliary personnel, cost of plant and medical equipment, medical supplies used up in the conduct of practice, and the amount of physician's time (hours per week) occupied "strictly on practice-related activities." Physicians' visits are totaled over three sites: office, home, and hospital. The Reinhardt-Yett study defined "returns to scale" as the relative increase in number of visits per physician associated with the same percentage increase applied to all input factors.

Without reference to mode of practice, their results were that the output (visits per week) of the individual physician showed the expected increasing returns to scale, if inputs were to be increased in relatively small private practices. Comparing solo practices to single-specialty group practices, they found that the latter produce "between 4 and 13 percent more patient visits than do solo practitioners at any given level of factor input." The report cautions that these results may be flawed because of the lack of data on total medical group output, instead of output of individual physicians. So little data were available on mixed-specialty groups that they decided to exclude all multi-specialty group data from the group-solo comparisons in this study. Furthermore, the preponderance of the single-specialty groups studied was very small, consisting of three to six physicians.

Included among the USC (1972) findings were these points: (a) "Solo practitioners tend to work fewer hours and employ fewer aides per physician than do their colleagues in groups or partnerships"; (b) quite apart from the longer hours worked, group practice physicians produced more visits per hour than those in solo practice—4.5 percent more for general practitioners, 6.2 percent for pediatricians, 13.8 percent for obstetricians-gynecologists, and 4.0 percent more for internists; (c) up to about four or five aides per physician, the total number of patient visits per week per physician increases with additional aides; and (d) adding more physician time as an input will increase patient units by a greater factor than an increase of proportionate size in any other input.

Another USC study by Kimbell and Lorant (c. 1970) used the responses to the Seventh Periodic Survey of Physicians by the American Medical Association as its data for analyzing production functions of solo physicians, and the data of the AMA's Survey of Medical Groups for analyzing group practice relationships. Economies of scale were measured in terms of *office* visits as a function of the inputs: physician time, number of allied personnel employed, and number of examining rooms (representing capital investment). Among their findings on solo practice were these: (a) an increase in physician time increases the number of office visits by a greater factor than an identical percentage increase of any of the other inputs—in fact, more than the increase in allied personnel and capital (examining rooms) combined (a given percentage increase in allied personnel will have a greater effect on office visits than the same percentage increase in examining rooms, although increases in the latter will also increase the output); (b) physicians who charge higher initial fees have a lower output of office visits; and (c) the total R^2 (the proportion of the total variation due to the "explanatory" variables) is only 0.13, so that other factors not in the analysis explain much more of the production than those included.

Regarding group practices, Kimbell and Lorant found that: (a) the most important factor in increasing office (as well as total) patient visits by far is still physician time input; (b) there are decreasing returns to scale in office visits (and total visits) for an increasing size of output (i.e., an increase of about 10 percent in input factors will increase output by only about 8 percent, although, for gross revenues, the return to scale is almost constant, tending to agree with Bailey's findings); and (c) practices using an incentive plan for income distribution "had 10 percent greater apparent efficiency" than practices applying completely equal sharing or salaries. "Efficiency" was measured by the degree to which the group practices produce above or below the output predicted by the model. The R^2 achieved by this analysis of group practices was about 0.80, so that the explanation of output by the input variables was much better than for solo physicians.

Another recently reported study on medical care productivity is that of Newhouse (1973). This paper addresses the question of costs per physician visit in different practice patterns, and a principal determinant was found to be whether or not the practice shared income equally or divided it among the members of the practice in proportion to the number of visits each doctor produced. It followed that solo, fee-for-service practice was found to yield the lowest overhead costs per visit, since this form of organization represents the most direct relationship between the income received by the physician and the visits produced by him. The sample studied comprised 20 practices, varying from 11 solo practices to two 5-physician groups, and three outpatient clinics of hospitals. Newhouse states "there is the obvious qualification that the sample is extremely small," and much of the paper is devoted to showing that equal income-sharing should theoretically lead to increased unit costs per visit.

Effects of size

In concluding this section on the literature dealing with economies of scale, a number of points must be noted. In using production functions in private fee-for-service practice, investigators have often considered patient visits as the key output measure. It would seem to be a questionable assumption, however, that more visits per hour are uniformly desirable. Clearly, the desirable number depends on patient care considerations, and flatly to equate an increasing number of visits per hour with greater efficiency cannot be excused by appealing to the assumption of "other things being equal." Studies of productivity which do not include some simultaneous observations on the content or quality of care are of doubtful usefulness at best, and may even be misleading.

Similar considerations hold in studying *economies of scale* in private fee-for-service practice. Assuming that physicians will keep unit (per visit) overhead costs down, if their income is directly tied to the net earnings of the visits they produce, might also imply that doctors would do almost anything they can "get away with" to maximize their net incomes. In a period of physician shortage, and in consideration of legal restrictions on competition entering the field, it would again seem to be questionable whether this type of motivation is widely operative.

Finally, with the preceding two points in mind, it might be germane to restate Klarman's 1972 summary on the research to date in the following manner: General economic theory, as outlined by Boan, Fein, and others, indicates that group practice should be more efficient than solo practice, all other things being equal, in terms of productivity. Monsma's theoretic formulation indicates that *prepaid* practice is expected to be more efficient than fee-for-service practice, in terms of avoidance of unnecessary utilization of expensive procedures. Research to date has not effectively proven these reasonable hypotheses false. In any event, the entire question of production efficiencies touches only one aspect of the HMO concept; other aspects of incentives to economy, when a fixed annual premium is paid for a broad scope of services, will be considered in the following sections.

Health Outcomes

PGP and health outcomes

The ultimate measure of HMO performance, as suggested earlier, is how healthy these organizations keep their members, compared with other patterns of medical care delivery. The sparsity of data on this crucial question, up to 1969, was evident in the review by Donabedian. It had been largely confined to the experience of the Health Insurance Plan of Greater New York and focused on mortality in the very young and the very old.

Since then, some little additional outcome data have been produced on this key question, but not always with conclusive results. A study by William I. Barton (1972), though based on a nationwide mortality study in 1964–1966, provides the first such nationwide data on infant mortality in relation to health insurance coverage. After adjustment for race, region, parental education, and live-birth order, the mothers with some health insurance coverage had significantly lower infant mortality rates than those not insured; when adjustment was made for family income, the infant mortality rate was still slightly lower for the insured childbirth cases (23.3 per 1,000 live births compared with 24.5), but the difference was not statistically significant. This study, unfortunately, does not come to grips with the HMO question. In fact, it was found, paradoxically, that mothers with more comprehensive health insurance coverage actually had *higher* infant mortality rates than those with more limited coverage; the author, however, speculates that this unexpected finding reflected characteristics of the mothers, rather than being attributable to the extent of insurance protection. He postulates that women with more complete insurance coverage were probably higher-risk mothers in the first place—in other words, a previous pregnancy complication had induced them to secure broader insurance protection.

The first American report applying sickness absenteeism as an outcome measure for comparing prepaid group practice with other patterns appeared in 1971. Robert L. Robertson (1971) studied work loss in 1966–1967 among schoolteachers covered under a

PGP-type of HMO, compared with teachers covered under a "Blue" plan. Although in this, as in other comparative studies, the effects of self-selection could not be completely eliminated (since membership in either type of insurance plan is the individual's own decision), the findings suggests a slightly lower råte of "work-loss from sickness or injury" for both men and women teachers covered by the HMO-type plan. The size of the differences varied with age level, and the greatest different characterized younger females. The overall age-standardized mean days of work loss were 3.88 days per year in the HMO-type plan for males compared with 4.01 days in the "Blue" plan; the parallel figures for females were 5.93 days compared to 6.41 days.

"Foundations" and health outcomes

With respect to the medical care foundation pattern of HMO, an as yet unpublished study from the UCLA School of Public Health (Newport and Roemer, 1973) examined perinatal mortality among mothers covered by Medicaid through the San Joaquin Foundation for Medical Care, compared with a closely matched county (Ventura) lacking a foundation and using traditional methods. Newport and Roemer found that, excluding county hospital births which are not influenced by MCF procedures, the perinatal death rates were lower in the foundation area for "white Anglo" childbirths, but higher for childbirths in black and Spanish-surname families. When ethnically standardized for the mix of these groups in the state-wide Medicaid population, the perinatal death rates in the foundation and matched comparison areas were virtually identical: 29.6 deaths per 1,000 total births in the former group and 30.1 in the latter. More interesting, perhaps, was the finding that in a third area, admittedly not matched to the foundation county, but lacking a foundation and having a strong county health department (with an active maternal and child health program), the perinatal death rate was *half* of that in either of the study counties, at 15.5 deaths per 1,000 births.

While these were the only recent health outcome studies with a direct bearing on evaluation of HMO performance, other investigations have been providing new approaches to the use of adjusted mortality data for evaluating the performance of complex organizations. Moses and Mosteller (1968) revealed large differences in the death rates for specified surgical operations made in large teaching hospitals throughout the country, even after adjustments for various patient characteristics. Roemer et al. (1968) developed a formula by which crude hospital death rates could be adjusted for average case-severity, so that adjusted death rates could serve as a basis for evaluating the overall quality of hospital performance. These methodologic studies may provide clues for evaluation of HMO performance on the basis of mortality outcomes.

Patient Attitudes

While more substantial data on health status outcomes is awaited, some idea of the quality of service in a medical care program may be validly inferred from the attitudes expressed by consumers or patients. Although consumer attitudes may be influenced by many factors in health service delivery unrelated to technical excellence, it is reasonable to consider that the speed and degree with which the service helps a person to recover from illness or to maintain his health is an important determinant of attitudes. This becomes more plausible as patients become better educated about health care requirements.

Since the Donabedian review, additional studies have reported relatively high degrees of satisfaction with health services associated with HMO patterns. The favorable population attitudes toward group practice in general, even when experience with such clinics was lacking, were noted earlier from the study by Metzner et al. (1972). Weinerman's paper (1964) on patient attitudes toward prepaid group practice plans showed a high degree of overall satisfaction in spite of many complaints about the impersonality of the doctor-patient relationship in a "clinic setting." His general summary of numerous studies up to 1964 is worth quoting (Weinerman, 1964:886):

> In general, the various investigations of attitudes of group health members suggest much appreciation for the technical standards of group health care, but less satisfaction with the doctor-patient relationship itself. In one way or another patients report disappointment with the degree of personal interest shown by the doctor and with the availability of his services when requested. Much more rarely is there criticism of the quality or the economics of group health care.

The dynamics of a sort of psychological trade-off—that is, tolerance of unsatisfactory doctor-patient relationships in return for judgment of good technical service and a "good buy" financially—in patient acceptance of the PGP pattern are reflected in the findings of Roemer et al. (reported in 1973, although based on a 1968 investigation). This study solicited the attitudes of health plan members along two dimensions: satisfaction with financial protection and with medical care received. Regarding financial protection, the preference for the PGP pattern, compared with open market plans, was overwhelming, prevailing in all types of family (large and small), in all religious categories, in all social classes, in families of either high or low geographic mobility, and whether or not the family had a history of chronic illness.

With respect to satisfaction of plan members with "the medical care received," the positive attributes of the PGP plans were not so impressive, although the occurrence of frank dissatisfaction was substantially *lower* in those plans, compared with private medical practice patterns. Definite dissatisfaction was reported by 8.6 percent of PGP plan families, compared to 17.4 and 20.3 percent in the commercial and "Blue" plan-types.

When these responses are analyzed by social groupings, some interesting differentials become evident. The low level of frank dissatisfaction with the PGP-type patterns, compared with the others, prevails in all social subgroups. For certain subgroups, however, the HMO-type plans also show the highest level of "very satisfied" members: these include (a) single-person family units (compared with larger units), (b) Protestants (compared with other faiths), (c) families with no history of chronic illness (compared with sicklier families), (d) adult men alone (compared with adult women), and (e) geographically mobile families (compared with relatively stable ones).

Similar general findings were reported by Greenlick (1972) regarding the Kaiser-Permanente Health Plan in Portland, Oregon. While his respondents indicated substantial general satisfaction with the plan, that satisfaction was most often attributed to the financial advantages ("reasonable premiums" for the benefits offered) and to the actual care received after the doctor was reached, but over 50 percent of the respondents complained about the time it took before they got an appointment—in other words, access to the doctor.

Another study of patient satisfaction (Leyhe and Procter,

1971) was focused on Medicaid recipients enrolled in a PGP plan in California, compared with other such persons getting care through traditional private doctor mechanisms. The investigators in that study concluded (Leyhe and Procter, 1971:II) that:

> No appreciable differences were found between responses of . . . [the PGP] enrollees and of those who used individual practitioners. . . . Medi-Cal enrollees of this private group practice apparently appraised their medical care as equivalent in almost all respects to that received from individual practitioners. This private (prepaid) group practice was not seen by the majority of the enrollees as having the objectionable features often attributed to public clinics.

Of the 51 questions used in this patient attitude survey, only four yielded significant differences between PGP and non-PGP respondents. In three of these questions, OAS (old-age security) Medicaid patients expressed the familiar objection that they had difficulty reaching a physician by telephone, could not see the same physician continuously, and did not get house call service. In the remaining question of these four, the *non-PGP* sample of AFDC (aid to families with dependent children) clients complained that they had difficulty obtaining ambulatory care because of problems with transportation—a service the PGP plan provided for its members.

One other conclusion of this study worth citing is that ". . . it became evident that patient education pertaining to the current source of care is extremely important." Since about 20 percent of the respondents reported that they had had no identifiable source for medical care before being accepted into the Medicaid program, this conclusion seems to suggest that a pattern of delivery with a clearly identified, physically accessible source for primary care is likely to be more successful in reaching previously underserviced populations with medical service.

Meaning of attitudes

Several comments are in order about patient attitudes toward prepaid group practice, typically associated with HMOs, as compared with traditional patterns. First, the policy of "dual" or "multiple choice" among plan types, always followed by the Kaiser-Permanente Plan and increasingly followed by other HMO-type plans, helps to assure that only persons willing to accept the "clinic pattern" of service will join such plans in the first place. Second, on the other hand, the clinic pattern clearly departs from traditional custom and experience among self-supporting families, and it is small wonder if the inevitable impersonalities, especially if the clinic is a large one, cause irritations or, at least, require psychological adjustment. Third, it must be realized that some of the dissatisfactions with PGP patterns are basically a result of the insufficient numbers of doctors in those programs—a situation which, in turn, relates to nationwide shortages; in light of the high incomes attainable in private practice, the PGP plans have understandably had difficulties in recruiting qualified physicians to fill all their posts.

Finally, it must be recognized that managerial problems are far from solved in most large-scale medical care organizations, whether for ambulatory or for impatient service. The hospital litera ture is full of reports about the "insensitivities" of patient care in large hospitals, whether or not prepayment is in the picture. There are obviously improvements needed in the efficiency of managing patient flow in organized medical care systems. In a sense, the most remarkable fact is the increasing degree of satisfaction that seems to be characterizing clinic services in spite of their departure from traditional patterns.

In regard to patient attitudes toward the medical care foundation pattern of HMO, compared with conventional private practice, there is little reason to expect much difference since conventional patterns of medical care are indeed applied by the foundations. The California PERS study (Medical Advisory Council, 1971) did, however, solicit three levels of satisfaction ("satisfied", "not entirely satisfied", or "dissatisfied") toward different aspects of the four plan-types used by these state government employees. The responses showed overwhelmingly high "satisfaction" in all plan-types across the three dimensions: plan administration, doctor's care, and hospitalization.

The differences were all very small, by these measures; but for the foundation plans, compared with the PGP model of HMOs, satisfaction levels appeared to be slightly higher for doctor's and hospital care, and slightly lower for plan administration. It is doubtful if these figures have any statistical significance. More important, they are bound to be strongly influenced by the general social settings, since, in California, the medical foundations operate in the smaller and more rural counties, while the PGP plans are largely concentrated in metropolitan counties.

Out-of-plan use

A reflection of patient attitudes toward the PGP pattern of HMO is bound to be given by the extent of out-of-plan use. Since the Donabedian review, the new data seem to suggest that this use is somewhat lower than reported in the earlier studies. Greenlick's report (1972) on the Portland branch of the Kaiser-Permanente Plan found that about 10 percent of persons had some out-of-plan use during the previous 12 months, but since this might have ranged from little to much service for these persons, he estimates that it would amount to under 10 percent of the total services.

Roemer et al. (1973) analyzed out-of-plan use separately for ambulatory doctor and hospital services. They found, through examination of medical records, that 12 percent of the ambulatory doctor contacts of PGP plan members during one year occurred with private doctors outside the plan; for hospitalizations, the out-of-plan admissions were 7.2 percent of the total. The relative lowness of these figures suggests that, in spite of some dissatisfactions, a decision of PGP plan members to seek care elsewhere (and pay privately—which may not be such a hardship, when premiums have been paid by employers, as is commonly true) is made relatively rarely. Moreover, even these low figures may be an overstatement, since the questionnaire used did not distinguish between outside care sought because of dissatisfaction (impatience for an appointment or the like) and such care sought in an emergency occurring outside the plan's geographic area—a type of care financially covered by "out-of-area" indemnity benefits.

In the previous section, it was noted that out-of-pocket outlays for doctor's and hospital services by PGP plan members were strikingly low, even though these figures included certain small in-plan copayments that are levied on certain membership groups in the HMO-type plans of the RHH study (Roemer et al., 1973). The general extent of out-of-plan use in PGP plans, by various measures of services or expenditures, would seem to be lower than in the earlier studies summarized by Donabedian (1969). It would seem reasonable to conclude that, as people have become more accustomed to the PGP model of medical care, they have been more inclined to stay with it, in spite of some difficulties; perhaps over the years there has also been improved efficiency in PGP operations. There still remain, nevertheless, obvious problems to solve in the sphere of plan-patient relationships within the HMO model.

HMOs and Planning

The whole HMO strategy has important implications for planning. In a sense, it shifts planning responsibilities from central governmental authorities to local voluntary bodies, within certain ground rules. It says that for a fixed monetary sum, the HMO must keep its customers happy, or at least sufficiently satisfied to stay with that HMO and not to leave it for the open market or to join another one. Within the constraints of money and membership expectations, the HMO would have wide leeway to provide health services in a variety of ways. The evidence so far suggests that, given a promotional boost by government "seed" grants, the potentials of HMOs, based on the PGP model, to provide good health service at relatively lower costs than the traditional open-market private medicine model are substantial. Reasonable interpretation, however, of the evaluative data on HMO performance, summarized above, requires certain "caveats."

Nearly all of the studies on effects, whether based on structure, process, or outcome, have been made on relatively large, stable, and well-established HMO models. It is altogether possible— and some of the recent California experience mentioned (Nelson, 1973) underscores the hazards—that some HMOs, especially the newer ones, may yield a very different performance record. As the American Public Health Association (1971) pointed out in an official policy statement, there are two principal hazards in the HMO concept: inequitable "risk" selection among enrollees and poor-quality care through underservicing.

Safeguards against both of these hazards are feasible through a process of public surveillance. Regarding risk selection or, more accurately, membership composition, standards with respect to age, sex, socioeconomic status, and past illness history could be set and applied to the actual enrollees of each HMO. Recurrent "open enrollment periods" are another device to help assure that every HMO is serving its fair share of high- and low-risk persons. Without such procedures, one or another HMO could offer competitively wider benefits or particularly low premiums simply by excluding or reducing its load of high-risk members.

Regarding the hazard of underservicing or other strategies for cutting HMO costs at the expense of quality, the surveillance procedures are more difficult and complex. There seems to be an increasing consensus that monitoring would be required along all principal channels of evaluation: input, process, and health outcomes. In January, 1972, a conference was sponsored by InterStudy and headed by Paul M. Ellwood (1973), who has done so much to promote the HMO concept, in order to grapple specifically with the problems of quality assurance under HMOs. The report of this conference suggests that the main emphasis was on the importance of developing sharpened measures of "clinical outcomes," as essential tools of a "Health Outcomes Commission" (in government) to promote quality assurance.

The general question of quality assurance has, of course, acquired greater national importance as collective financing of medical care (both through government and voluntary insurance) has increased—quite aside from the issue of HMOs. In January of 1973, still another major national conference was held on this question (U.S. Department of Health, Education, and Welfare, 1973), again stressing the importance of developing reliable measurements of both medical care process and outcome. The enactment of P.L. 92–603, the 1972 amendments to Medicare and Medicaid, adds further impetus to the need for quality criteria, with the new legal requirement of "professional standard review organizations" (PSROs) to blanket the nation. More research on formulating readily applicable measurements of both medical care process and outcome is obviously needed.

With several bills pending in the U.S. Congress for promotion of HMOs, including versions backed by both major political parties, it is a fair guess that the future holds expansion of HMO patterns of both major types—the PGP and the medical care foundation models. In the light of both continuously rising health care costs and the agreed-upon persistent need for comprehensive health planning (one item in the 1973–1974 Presidential budget contemplated for expansion, in contrast to the cutbacks in so many other sectors of the health field), one may reasonably look upon the HMO strategy as a peculiarly American approach to planning, in which responsibilities are delegated to numerous local mini-systems, in contrast to the usual European strategy of centralized controls. The private sector, through HMO development, would be vested with responsibilities and incentives to regulate itself and to meet the health needs of the population. As we have seen from the accumulated evidence, there is much reason to have confidence in the soundness of this strategy. Yet, as we have also seen, when and if HMOs become more a "mainstream" than a "vanguard" phenomenon, there will be enormous needs for continuing vigilance to protect the interests of consumers both inside and outside of health maintenance organizations.

Milton I. Roemer, M.D.
University of California
School of Public Health
405 Hilgard Ave.
Los Angeles, California 90024

William Shonick, PH.D.
University of California
School of Public Health
405 Hilgard Ave.
Los Angeles, California 90024

Prepared at the invitation of the National Academy of Sciences, Institute of Medicine (Washington, D.C.).

References

American Hospital Association
  1972 Review of 1971 Certificate-of-Need Legislation. Survey report. Chicago: American Hospital Association.

American Public Health Association
  1971 "Health maintenance organizations: a policy paper." American Journal of Public Health 61 (December): 2528–2536.

Avnet, Helen H.
  1967 Physician Service Patterns and Illness Rates. New York: Group Health Insurance.

Bailey, Richard M.
1968 "A comparison of internists in solo and fee-for-service group practice in the San Francisco Bay area." Bulletin of the New York Academy of Medicine 44 (November): 1293–1303.

Barton, William I.
1972 "Infant mortality and health insurance coverage for maternity care." Inquiry 9 (September): 16–29.

Bechtol, Thomas A.
1972 (General manager of the Physicians' Association of Clackamas County, Oregon) Personal communication, July 10.

Berkanovic, Emil
1973 Prepayment vs. Fee-for-Service for Medicaid Recipients. Unpublished data, University of California Survey Research Center.

Boan, J. A.
1966 Group Practice. Ottawa: Royal Commission on Health Services, Queen's Printer.

Breslow, Lester
1972 "Health maintenance services in health maintenance organizations." Association of Teachers of Preventive Medicine Newsletter 19 (Winter): 2.

Brook, Robert H.
1972 A Study of Methodologic Problems Associated with Assessment of Quality of Care. Doctoral dissertation, Johns Hopkins School of Hygiene (May, processed).

Bunker, John P.
1970 "Surgical manpower: a comparison of operations and surgeons in the United States and in England and Wales." New England Journal of Medicine 282 (January 15): 135–144.

Cauffman, Joy G., and Milton I. Roemer
1967 "The impact of health insurance coverage on health care of school children." Public Health Reports 82 (April): 323–328.

Committee on the Costs of Medical Care
1932 Medical Care for the American People. Chicago: University of Chicago Press.

Cook, Wallace H.
1971   "Profile of the Permanente physician." P. 104 in Somers, Anne R. (ed.), The Kaiser-Permanente Medical Care Program. New York: Commonwealth Fund.

Dickinson, Frank G., and C. E. Bradley
1952   Discontinuance of Medical Groups 1940–49, Bulletin No. 90. Chicago: American Medical Association, Bureau of Economic Research.

Donabedian, Avedis
1969   "An evaluation of prepaid group practice." Inquiry 6 (September): 3–27.

Du Bois, Donald M.
1970   "Organizational viability of group practice." Pp. 378 414 in Roemer, Milton I., Donald M. Du Bois, and Shirley W. Rich (eds.), Health Insurance Plans: Studies in Organizational Diversity. Los Angeles: University of California School of Public Health.

Egdahl, Richard E.
1973   "Foundations for medical care." New England Journal of Medicine 288 (March 8): 491–498.

Ellwood, Paul M., et al.
1973   Assuring the Quality of Health Care. Minneapolis: InterStudy.

Gartside, Foline E.
1971   The Utilization and Costs of Services in the San Joaquin Prepayment Project. Los Angeles: University of California School of Public Health (January, processed).

Gartside, Foline E., and Donald M. Procter
1970   Medicaid Services in California under Different Organizational Modes: Physician Participation in the San Joaquin Prepayment Project. Los Angeles: University of California School of Public Health (January, processed).

Glasgow, John M.
1972   "Prepaid group practice as a national health policy: problems and perspectives." Inquiry 9 (March): 3–15.

Greenberg, Ira G., and Michael L. Rodburg
1971   "The role of prepaid group practice in relieving the medical care crisis." Harvard Law Review 84 (February): 887–1001.

Greenlick, Merwyn
  1972 "The impact of prepaid group practice on American medical care: a critical evaluation." The Annals of the American Academy of Political and Social Science 399 (January): 100–113.

Haley, Thomas W.
  1971 "Physicians' Association of Clackamas County." Hospitals 45 (March): 8.

Hill, Daniel B., and James E. Veney
  1970 "Kansas Blue Cross–Blue Shield out-patient benefits experiment." Medical Care 8 (March–April): 143–158.

Kelly, Denwood N.
  1965 "Experience with a program of coverage for diagnostic procedures provided in physicians' offices and hospital out-patient departments—Maryland Blue Cross and Blue Shield plans (1957–1964)." Inquiry 2 (November): 28–44.

Kimbell, Larry J., and John H. Lorant
  c.1970 Production Functions for Physician Services. Los Angeles: University of Southern California, Human Resources Research Center (undated, processed).

Klarman, Herbert E.
  1963 "The effect of prepaid group practice on hospital use." Public Health Reports 78 (November): 955–965.

  1970 "Economic research in group medicine." Pp. 178–193 in Beamish, R. E. (ed.), New Horizons in Health Care. Winnipeg, Canada: First International Congress on Group Medicine.

  1971 "Analysis of the HMO proposal—its assumptions, implications, and prospects." Pp. 24–38 in Health Maintenance Organizations: A Reconfiguration of the Health Services System. Chicago: University of Chicago Center for Health Administration Studies.

Kovner, Joel W., L. Brian Browne, and Arnold I. Kisch
  1969 "Income and use of outpatient medical care by the insured." Inquiry 6 (June): 27–34.

Leyhe, Dixie L., and D. M. Procter
  1971 Medi-Cal Patient Satisfaction under a Prepaid Group Practice and Individual Fee-for-Service Practice. Los Angeles: University of California School of Public Health (June, processed).

Mechanic, David
c.1972   Physician Satisfaction in Varying Settings. University of Wisconsin (mimeographed, undated).

Medical Advisory Council to the California Public Employees Retirement System
1971   Final Report on the Survey of Consumer Experience under the State of California Employees Hospital and Medical Care Act. Sacramento: Medical Advisory Council, California Public Employees Retirement System.

Metzner, Charles A., Rashid L. Bashshur, and Gary W. Shannon
1972   "Differential public acceptance of group medical practice." Medical Care 10 (July–August): 279–287.

Monsma, George N.
1970   "Marginal revenue and demand for physicians' services." Pp. 145–160 in Klarman, Herbert E. (ed.), Empirical Studies in Health Economics. Baltimore: Johns Hopkins Press.

Moses, Lincoln E., and Frederick Mosteller
1968   "Institutional differences in post-operative death rates: commentary on some findings of the National Halothane Study." Journal of the American Medical Association 203 (February 12): 7.

Moustafa, A. Taher, Carl E. Hopkins, and Bonnie Klein
1971   "Determinants of choice and change of health insurance plan." Medical Care 9 (January–February): 32–41.

National Advisory Commission on Health Manpower
1967   Report. Vol. 11:197–228. Washington: Government Printing Office.

Nelson, Harry
1973   "Investigation of prepaid health programs asked: possible fraud in some cases hinted by L.A. County unit." Los Angeles Times, February 24:1.

Newhouse, Joseph P.
1973   "The economics of group practice." The Journal of Human Resources 8 (Winter): 37–56.

Newport, John, and Milton I. Roemer
1973   "Health service outcome under medical care foundations: perinatal mortality in Medicaid childbirths covered by a county medical foundation compared to other delivery models." Publication pending.

Perrott, George St. J.
  1971   Federal Employees Health Benefit Program: Enrollment and Uti-
         lization of Health Services 1961–1968. Washington: Department
         of Health, Education, and Welfare, Public Health Service.

Peterson, Malcolm L.
  1971   "The first year in Columbia: assessments of low hospitalization
         and high office use." Johns Hopkins Medical Journal 128 (Janu-
         ary): 15–23.

Prybil, Lawrence D.
  1971   "Physician terminations in large multi-specialty groups." Medical
         Group Management 18 (September): 4–6, 23–25.

Reinhardt, Uwe E., and Donald E. Yett
  1972   Physician Production Functions under Varying Practice Ar-
         rangements. Technical Paper Series No. 1. Washington: U. S. De-
         partment of Health, Education, and Welfare, Community Health
         Service.

Robertson, Robert L.
  1971   "Economic effects of personal health services: work loss in a
         public school teacher population." American Journal of Public
         Health 61 (January): 30–45.

Roemer, Milton I.
  1958   "The influence of prepaid physician's service on hospital utiliza-
         tion." Hospitals 16 (October): 48–52.

Roemer, Milton I., and Donald M. Du Bois
  1969   "Medical costs in relation to the organization of ambulatory
         care." New England Journal of Medicine 280 (May): 988–993.

Roemer, Milton I., and Foline E. Gartside
  1973   "Peer review in medical foundations: its effect on qualifications
         of surgeons." Health Services Reports. University of California
         School of Public Health (December).

Roemer, Milton I., Robert W. Hetherington, Carl E. Hopkins, Arthur
E. Gerst, Eleanor Parsons, and Donald M. Long
  1973   Health Insurance Effects: Services, Expenditures, and Attitudes
         under Three Types of Plan. Ann Arbor: University of Michigan
         School of Public Health.

Roemer, Milton I., A. Taher Moustafa, and Carl E. Hopkins
1968   "A proposed hospital quality index: hospital death rates adjusted for case severity." Health Services Research 3 (Summer): 96–118.

Roemer, Milton I., and Max Shain
1959   Hospital Utilization under Insurance, Monograph Series No. 6. Chicago: American Hospital Association.

Ross, Austin, Jr.
1969   "A report on physician terminations in group practice." Medical Group Management 16: 15–21.

Shapiro, Sam
1971   "Role of hospitals in the changing health insurance plan of Greater New York." Bulletin of the New York Academy of Medicine 74 (April). 374–381.

Social Security Administration
1971   Medicare Experience with Prepaid Group Practice Enrollees. Washington: Social Security Administration Office of Research and Statistics (March, processed).

U. S. Department of Health, Education, and Welfare
1973   Quality Assurance of Medical Care. Monograph. Washington: Regional Medical Programs Service (February, processed).

Weinerman, E. Richard
1964   "Patients' perceptions of group medical care." American Journal of Public Health 54 (June): 880–889.

1969   "Problems and perspectives in group practice." Group Practice 18 (April): 30.

Williamson, John W.
1971   "Evaluating quality of patient care." Journal of the American Medical Association 218 (October 25): 4.

Yankauer, Alfred, John P. Connelly, and Jacob J. Feldman
1970   "Physician productivity and delivery of ambulatory care: some findings from a survey of pediatricians." Medical Care 8 (January–February): 35–46.

Yett, Donald E.
1967   "An evaluation of alternative methods of estimating physicians' expenses relative to output." Inquiry 4 (March): 3–27.

Assessing the Evidence
on HMO Performance

HAROLD S. LUFT

Health Policy Program,
University of California,
San Francisco

P REPAID MEDICAL SERVICE PLANS HAVE EXISTED ON
the American scene for over a century. Because most of these
early plans catered to defined populations—usually on a religious, ethnic, or employment basis—they operated in relative obscur-
ity until the Depression. Then, in 1932, the Committee on the Costs
of Medical Care recommended that health care be furnished by organized groups of health professionals, preferably in a hospital setting,
on a group payment basis. Prepaid health delivery plans came into
public view, with special prominence given to such innovative programs as those established by the Ross-Loos Medical Group in Los
Angeles, the Farmer's Union Co-operative Hospital of Elk City, Ok-
lahoma, and the Trinity Hospital and Clinic in Little Rock, Arkansas.
In an era when most Americans were without any form of health
insurance coverage and when private health care was too costly for a
large segment of the population, prepaid health services were touted
as a means of enabling families of average income to afford preventive,
diagnostic, and therapeutic care at a predetermined cost. Prepayment
applied insurance principles of spreading risks, and financing by
budgeted premiums payable over time (of wellness, and not only at
time of illness).

Milbank Memorial Fund Quarterly/*Health and Society,* Vol. 58, No. 4, 1980
© 1980 Milbank Memorial Fund and Massachusetts Institute of Technology
0160/1997/5804/0501-37 $01.00/0

In the fifty years that have ensued since the study by the Committee on the Costs of Medical Care, health insurance has become widely available to most Americans and third-party payers have assumed responsibility for a major portion of most health bills. The growth of the health sector has been spurred by federal programs that have funded hospital construction, expanded the number and size of professional schools, fostered the development of new technologies, and encouraged the spread of health insurance. During the same period, national health expenditures have risen precipitously, from 4.1 percent of the gross national product in 1935 to 9.0 percent in 1979 (Gibson, 1979; Health Care Financing Administration, 1980). In response to an ever-increasing health budget, the focus of national health policy began to shift in the 1970s from guaranteeing accessibility of health services to cost containment. Once again, prepaid health services became the focus of national attention.

Revived federal interest in prepaid health plans dates back to 1970 when the term "health maintenance organization" (HMO) was coined by Paul Elwood, Jr., in an attempt to encourage the Nixon administration to accept the principle of prepayment in combination with coordinated organization of services. Since that time, the HMO concept has been espoused by a variety of political activists concerned with such divergent goals as cost containment, consumerism, and limits on government involvement in the health care system. HMOs have been viewed as more cost efficient than traditional fee-for-service forms of coverage, while providing medical care of comparable or better quality; HMOs have also been seen as stimulating competition within the health industry by encouraging traditional providers to adopt cost-containment programs and to develop new premium and benefit structures. Since 1973, federal policy has encouraged the development and growth of HMOs through a program of grants and loan guarantees; the HMO Act of 1973, P.L. 93-222 (Section 1310), has also sought to improve the marketability of HMO plans by requiring certain categories of employers to expand their health benefit programs to include HMO options. Whether and how public policy should continue to encourage the growth of health maintenance organizations depends upon the extent to which the experience with HMOs confirms widespread expectations as to their performance.

This paper will report on the available evidence concerning HMO performance. To lay a foundation for the discussion, the first section will begin with a generic definition of HMOs, followed by a discussion of the diversity of HMOs; the next section will summarize major findings concerning HMO performance vis-a-vis their own enrollees; and the third section will explore possible implications of competition in the health industry, particularly in terms of the influence of HMO activity upon fee-for-service providers. A final section will discuss unanswered policy questions.

Definition and Scope of the HMO Concept

Reflecting its political origins, the term health maintenance organization has been used to refer to a variety of plans. Some people use the term to mean the prepaid group practices that have existed for decades, such as the Kaiser-Permanente plan. In contrast, the federal HMO Act of 1973 restricts application of the term to organizations that comply with an extensive array of requirements. Individual as well as group practices can qualify as HMOs under the act, but some HMO-type organizations have chosen not to seek federal qualification.

Each of these definitions is too narrow to permit comprehensive analysis of HMO performance. For purposes of analysis, we define HMOs in terms of a set of essential behavioral characteristics:

1. The HMO assumes a *contractual responsibility* to provide or ensure the delivery of a stated range of health services, including at least physician and hospital services.

2. The HMO services an *enrolled, defined* population.

3. The HMO has *voluntary enrollment* of subscribers.

4. The HMO requires a *fixed periodic payment* to the organization that is independent of use of services. (There may be small charges related to utilization, but these are relatively insignificant.)

5. The HMO assumes at least part of the *financial risk* and/or *gain* in the provision of services.

Contractual responsibility implies that the HMO member has the legal right to medical care provided by the HMO. This situation is in contrast with the conventional one in which the medical care provider has the right to decide whether to accept the patient and is under no obligation, other than an ethical one, to provide treatment. The existence of an *enrolled, defined population* means that the HMO knows its obligations and can estimate the probable demand for its services. *Voluntary enrollment* implies that consumers can choose either the HMO or a conventional insurer; mandatory enrollment could include within the definition settings such as military and student health clinics. The *fixed periodic payment,* independent of the quantity of services provided, implies that, for a given enrollee, the HMO does not gain any substantial revenue by providing more services. In fact, the fewer services the HMO provides, the more the HMO will increase its net revenue after expenses. (In the long run, of course, the HMO may gain more enrollees by offering more services, and it will lose members if it noticeably underserves them.) Finally, *financial risk* implies that the HMO will suffer or benefit financially from its decisions to provide services. The presence of risk creates the incentives for cost containment that have made HMOs so attractive to policy makers.

This definition purposely allows considerable latitude for the organizational characteristics of HMOs. Note that the definition did not specify any restrictions on the method by which individual physicians are paid or on whether services are offered in a single group setting or dispersed over a large number of practitioners' offices.

There are basically two types of HMOs: the group/staff model, sometimes referred to as prepaid group practices (PGPs), and individual practice associations (IPAs).[1] Although there are many important exceptions, most group or staff model plans pay their physicians on a salary or capitation basis, and most individual practice associations are composed of physicians in private offices who bill the HMO on a fee-for-service basis. (The group model HMO involves an independent medical group that contracts with the HMO; in the staff model the physicians are hired directly by the HMO.)

Health maintenance organizations also vary in the extent to which they meet the five criteria of the overall HMO definition. The comprehensiveness of guaranteed services varies widely among plans and beneficiaries. The Kaiser Foundation Health Plan of Southern

---

[1] Foundations for medical care are sometimes considered synonymous with IPAs, although not all IPAs are foundations, nor all foundations IPAs. See Egdahl (1973) and Edgahl et al. (1977).

California, for example, reported at least five different basic benefit packages in 1971, with monthly premiums ranging from $7.82 to $16.00 per subscriber (Somers, 1971). Groups also may purchase special coverages for eyeglasses, drugs, mental health care, and other benefits. Federally qualified HMOs must offer a basic benefit package but additional services may be tailored to the enrollee group.

The defined populations served by HMOs also vary widely. For instance, HMOs vary in size from 3,000 to more than 1 million enrollees. In some cases, enrollees are a homogeneous population, such as a university faculty. In other cases, the population is heterogeneous. The geographic base of enrollment may be concentrated in a single town (such as Columbia, Maryland, or Marshfield, Wisconsin), or widely dispersed through several metropolitan areas (such as the Kaiser plans in California), or a large rural region (such as the San Joaquin Foundation in California). Furthermore, although the enrolled population at any time is known, because of the capitation method of payment, enrollee turnover may vary from under 5 to over 75 percent per year (Cutler et al., 1973; Breslow, 1975). Finally, the population enrolled on a prepaid basis may represent a wide range (2 to 90+ percent) of the patients seen by a group of physicians.

The degree of freedom of choice in enrollment also varies, not because of requirements for membership, but because of limited access to other providers or modes of insurance. An effective HMO monopoly can occur in underserved areas, such as inner cities and rural communities, particularly when public financing programs, notably Medicaid, set reimbursement levels so low that private practitioners refuse to participate in them.

The structure of HMO coverage also shows great variation. Health maintenance organizations may use cost-sharing to varying degrees, and several types of cost-sharing may be involved. In the early 1970s, California state employees were enrolled in HMOs that had coinsurance rates of zero, 20 percent, and 25 percent, and deductibles of zero and $2 per visit, or $25 per illness (Dozier et al., 1973). Some plans currently include copayments and maximum out-of-pocket provisions (Miller, 1980).

The exposure to risk also varies among HMOs. The Health Insurance Plan of Greater New York (HIP) and other plans that use conventional insurance for hospital care are not at risk for hospital expenses. Even when an HMO is at risk for all services, risk can be allocated in a variety of ways among three functional (and sometimes legally distinct) parts of an HMO: 1) the "plan," which contracts with enrollees; 2) the physicians, who provide medical services; and 3) the hospital, which provides inpatient services. Zelten (1979) has described eight models of HMO organization that, in turn, can be aggregated into two groups: those that own their own hospitals and those that contract with community hospitals for inpatient services. Zelten's classification of HMOs ranges from the most highly integrated HMO form, where the HMO owns or controls its hospital facilities and hires physicians on a salaried basis, to the most loosely structured form in which the HMO contracts with community hospitals and with a physician-sponsored entity, the individual practice association (IPA). In addition to the models described by Zelten, two other models are noteworthy: the "Safeco" (United Healthcare) model, in which the HMO establishes a primary care network with each primary care physician responsible for specialty referral, emergency room use, and hospital admissions (Moore, 1979); and proposed hospital capitation experiments, in which an insurance entity or Medicaid agency contracts directly with hospitals to provide care to a defined population on a capitation basis.

HMOs differ not only in terms of organizational structure, but also in terms of their sponsorship. HMOs have been sponsored by universities, large commercial insurers, unions, employers, multispecialty groups, hospitals, consumer groups, municipal agencies, and for-profit management firms. In turn, sponsorship influences the selection of the professional staff and, ultimately, plan performance. For instance, a consumer-run HMO is unlikely to attract or hire physicians whose primary motivation is income maximization. A multispecialty medical group with a tradition of emphasizing high-quality secondary and tertiary care may be ill prepared to provide primary care to HMO subscribers. A university-sponsored plan may attract physicians who give precedence to the educational aspects of diagnosing and treating patients rather than to potential cost implications.

Because of the diversity of plans classified under the label "HMO," an evaluation of HMO performance must identify major variations in plan structure and sponsorship whenever possible. It must be remembered that because every HMO has some unique features, no evaluation can fully identify to what extent the performance of a specific

HMO relates to its general characteristics and to what extent to its special features.

Claims and Evidence on HMO Performance

In evaluating the evidence on HMO experience, four important caveats must be kept in mind. The first stems from the diversity of HMOs. To understand the published findings, one must take each HMO as a unique case. Yet, to be useful for policy makers, results must be generalizable; thus the findings of many studies may have to be lumped together, all but the most obvious differences being ignored.

The second caveat relates to the availability of data. A recently completed comprehensive review of the published evidence on HMO performance indicates that available data vary in depth, breadth, and quality (Luft, 1980c). For example, more than fifty comparisons of hospitalization are available, but for some dimensions of performance only a single study has been published.

The third caveat relates to the source of published findings on HMO performance. By far the bulk of the studies relate to a handful of large, well-established plans. Most of these are hospital-based prepaid group practices and almost all relate to plans developed before the "new wave" of HMOs in the mid to late 1970s.

Finally, there have been no randomized, controlled experiments that involve the assignment of a representative group of people to a wide range of health insurance plans and health maintenance organizations. Therefore, while we can say that costs (or utilization, or satisfaction) are lower in one situation than in another, we cannot really determine whether the differences are attributable to general characteristics of the plans, to unique features of the providers and administrators, or to subtle differences among the people selecting each plan.

HMO Costs

Health maintenance organizations are intuitively attractive as a means for cost control because they alter the usual economic incentives in medical care and give providers a stake in holding down costs. The evidence supports this theory, particularly when the response to HMO incentives is compared with the prevailing system of extensive third-party reimbursement for providers. In all instances, the total cost of medical care (premium plus out-of-pocket costs) for HMO enrollees is lower than for comparable people with conventional insurance coverage (Luft, 1978a; Wersinger and Sorensen, 1980). The lower costs are clearest for enrollees in prepaid group practices, where total costs range from 10 to 40 percent below costs for conventional insurance enrollees. Although the evidence is scanty, costs for enrollees in individual practice associations appear no lower than for enrollees in conventional plans.

Although there is substantial evidence of lower costs for HMO enrollees, there is little evidence that costs in HMOs are growing less rapidly than in the overall medical care sector (Luft, 1980a). This is not to belittle the importance of a 10–40 percent cost difference, but it suggests that HMOs may not have the solution to the dynamic of escalating medical costs within a predominantly third-party, cost reimbursement medical system.

Knowing that costs are lower for HMO enrollees is only the first step. Total costs can be divided into the cost per unit of service and the number of services of each type provided by the system. Differences in total costs, then, theoretically could reflect differences in each of these elements. If lower HMO costs did reflect lower costs per unit, HMO input prices would have to be lower, or HMO production more efficient. Because HMOs generally pay the going rate for the people they hire, and their physicians have earnings comparable to those in fee-for-service practice, attention must be focused on the issue of HMO efficiency, as related to physician productivity, use of auxiliary personnel, administrative services, and duplication of facilities.

The question of whether group practice leads to economies of scale has long been a subject of debate. It is important to recognize that this debate has little to do with the performance of HMOs as a unique organizational form; whatever economies of scale exist should be equally obtainable by both fee-for-service and prepaid medical groups. Unfortunately, measurement of returns to scale is confounded by disagreement on measures of outputs or inputs and the paucity of data available for analysis.

Studies of economies of scale have reflected these analytical problems and produced mixed results. Most agree that economies of scale may occur as practice size increases, but that these economies peak at a relatively low scale, between two and five practitioners. Whether productivity per physician remains constant or even declines beyond that point is hard to evaluate. Thus there is no real support for the claim that large prepaid group practices realize substantial economies of scale in ambulatory care (Held and Reinhardt, 1979).

Size has an effect on physician productivity as well as on organizational output. There is a substantial body of theoretical literature that argues that the rewards for efficient practice are inversely related to the size of the group, thereby encouraging reduction in physicians' work effort as the size of their practices rises (Newhouse, 1973; Sloan, 1974). Data problems exist here as well, but the empirical evidence suggests that physician productivity in ambulatory care is higher in small groups than in large groups, whether the financing for the large groups is prepaid or fee-for-service. Thus group size, not the unique financial characteristics of the HMO, appears to be the critical factor in physician productivity. The relation between size and productivity may reflect the attraction of different types of physicians to solo, small group, and large group practices. For instance, physicians in relatively large groups have been found to desire such benefits as longer vacations, more time for educational leave, and reduced patient loads. In one study that did compare fee-for-service groups with prepaid groups, the prepaid physicians were found to spend approximately 11 percent less time seeing patients than their fee-for-service counterparts (Held and Reinhardt, 1979).

Another potential source of increased efficiency is the use of allied health professionals (AHPs) in large group practices. It has been argued that people with special skills (e.g., physicians' assistants, nurse practitioners, orthopedic technicians, and nurse midwives) can provide care at lower costs than physicians. To the extent that there are indivisibilities associated with task delegation, large group practices will be better able to employ AHPs. On the other hand, if the teamwork and role definition implied in the use of AHPs is threatening to the physician staff, efficient use of AHPs cannot be achieved. As pointed out in a Mathematica Policy Research Study (Held and Reinhardt, 1979) the actual delegation of tasks in the prepaid and in fee-for-service groups was quite similar. Effective integration of AHPs into the practice setting may be more directly related to the age of the group than to size or financial structure, with newly developed groups being able to design the work flow from the ground up, rather than having to contend with a modification of existing practice patterns.

Another possible economy relates to enrollment size. For a long time, one of the widely accepted generalizations about HMOs was that 30,000 members were necessary before a plan could break even financially (that is, arrive at a point where revenues equaled expenditures on a current, rather than a cumulative basis). As noted by Zelten (1979), the 30,000 figure was not the result of careful research into HMO operations, but rather the casual acceptance of a frequently quoted figure as to the optimal size for planning group facilities.

Theoretically, an HMO that grows large enough to be able to control or own hospital facilities should be able to achieve greater efficiency, since the most expensive part of medical care occurs in the hospital. On this point data are available only for the largest of plans because, until recently, only the Kaiser plans and Group Health Cooperative of Puget Sound controlled their own hospitals. Data for Kaiser hospitals in California and Oregon, as well as for the Group Health Cooperative of Puget Sound hospital, can be compared with data from a matched sample of hospitals of similar size in the same regions. The data show no consistent differences in cost per patient day, although lengths of stay are shorter, and thus costs per case are lower in the HMO-controlled hospitals (Luft, 1980c). A detailed examination of hospital costs for people in Group Health Cooperative of Puget Sound and those in a comprehensive Blue Cross-Blue Shield plan in Seattle indicates that the hospital costs for the HMO members were about 25 percent lower. Almost all this difference, however, was attributable to lower utilization rates; the unit costs for drugs, X-rays, laboratory and other services were comparable (McCaffree et al., 1976).

Health maintenance organizations also may increase their relative efficiency by avoiding duplication of facilities. It has often been pointed out that community hospitals compete for physicians by purchasing special equipment that may subsequently be underutilized (Lee, 1971; Cohen, 1978; Holoweiko, 1980). HMO-controlled hospitals should not face this problem; Kaiser, for example, appears to centralize its services and to have less duplication of facilities than do conventional hospitals (Luft and Crane, 1980).

To summarize the evidence on costs, existing prepaid group practices clearly have been able to provide medical care for their enrollees at costs 10 to 40 percent lower than those in conventional plans. The lower costs do not appear to stem from substantially lower costs per unit of service. Although large systems such as Kaiser do appear to reduce duplication of facilities, there are few real economies of scale. Instead, we must look to differences in the utilization of services to explain observed cost differences.

Utilization of Services

In contrast to the relative paucity of data on costs, there is ample evidence on both inpatient and ambulatory care utilization by enrollees in HMOs and in conventional plans. Differences are likely to be concentrated in hospital rather than in ambulatory care. Hospital use is easier to control. The consumer can directly initiate an ambulatory visit, but only a physician can authorize a patient's admission to a hospital. Furthermore, HMOs typically lower financial barriers to ambulatory usage and may attempt to substitute ambulatory for inpatient care.

A review of more than two dozen studies indicates somewhat more ambulatory visits for HMO enrollees, particularly those in individual practice associations, than for patients in the fee-for-service system. Differences are greater for hospitalization. Based on more than fifty observations over a twenty-five-year period, those studies with good data almost unanimously support the claim that enrollees in prepaid group practices have lower hospitalization rates than do people with conventional insurance. The results for individual practice association enrollees are more mixed. Average differences in utilization by enrollees in HMOs and by people who rely on fee-for-service medical care are substantial, with about 30 percent fewer hospital days for enrollees in prepaid group practices, and 20 percent fewer days for enrollees in individual practice associations. HMO enrollees have a somewhat shorter stay than do people in conventional plans, but most of the overall utilization difference stems from lower admission rates.

If we ignore the impact of specific organizational features, there are two primary explanations for these lower admission rates: 1) that HMOs identify and screen out cases that really do not require hospitalization—the discretionary or "unnecessary" cases; and 2) that

HMOs achieve a lower hospitalization rate without any apparent discrimination among cases according to obvious "necessity."

The best available data from a broad range of HMOs tend to support the second explanation rather than the first. HMOs do not achieve a disproportionate share of their lower admission rates by "reducing" surgical as opposed to medical cases; instead, admissions seem to be lower across the board. Similarly, although admissions for certain "discretionary procedures," such as hernia repair and hysterectomy, are lower in HMOs than in comparison plans, the figures for discretionary procedures do not appear disproportionately lower than the figures for all surgery. One must immediately point out, however, that the measures of "discretionary" care are very rough approximations that mask the fine distinctions in patient care. It is highly likely that many so-called discretionary admissions are actually essential, and that many "nondiscretionary" admissions are actually optional.

Recognizing the complexities of evaluating admissions, and assuming a scattering of discretionary cases in all patient categories, we find four possible, but not mutually exclusive, interpretations of the reasons for lower hospital admissions in HMOs: 1) Rather than reducing admissions for broad categories of patients identified as "discretionary," an effective HMO reduces admissions that case management reveals as "discretionary." In other words, a good physician can, if pressed, triage patients on a one-by-one basis and decide who really needs admission and who can be treated on an ambulatory basis. 2) Self-selection among HMO enrollees may result in lower admission rates; that is, better health or greater aversion to hospital admissions among HMO enrollees may contribute to the differential between HMO and fee-for-service (FFS) admission rates. 3) HMOs may provide preventive care that reduces the occurrence of health problems that require hospital admissions. 4) HMOs may undertreat, or traditional providers overtreat, nondiscretionary cases. To test this hypothesis, we must examine quality of care in HMOs.

As pointed out by Blumberg (1980), the preceding discussion tacitly assumes that the fee-for-service sector is the norm against which HMO hospitalization should be compared; if the perspective is reversed, and the higher hospitalization rate by FFS providers is examined, the following explanations appear: 1) Because physicians' fees and other components of hospital care are more completely covered by conventional third parties than are ambulatory services,

FFS patients are less sensitive to hospital costs than to prices for office care. 2) Physician services in the hospital result in little practice expense to physicians and hence yield greater net revenue and greater incentive to hospitalize. 3) PGP physicians have little or no personal economic incentive to hospitalize since individual incomes do not depend on the location where care is provided. 4) Since HMO patients have negligible out-of-pocket costs, regardless of where care is provided, their concern may be more in terms of indirect costs (e.g., family convenience).

Returning to our focus on HMOs, however, we can examine in the following sections the available evidence with respect to consumer selection, preventive services, and quality of care.

Factors Affecting Consumer Selection of an HMO

People are not randomly assigned to health maintenance organizations or to conventional medical care plans. HMO enrollees generally choose HMO membership over other delivery options. The HMO literature about self-selection has been somewhat ambivalent. The theory of consumer preference (often identified in this instance as the "risk-vulnerability hypothesis") argues that people most concerned about the expected costs of medical care will choose the HMO option. In fact, HMOs have been concerned that self-selection on this basis through open enrollment periods will leave them with those people who are sickest. Conversely, it has been argued that low HMO utilization rates prove that HMO members were healthier at the time they chose to enroll. Sociological factors (e.g., attitudes toward illness and medical care) and demographic factors (e.g., age, sex, and marital status) also influence the HMO choice. Some studies have concluded that people who join health maintenance organizations are likely to be older than people with conventional coverage, to be married, and to have young children. But other studies do not indicate any statistically significant differences between HMO members and people with conventional third-party coverage (Berki and Ashcraft, 1980). A second level of analysis compares perceived measures of health status for HMO members and nonmembers. Some studies have indicated no differences in perceptions of health status. Others that have focused on chronic and acute conditions indicate either no differences or mixed results, with HMO members reporting more of certain types of illnesses and no differences in other measures (Berki and Ashcraft, 1980).

Roghmann and associates (1975) provide data relating more explicitly to the risk-vulnerability hypothesis by examining out-of-pocket medical expenses of people who later chose to stay with conventional coverage or to join various prepaid plans. Although differences in total expenditures were not statistically significant, families who stayed with Blue Cross-Blue Shield (BC-BS) averaged lower total expenditures ($281) than did those who joined prepaid plans ($332). Moreover, families who stayed with BC-BS had statistically significant lower expenses for physician, laboratory, and X-ray services. Another study (Roghmann, Sorensen, and Wells, 1980) shows that in the year before the enrollment the hospitalization rate for people who left BC-BS to join the prepaid group practices was only half the rate for people who stayed with BC-BS.

Studies of enrollment choices between HMOs and conventional insurance (dual or multiple choice) indicate that people who have good relationships with their physicians are unlikely to give them up to join a prepaid group practice (Berki et al., 1977). Patients currently under treatment also would not be expected to switch physicians. (This is not an issue if the choice lies between a conventional insurer and an individual practice association that includes those physicians.) People who have no close relationship with a physician, or who perceive substantial financial benefits from the prepaid group practice, are thus the most likely enrollees in HMOs.

What are the advantages an HMO offers individuals already covered by conventional insurance? Conventional coverage offered in dual-choice situations usually includes reasonably comprehensive hospitalization benefits that, with the exception of maternity coverage, are comparable to HMO protection. The major financial advantage of HMOs is their coverage of ambulatory visits. Enrollment in HMOs is therefore most likely among people who anticipate a large number of ambulatory visits.

Differentials in coverage for maternity care appear to affect the choice of an HMO, and, in turn, hospital utilization, although recent changes in federal law mandating maternity coverage may in the future diminish this effect. In the multiple-choice situation in Rochester, New York, Blue Cross-Blue Shield offered only $155 toward maternity costs that averaged $850 to $1,000, while the prepaid plans offered complete coverage. The subsequent general fertility of Blue Cross members was 30.9 births per 1,000 women aged 15 to 44, while the rates in three prepaid plans were 75.1, 81.5, and 148.8 (Wersinger, 1975).

Lower hospital admission rates for HMOs also might reflect members' tendency to disenroll from the plan or to obtain outside care if they seek hospitalization. If the HMO encourages its physicians to avoid hospitalization, then the patient may well seek outside opinions or treatment or, in a dual-choice situation, switch coverage at the next open enrollment period. Theoretically, a relatively small number of "switchers with hospitalization in mind" can have a substantial effect on hospitalization rates. Unfortunately, this phenomenon is difficult to measure, and no evidence is available on its occurrence.

It is crucial to point out that differential selection is likely to be most important when an employed population is first offered a multiple-choice option with prepaid group practices and other plans. Eventually, the people who lacked physician ties and joined the PGP will develop ties to PGP physicians, the young will age and their health will deteriorate. Thus, the selection effect will be reduced over time. Following this logic, the selection effect is likely to be more important in the brand-new Rochester plans than in the Kaiser plans in California, the majority of whose enrollees have been members for quite some time (Blumberg, 1980). Moreover, although we can say that a selection effect occurs in certain circumstances, we do not know whether it accounts for a large or a small fraction of the observed differential in any particular study, let alone know its importance in general.

Self-selection in HMO membership has important consequences for the evaluation of HMO performance. If the lower hospital utilization and associated lower costs of health maintenance organizations are a function of their membership rather than of their structure or financial incentives, then expectations about the effect of HMO expansion may require substantial adjustment. Rather than promoting efficiency in the overall delivery system, increased HMO membership might simply alter the distribution of medical costs. The expansion of dual choice and of HMOs might draw low users of hospital care into HMOs and leave high users in conventional insurance plans. On the other hand, if HMOs attract persons who are high users of some services and lower users of other services, there may be little effect from self-selection.

Use of Preventive Services

Studies concerning the provision of preventive services can be divided into two groups that appear to offer contradictory findings (Luft, 1978b). The first group supports the hypothesis that HMO enrollees receive more preventive services than do people with conventional health insurance. The second group suggests that there are no differences in the use of preventive services, or that the HMO enrollees receive even fewer services than do people with conventional coverage. In fact, the two sets of studies are not really in conflict. With a few exceptions, the different results can be explained by focusing not on the distinction between HMO and other forms of coverage, but on the presence or absence of coverage for preventive visits. Such coverage is almost universal with HMOs, but it is rare with conventional insurance. Thus, those studies that involve a comparison between HMO enrollees and people with conventional insurance coverage (the first group above) are actually testing two variables: 1) an HMO health maintenance effect, and 2) the differential financial coverages for preventive care. In the few instances in which the third party covers preventive visits (the second group of studies), the second (insurance) variable is held constant and there appears to be little or no HMO health maintenance effect. Studies comparing HMO enrollees with people having conventional coverage for preventive services typically produce ambiguous results: the HMOs provide more preventive care of some types and less of others. These results may reflect recent skepticism in the medical community concerning the efficacy of many "preventive services," such as tests, screenings, and checkups (Collen et al., 1973; Sagel et al., 1974; Cochrane and Elwood, 1969; Foltz and Kelsey, 1978).

Quality of Care

Improved health status or outcome is the ultimate objective of medical care. Unfortunately, outcomes are very difficult to measure. Health services researchers, therefore, rely on other measures of medical care quality, such as the presence of "appropriate" resources (structural measures) and the use of "appropriate" procedures for given cases (process measures). There is unfortunately little evidence that structure, process, and outcome measures correlate well with each other or with what people might recognize as "quality" (Brook, 1973a, 1973b; McAuliffe, 1979).

In terms of "structural" measures, the available data generally support the argument that health maintenance organizations have resources at least as good as those of the conventional system. HMOs tend to have higher proportions of more highly trained physicians and are more likely to use accredited hospitals, but there are a number of important exceptions. Some HMOs have not been able to get ready access to the "better" hospitals and others apparently have chosen not to emphasize specialists and accredited, nonprofit facilities.

Finally, group practice is not essential to peer review; physicians in group practice do have the advantage of physical proximity, but individual practice associations and fee-for-service practices allow the development and use of practice profiles for evaluating physicians.

Although HMOs tend to score higher than conventional practitioners when process measures (especially laboratory tests and procedures) are used, this differential appears to reflect comprehensiveness of coverage rather than organizational characteristics. Large prepaid group practices often exhibit higher quality than do average fee-for-service providers, but the quality is not noticeably higher than what large fee-for-service groups provide.

Outcome measures are most important in quality evaluation, but the available studies focus on narrowly defined mortality-morbidity measures or on broad outcomes such as disability days. The early studies of the Health Insurance Plan of Greater New York (HIP) showed lower prematurity and mortality rates for HMO enrollees (Shapiro, Weiner, and Densen, 1958; Shapiro et al., 1960, 1967). Few subsequent studies offer conclusive evidence in any direction. In general, the available data suggest that outcomes in HMOs are much the same as or somewhat better than those in conventional practice.

In sum, although the quality question remains unresolved, there is no evidence that HMOs achieve their utilization and cost savings by offering substantially lower-quality care than the fee-for-service system. In fact, there is some suggestion of higher quality in health maintenance organizations, as shown in the Cunningham and Williamson (1980) review of the literature.

Consumer Satisfaction

The most important features of HMOs for which evidence on consumer satisfaction is available are access, financial coverage, continuity of care, communication, and perceived quality. Among a broad range of access measures, prepaid group practices offer shorter waiting times, but longer waiting periods to obtain an appointment. The relative value of these two measures of access will vary among individuals. The PGP pattern is probably best for people with routine problems that can be scheduled, such as checkups and periodic visits for chronic conditions. People with "semiurgent" acute problems who can afford the time to wait in the office are more likely to prefer fee-for-service practitioners and the guarantee of eventually seeing their own physicians.

HMO members almost universally express greater satisfaction with the financial coverage provided than do people with other insurance coverage.

HMOs and fee-for-service arrangements also seem to differ with respect to physician-patient relationships (Mechanic, 1976). Prepaid group practices appear to offer less continuity of care when that care is measured by consumer identification with a single physician. But when care is measured in terms of availability of patients' records, a group may be able to provide more continuity of care. However, the role of doctor-patient ties in choice of plan suggests that continuity of provider may be less important for people choosing prepaid groups than are financial incentives.

People enrolled in prepaid group practices seem less happy about their ability to communicate with physicians than do fee-for-service patients or people enrolled in individual practice associations. The general view is that PGP physicians are less willing than individual practitioners to spend time with patients. In turn, physicians in prepaid group practices are reported to be dissatisfied with the degree of communication they have with their patients (Mechanic, 1975).

Another approach to measuring consumer satisfaction relates to the extent to which PGP subscribers continue to use services outside the plans. However, it is not generally known to what extent such services substitute for, rather than supplement, services available within the plans. Between 5 and 20 percent of prepaid group practice members are regular outside users, and a comparable proportion of different members each year use an occasional service outside the plan. Overall, outside use accounts for 7 to 14 percent of all services members receive. If outside use represents dissatisfaction, the extent of outside use is comparable to the proportion of members who when interviewed reported substantial dissatisfaction. To a certain degree, outside use may also be a reflection of duplicate coverage. According to a 1980 Kaiser study, approximately 14 percent of HMO enrollees had duplicate coverage; added to this number are Medicare beneficiaries who retain the ability to seek consultations or treatment outside the HMO system (Blumberg, 1980). Unknown is the percentage of enrollees who primarily seek treatment outside the HMO but look upon HMO benefits as a form of "catastrophic coverage."

The dual-choice arrangements available to most HMO members offer what may be the best single *objective* measure of overall satisfaction. The impressive record of long-term growth in the HMO share within given enrollee groups implies that the levels of dissatisfaction are relatively low and have an insignificant effect on membership. Among every group of new enrollees, a small proportion, perhaps 5 to 10 percent, find that they really do not like the HMO. Others become dissatisfied for one reason or another and leave. These withdrawals, however, are more than offset by new members coming in from conventional plans.

The coexistence of dissatisfaction in face of growing HMO membership reflects the decision-making process in the dual-option setting. In choosing between HMOs and traditional coverage, potential HMO enrollees must weigh various factors, such as financial coverage, premiums, perceived quality, and access. For some people, the benefits of the HMO option outweigh the disadvantages. Hence, HMO members like the short waits and comprehensive coverage, but are dissatisfied with the amount of time it takes to get an appointment, their inability to see their usual physician for urgent visits, and the limited communication and warmth in their patient-physician relationship. However, when offered the opportunity to switch out of the HMO in open enrollment periods, most choose to stay in the HMO.

Evidence on consumer satisfaction, then, like evidence on other elements of HMO experience, is not clear-cut. It seems fair to conclude that HMO costs tend to be lower than fee-for-service costs for broadly comparable populations; that lower costs primarily reflect lower hospital utilization; and that, although we cannot identify the causes of these lower rates, they appear to be neither a product of poor-quality care nor a source of significant consumer dissatisfaction.

Physician Satisfaction

By tradition and law, physicians are the pivotal element in medical care delivery. HMOs must be able to attract physicians in sufficient number and with suitable training and qualifications to compete effectively with the fee-for-service system. A national sample of pediatricians and general practitioners, in solo, group, and prepaid group practice, has shown that physicians in prepaid practice work shorter hours and earn less (Mechanic, 1975). Most prepaid groups have some form of income-sharing that results in a general leveling of income differences across specialties. Physician dissatisfaction with work overload has been reported in several studies (Freidson, 1973; McElrath, 1961) but national surveys of physicians in general show substantial dissatisfaction with a lack of free time (Owens, 1977, 1978). Some of the dissatisfaction of HMO-based physicians may be attributed to the contractual nature of prepaid systems; whereas fee-for-service physicians can refuse to treat or refer out patients they see as neurotic or overly demanding, all HMO subscribers have the right to receive medical treatment within the system. On the other hand, HMO coverage allows physicians to practice high-quality medical care without having to be concerned about a patient's ability to pay (Cook, 1971; Hetherington, Hopkins and Roemer, 1975).

Physician satisfaction with HMOs can also be measured in terms of the ability of plans to recruit new physicians and to keep turnover to a reasonable level. Whereas prepaid groups had difficulty recruiting physicians in the 1950s and early 1960s because of the opposition of the medical establishment, the situation has now changed and positions are readily filled, with the exception of certain subspecialty areas (e.g., orthopedics, neurosurgery) in which physicians in private practice can command exceptionally high incomes (Saward and Greenlick, 1972; Lum, 1975; Smillie, 1976). Turnover rate for physicians tends to be significantly higher during the first two years of "probationary" employment than it is for more senior PGP physicians who have achieved partnership status. For instance, at the Permanente Medical Group (Northern California Kaiser), the termination rate among employed physicians ranged from 7.7 to 16.2 percent between 1968 and

1975, with an average of 12.0 percent; for partners, the rate ranged from 1.3 to 4.8 percent, with a mean of 2.6 percent, of which two-fifths was due to death or disability (Smillie, 1976).

To date, physician satisfaction has been measured largely in terms of the practice setting within well-established prepaid groups. The attitudes of physicians in newly formed groups or IPAs—particularly during the start-up stages—need to be examined, since the incentives, work load, and income base of the new plans may vary significantly from those of the often studied plans such as Kaiser, HIP, and Group Health Cooperative.

Meeting the Needs of the Poor, Aged, and Rural Populations

Most HMOs have been designed for the middle and working classes, usually within an urban or suburban environment. In 1979, 4.3 percent of HMO enrollment comprised Medicare subscribers, whereas Medicare enrollees account for roughly 10 percent of the American population (National HMO Census, 1979). This low participation rate is the result of two factors: 1) HMOs can not use the savings resulting from lower hospital use to attract Medicare beneficiaries through better coverage; and 2) complex Medicare reimbursement policies fail to provide an incentive for HMOs to seek out Medicare beneficiaries (Luft et al., 1980; Strumpf, 1979). Basically, HMOs can receive payment from the Health Care Financing Administration either according to a cost-reimbursement system or on a capitation basis. Cost reimbursement produces increased administrative costs for HMOs which, instead of providing a full range of services for a fixed predetermined amount, must keep track of deductibles, of Medicare-covered services, and of the costs associated with each individual service. Annual capitation rates for at-risk HMOs are equal to the adjusted average per capita cost (AAPCC) provided to Medicare beneficiaries who receive fee-for-service care; any savings generated by the HMOs are shared with the government, while deficits must be absorbed or carried forward to be offset against future savings. As a result of these disincentives, by 1978 only one plan had contracted with Medicare on a risk basis (Group Health Cooperative of Puget Sound).

In 1979, discontent with Medicare policy led to various proposals in Congress to restructure HMO reimbursement. Included in the proposals were the following: development of risk contracts that would pay HMOs prospectively at 95 percent of the AAPCC; use of the HMOs' community rate, adjusted for Medicare utilization, for comparison with the AAPCC; and the difference between the AAPCC and the HMOs' community rate, to be returned to Medicare enrollees in the form of reduced premiums and/or expanded service benefits. Several capitation experiments, using the 95 percent formula, are currently being funded by the Health Care Financing Administration, but the results of the experiments are not yet available.

As with the Medicare program, participation by HMOs in the Medicaid program has also been extremely restricted. As of June 1979, 246,268 persons, or approximately 3 percent of all HMO enrollment, were Title XIX (Medicaid) eligibles, whereas they comprised approximately 10 percent of the U.S. population. Originally, when the HMO concept was formulated in the early 1970s, HMOs were seen as a means of improving the health care of the poor while providing an alternative to the open-ended costs of the fee-for-service system. By 1973, some 62 prepaid health plans (PHPs) in twelve different states were providing care to slightly over 200,000 individuals (Strumpf, 1979). Then came a series of scandals associated with the Medicaid program. Medicaid "mills," operating on a fee-for-service basis in large urban centers, such as New York City, were discovered to be delivering shoddy care and to be using fraudulent billing practices. In California, the PHPs were accused of questionable marketing and enrollment procedures, of delivering poor-quality care, of restricting access to medical personnel, and of siphoning funds from non-profit HMO entities into for-profit subsidiaries (Goldberg, 1976; California Department of Health, 1975; Chavkin and Treseder, 1977). Analyses of the California situation revealed that the problem was not in the concept of prepayment, but in the design and administration of the PHP program within the state government. The California experience, however, led to a major restructuring of Medicaid HMO contracts by Congress. PL 94-460 (1976) specified that prepaid plans thereafter had to meet the standards of federally qualified HMOs (with certain exceptions granted to public agencies and rural facilities) and that private-pay enrollees (non-Medicare and non-Medicaid) had to comprise at least 50 percent of the subscribers within a specified time period.

To date, the number of Medicaid contracts has not increased significantly above the 1973 level. Appropriate incentives do not currently exist for Medicaid enrollees to seek out prepaid plans; conversely, prepaid plans do not have any financial incentives to develop Medicaid contracts. For instance, if an individual Medicaid recipient stays within the fee-for-service system, he/she is in a position to choose any physician desired (given availability). The HMO represents a narrowing of that choice to those physicians who work within the prepaid system. Moreover, under Medicaid, copayments for ambulatory services are prohibited, thereby eliminating a major financial incentive used by HMOs to attract the middle class. For HMOs, negative factors associated with the signing of a Medicaid contract include the increased costs associated with administration and marketing of the program, high turnover of Medicaid enrollees because of loss of Title XIX eligibility, unrealistic capitation rates, as well as the possibility of increased utilization of medical services by the needy.

Whereas most HMOs do not maintain inner city locations and therefore accessibility may be a problem for Medicaid recipients, in rural areas the problem is even more aggravated. In particular, nonmetropolitan areas with stable or declining populations have the greatest difficulty attracting and retaining physicians (Cotterill and Eisenberg, 1979). For the poor and aged, geographic access is further complicated by financial constraints and by the small number of physicians who accept Medicare and Medicaid patients. Open-panel IPAs have been viewed as one way of implementing prepaid coverage for rural populations; another method calls for networks of primary care physicians, operating in conjunction with HMOs in urban settings. The feasibility of new group practices is more open to question, as researchers have found that physicians seek out areas with a reasonably rapid population growth and relatively rapid access to metropolitan areas (Cotterill and Eisenberg, 1979).

Thus, HMOs have only just begun to deal with the needs of the poor, the aged, and rural populations. In speaking of HMOs, this paper has described prepaid systems largely in terms of the generic definitions, without specifying the organizational variables that can affect performance. For instance, sponsorship of an HMO may influence the decision of an HMO to provide care to the needy or the aged; a consumer-sponsored plan is more likely to place social goals above financial considerations, whereas a for-profit plan operated by an investor group will have different priorities. Performance of a plan can vary in terms of external or environmental factors, such as the legal and regulatory constraints of state laws and the structure of the local health care market. The internal organization of the plan, in terms of professional staffing ratios, administrative structure, physician reimbursement, risk-sharing arrangements, and availability of stop-loss insurance, ownership of hospitals or negotiation of bed rates, may also affect plan growth and quality of care. Unfortunately, most research about HMOs has examined performance largely in terms of the group/staff versus IPA dichotomy, rather than looking at specific organizational variables. Although some evidence exists on each of these issues, there are few studies available and the material should be considered at best exploratory (Luft, 1980c). From a research perspective, there are several times as many explanatory variables as there are observations. However, the increased awareness among researchers that HMOs differ is beginning to lead to more concern with the factors that explain HMO performance.

The Competitive Impact of HMOs

Perhaps the most important potential role for HMOs is in promoting competition within the health care system; by stimulating conventional providers to restructure medical practice and insurance benefits, HMOs function as catalysts for cost containment. Alain Enthoven's (1978) "Consumer Choice Health Plan" is based on this premise, as are a variety of procompetition proposals introduced in Congress, beginning in 1979. Unfortunately, only a handful of studies deal with this crucial problem and the available evidence is mixed (Luft, 1980b).

A 1977 study by the Federal Trade Commission (FTC) argues that the entry of HMOs is responsible for lowering the hospital utilization of people in conventional plans. Goldberg and Greenberg (1977) rest their case on two types of analysis: 1) regressions of hospital utilization by Blue Cross members as a function of HMO market share and other variables; and 2) interviews in various HMO market areas. Unfortunately, the regressions are dominated by four states on the West Coast: California, Washington, Oregon, and Hawaii, all of which have both high HMO market shares and low utilization rates. If these four states are omitted, the negative relation is no longer significant. The interviews indicate clear competitive reactions by Blue Cross of Northern California to Kaiser's growth, beginning in the 1950s, but little supporting evidence in other areas. Also, for the California story, the FTC investigators ignored overall developments in the insurance market (e.g., the split between Blue Cross and Blue Shield and the entrance of commercial insurers); thus, the decline in hospital utilization in California, which appeared during a period of substantial HMO growth, cannot be used as prima facie evidence of an "HMO effect."

Other situations that have been used in support of the competitive model also produce equivocal results. For instance, in Rochester, New York, there has been intense competition between several HMOs and the local Blue Cross/Blue Shield plan. There the inpatient medical-surgical utilization rate for BC/BS members under 65 years of age was relatively constant from 1974 to 1977 at about 625 days, then dropped precipitously to 547 by mid-1979, a decline much larger than for any other eastern Blue Cross Plan. Blue Cross of Rochester attributes much of this decline to a competitive effect (Finger Lakes Health Systems Agency, 1980). There are a number of alternative explanations, however. First, Rochester has had aggressive health planning since the late 1940s, and traditionally has had a very low ratio of beds per capita. It also has an actively interested group of large employers who are encouraging innovation and cost control. A rather unusual regional budgeting strategy is being implemented (Sorensen and Saward, 1978). Finally, changes in New York State policies toward nursing home reimbursement have made it more difficult to transfer Medicare and Medicaid recipients out of hospitals. Given the tight bed supply, this could force down the BC/BS utilization rate by limiting the number of beds available to those who are not elderly and not poor (Wersinger, 1979).

In Hawaii there is very low hospital utilization in both Kaiser and the Hawaii Medical Service Association (HMSA). Although HMSA is nominally a Blue Shield plan, it exercises rather stringent controls over utilization and thus acts like an IPA or a cost-conscious alternative delivery system (McClure, 1978). But the history of HMSA, beginning with its founding by local social workers, the Hawaii heritage of plantation-provided medical care, and Hawaii's unique ethnic mix suggest that the HMSA behavior may have more to do with its special history than with competition with Kaiser (Bailey, 1971). Christianson and McClure (1979) offer a detailed description of competition among seven HMOs in Minneapolis-St. Paul. All but one of these HMOs were formed within the past five years, however, and the Christianson-McClure focus is primarily on the behavior of the HMOs, rather than on the long-term responses of conventional providers. An InterStudy report has documented a drop in the rate of increase of total per capita hospital expenditures, presumably because of decreased hospital utilization. Medicare data compiled by the professional standards review organization (PSRO) in the Twin Cities showed a larger drop in hospital admissions for the over-65 population in 1977 (−6.5 percent) than for any other PSRO in the country (Ellwein, 1979). Again, it is difficult to separate out the causes for the decline in hospital utilization. For example, utilization review programs used by the PSRO and the individual hospitals may have had some effect; similarly, pressure from large corporate employers to hold down health-benefit costs also may be important.

To date, "the HMO effect" has been discussed largely in terms of an effect upon hospitalization rates, insurance premium costs, benefit packages, and the pricing of professional and hospital services. Little attention has been devoted to the issue of overall health expenditures. If competition between HMOs and conventional providers does affect overall costs, one might expect this situation to appear in California with its massive Kaiser plans, its competing HMOs, and a documented history of Blue Cross concern. By some standards the mix of medical services bought by Californians may be more efficient than elsewhere, because hospital use is low and physician use is high, but there is no evidence that massive HMO enrollment has resulted in overall cost containment. In fact, per capita medical care expenditures by all Californians and by Medicare beneficiaries in California are among the highest in the nation (Social Security Administration, 1971; Cooper, Worthington, and Piro, 1975).

Policy Questions

The previous sections of this paper have attempted to describe what is known about the performance of HMOs. Unfortunately, there is a great deal that is not known about HMO performance. The answers to some unanswered questions may be useful to planners, the designers of HMOs, or others, but are not particularly relevant to federal and state policy makers. Examples of such questions are whether HMOs are efficient users of allied health personnel, or whether they adopt medical technology wisely. The answers to other questions, however, may have a direct bearing on policy decisions. This section will outline some of these policy-relevant areas that require further investigation.

The Federal HMO Qualification and Monitoring Process

To obtain federal funding for planning, development, and start-up costs, and to qualify for the employer-mandating provisions, health plans must conform to a narrowly defined set of criteria. Some well-established plans have either delayed or intentionally not sought federal qualification. Criticism has centered largely around the mandatory open-enrollment period, the specification of the maximum benefit package, and the community rating requirement. Which of these and other features cause the most difficulties for HMOs?

The Office of Health Maintenance Organizations has a policy of restricting the number of loans and grants in each market area so as not to encourage too much competition for plans it has already helped support. At what level does an increase in the number of HMOs begin to pose serious competitive threats to other HMOs? Are there ways to identify among the applicants the strongest potential survivors, so that support is not allocated solely on a first-come, first-served basis? Is it possible to establish a system with competitive renewals, whereby early support for a plan with little likelihood of success will not preclude support for a later, but much more promising plan? Does the entry of for-profit firms, through the purchase of subsidized, not-for-profit HMOs, subvert the intent of the HMO act or strengthen it by resulting in a stronger and more viable HMO presence? What techniques can be used to predict more accurately which markets are ripe for HMO development and which plans are likely to succeed?

What are the advantages and disadvantages of relatively independent state and federal reporting requirements and monitoring? That is, are some state requirements or techniques substantially more useful in validating data and identifying and correcting problems? If so, how might the two systems be better integrated to retain the benefits of each while reducing unnecessary duplication? What types of quality assessment can be implemented effectively and yet offer reasonable protection to the public?

What is the impact of an HMO failure on its enrollees and on other HMOs? Should other HMOs in the area be required to accept the former enrollees of the failed HMO? What types of reinsurance should be provided (and by whom) to protect enrollees in the case of a plan's insolvency? What effect does the fear by employers and potential enrollees of plan insolvency have on marketing of new plans?

In some areas, prepaid systems have developed that have certain HMO features (i.e., hospital-sponsored capitation plans or primary care networks) but do not meet all the requirements for HMO qualification. In other areas, plans that fit the federal definition have chosen not to seek federal qualification. Although this precludes federal assistance and use of the employer-mandating provision, such plans can tailor their benefit packages and experience-rate employee groups. What are the implications of this type of competitive setting? Do the federally qualified HMOs "open up the market," only to lose it later to experience-rated plans? Does the wider range of alternatives improve the market for everyone? Should all plans, if state-licensed, be allowed to make use of the mandating process? Are there other incentives that can induce plans to become federally qualified?

HMOs and the Health Insurance Market

HMOs compete not only with each other but also, what is more important, with conventional insurers. The federal qualification process and many state regulations impose restrictions on HMOs and other prepaid systems that are not applied to conventional health insurers. What are the implications of this double standard? In particular, how important are experience-rating and the selection of benefits? What is the effect of the increasing similarity of benefits resulting from the expansion of maternity coverage through the Civil Rights Amendments of 1978, and state-mandated coverage for certain problems of mental health and drug abuse? Many conventional carriers are entering the HMO market by establishing new HMOs or purchasing existing plans. From one perspective this is desirable because of the wealth of expertise and financial support they can bring to bear. From another perspective, one might fear anticompetitive behavior designed to protect the carrier's primary business. To what extent should conventional carriers be encouraged in or discouraged from establishing HMOs?

Some current legislative proposals are designed to alter the tax code to make employees more sensitive to the cost of their health insurance and to encourage HMOs. Does the experience of employee groups with multiple-choice options support the notion of rational decision-making? How important a problem is enrollment by people to obtain a set of expensive services under high-option coverage one year, who switch to the low-option plan the next? What is the impact of the increasing proportion of people with duplicate health insurance coverage through other family members?

Much of the impetus for changes in the tax law is based on the belief that increased competition between HMOs and the conventional system will lead to cost-containing responses by the latter. As was pointed out, there is some evidence supporting this notion, but there are almost always alternative explanations for each set of findings. Thus, we need to know much more about the competitive effects of HMO development. Furthermore, it is likely that HMOs engender beneficial competitive responses in some settings, little response in others, and perhaps detrimental responses in others. (For instance, the California Prepaid Health Plan scandals poisoned the waters for many legitimate HMOs.) What factors characterize and influence the type of effects HMOs may have?

Much of the HMO discussion envisions separate prepaid group practices, networks of clinics, or small IPAs. What happens when several HMOs contract with the same set of providers? For instance, a fee-for-service group may see conventionally insured patients, be part of a network of groups, and have contractual relationships with several IPAs or carrier-sponsored alternative delivery systems. Are there significant cross-subsidies among patients, and are there conflicts of interest? In another situation, what are the implications of a large IPA that dominates a medical care market and controls costs, in part, by excluding certain physicians or hospitals? How does one balance the efficiency against the antitrust implications?

Medicare and Medicaid

Most of the recent HMO policies have been focused on improving the HMO option for employed populations. Although a substantial number of Medicare beneficiaries belong to HMOs, most have "aged in"—having been members before retirement. Moreover, with the exception of some experimental programs, Medicare legislation has not allowed capitation payments that are attractive to HMOs. Thus Medicare beneficiaries are treated by HMO providers on what is essentially a fee-for-service arrangement. One current proposal would allow the Health Care Financing Administration (HCFA) to pay HMOs a capitation equal to 95 percent of the average adjusted cost for fee-for-service Medicare beneficiaries in the area. If this were to occur, would HMOs change their style of practice for their current Medicare beneficiaries? How would the beneficiaries react to limits on coverage for outside use? Would new Medicare enrollees be "good" or "bad" risks and what factors might influence such selective enrollment? How well can the capitation payment be adjusted to reflect the differential enrollment of certain types of people? What are the implications of returning savings to enrollees in increased benefits or reduced costs?

For Medicaid beneficiaries the situation is rather different. State agencies have the option of contracting with HMOs and several have done so, with a wide range of success. Several problems occur in linking HMOs and the poor: 1) The intermittent eligibility of many beneficiaries and fluctuating state policies make Medicaid contracts far less desirable than employee groups to most HMOs. 2) Medicaid coverage is usually extensive and allows no copayments, so that the financial savings available to the typical HMO enrollee can not be used as an enrollment incentive. 3) Since the poor are often concentrated geographically, it is difficult for an HMO to enroll a significant number of the poor without becoming a Medicaid-only plan. The solutions to these problems will require substantial experimentation. Perhaps the maximum of 50 percent federally funded enrollees should be waived in certain instances. Can HMO-type plans be designed to meet the health needs of the most severely ill Medicaid beneficiaries with chronic health problems, or who need long-term care? How well do voucher systems work for a poverty population? What types of quality controls and marketing surveillance are feasible and appropriate? What systems can also provide services to the near-poor not covered by employer or union sponsored plans?

Local Health Planning and Regulation

Health care planning and regulation through health systems agencies, certificate-of-need regulations, and hospital rate-setting are designed to correct perceived problems with the conventional medical care system. HMOs operate with a markedly different set of incentives and have been exempted from some of these restrictions, such as certificate of need. Has this exemption worked as planned, to allow HMOs to grow and purchase existing facilities? Or is it occasionally used as a loophole to build facilities that are then used or taken over by conventional providers? Does the 50,000 enrollment minimum too severely limit the exemption to selected plans or is it reasonable? What happens to resources in conventional hospitals as HMOs get their own equipment and facilities? Do HMOs use their bargaining power to encourage more efficient performance by contracting hospitals? Or do they use it to extract favorable rates that are then subsidized by other patients?

Posing questions for further research is a relatively easy but quite humbling undertaking, as it points out how little we know. In some instances, the answers can be developed through carefully designed and executed research studies of the existing system. In other areas, one cannot merely look before leaping, one must carry out some experiments to test new organizational forms and to see how people and institutions react under altered incentives. Understanding the structure and operation of the medical care system is a relatively recent phenomenon, with much of the work having taken place in the fifteen years since Medicare and Medicaid. Although policy initiatives will not await firm research findings, policies should be designed with the understanding that they may need to be changed as we learn more about their effects and about how the medical care system responds to a changing environment.

References

Bailey, R.M. 1971. *Medical Care in Hawaii: 1970.* Berkeley: University of California, Institute of Business and Economic Research.

Berki, S.E., Ashcraft, M.L.F., Penchansky, R., and Fortus, R.S. 1977. Enrollment Choice in a Multi-HMO Setting: The Roles of Health Risk, Financial Vulnerability, and Access to Care. *Medical Care* 15 (February): 95–114.

———, and Ashcraft, M.L.F. 1980. HMO Enrollment: Who Joins What and Why: A Review of the Literature. *Milbank Memorial Fund Quarterly/Health and Society* 58 (Fall): 588–632.

Blumberg, M.S. 1980. Health Status and Health Care Use by Type of

Private Health Coverage. *Milbank Memorial Fund Quarterly/ Health and Society* 58 (Fall): 633–655.

Breslow, L. 1975. Statement for Senate Permanent Subcommittee on Investigations of the Committee on Government Operations, March 12, 1975. In U.S. Senate, Committee on Government Operations, Permanent Subcommittee on Investigations, *Prepaid Health Plans,* Hearings, March 13–14, 1975, 94th Congress, 1st Session. Washington, D.C.: Government Printing Office.

Brook, R.H. 1973. Critical Issues in the Assessment of Quality of Care and Their Relationship to HMOs. *Journal of Medical Education* 48 (April, Part 2):114–134.

———. 1973b. *Quality of Care Assessment: Comparison of Five Methods of Peer Review.* National Center for Health Services Research and Development. Washington, D.C.: Government Printing Office.

California Department of Health. 1975. Prepaid Health Plans: The California Experience. In U.S. Senate, Committee on Government Operations, Permanent Subcommittee on Investigations, *Prepaid Health Plans,* Hearings, March 13–14, 1975, 94th Congress, 1st Session. Washington, D.C.: Government Printing Office.

Chavkin, D.F., and Treseder, A. 1977. California's Prepaid Health Plan Program: Can the Patient Be Saved? *Hastings Law Journal* 28 (January): 685–760.

Christianson, J.B., and McClure, W. 1979. Competition in the Delivery of Medical Care. *New England Journal of Medicine* 301:812–818.

Cochrane, A.L., and Elwood, P.C. 1969. Screening: The Case against It. *Medical Officer* 121 (January):53–57.

Cohen, H. 1978. Testimony. In *Technology and the Cost of Health Care,* Hearings before the U.S. House, Committee on Science and Technology, September 26, 27, October 6, 1978. Washington, D.C.: Government Printing Office.

Collen, M.F., Dales, L.G., Friedman, G.D., Flagle, C.D., Feldman, R., and Siegelaub, A.B. 1973. Multiphasic Checkup Evaluation Study: 4. Preliminary Cost Benefit Analysis for Middle-Aged Men. *Preventive Medicine* 2 (June):236–246.

Cook, W.H. 1971. Profile of the Permanente Physician. In Somers, A.R., ed., *The Kaiser-Permanente Medical Care Program: A Symposium.* New York: Commonwealth Fund.

Cooper, B.S., Worthington, N.L., and Piro, P.A. 1975. *Personal Health Care Expenditures by State.* DHEW Publication No. (SSA) 75–11906. Washington, D.C.: Government Printing Office.

Cotterill, P.G., and Eisenberg, B.S. 1979. Improving Access to Medical Care in Underserved Areas: The Role of Group Practice. *Inquiry* 16 (Summer):141–153.

Cunningham, F.C., and Williamson, J.W. 1980. How Does the Quality of Health Care in HMOs Compare to That in Other Settings? An Analytic Literature Review: 1958 to 1979. *Group Health Journal* 1 (Winter):4–25.

Cutler, J.L., Ramcharan, S., Feldman, R., Siegelaub, A.B., Campbell, B., Friedman, G.D., Dales, L.G., and Collen, M.F. 1973. Multiphasic Checkup Evaluation Study: 1. Methods and Population. *Preventive Medicine* 2 (June):197–206.

Dozier, D., Harrington, D.C., Krupp, M.A., Schwarberg, C.F., Jr., and Yedidia, A. 1973. 1970–71 Survey of Consumer Experience: Report of the State of California Employees' Medical and Hospital Care Program, prepared under the policy direction of the Medical Advisory Council to the Board of Administration of the Public Employees' Retirement System. Sacramento, Calif.

Egdahl, R.H. 1973. Foundations for Medical Care. *New England Journal of Medicine* 288:491–498.

———, et al. 1977. The Potential of Organizations of Fee-For-Service Physicians for Achieving Significant Decreases in Hospitalization. *Annals of Surgery* 186:388–399.

Ellwein, L.K. 1979. *Health Care Trends: Minneapolis/St. Paul Summary Highlights.* Excelsior, Minn.: InterStudy.

Enthoven, A.C. 1978. Consumer Choice Health Plan. *New England Journal of Medicine* 298:650–658 and 709–720.

Finger Lakes Health Systems Agency. 1980. *Health Maintenance Organizations in Rochester, New York: History, Current Performance, and Future Prospects.* Rochester: Finger Lakes Health Systems Agency, Task Force on Prepaid Health Care.

Foltz, A.-M., and Kelsey, J.L. 1978. The Annual Pap Test: A Dubious Policy Success. *Milbank Memorial Fund Quarterly/Health and Society* 56(Fall):426–462.

Freidson, E. 1973. Prepaid Group Practice and the New Demanding Patient. *Milbank Memorial Fund Quarterly/Health and Society* 51 (Fall):473–488.

Gibson, R.M. 1979. National Health Expenditures, 1978. *Health Care Financing Review* 1(1):1–36.

Goldberg, L.G., and Greenberg, W. 1977. *The HMO and Its Effects on Competition.* Washington, D.C.: Federal Trade Commission, Bureau of Economics.

Goldberg, V.P. 1976. Some Emerging Problems of Prepaid Health Plans in the Medi-Cal System. *Policy Analysis* 1(1):55–68.

Health Care Financing Administration, Office of Research Demonstrations and Statistics. 1980. National Health Expenditures and Related Measures. *Health Care Financing Trends* 1(2):1–6.

Held, P.J., and Reinhardt, U., eds. 1979. *Analysis of Economic Perfor-*

mance in Medical Group Practices: Final Report. Princeton: Mathematica Policy Research.

Hetherington, R.W., Hopkins, C.E., and Roemer, M.I. 1975. *Health Insurance Plans: Promise and Performance.* New York: Wiley-Interscience.

Holoweiko, M. 1980. Why Hospitals May Be Giving Your Colleagues an Edge. *Medical Economics* (January 21):85–88.

Lee, M.L. 1971. A Conspicuous Production Theory of Hospital Behavior. *Southern Economic Journal* 38 (July):48–58.

Luft, H.S. 1978a. How Do Health Maintenance Organizations Achieve Their "Savings"? Rhetoric and Evidence. *New England Journal of Medicine* 298:1336–1343.

————. 1978b. Why Do HMOs Seem to Provide More Health Maintenance Services? *Milbank Memorial Fund Quarterly/Health and Society* 56 (Spring):140–168.

————. 1980a. Trends in Medical Care Costs: Do HMOs Lower the Rate of Growth? *Medical Care* 18(1):1–16.

————. 1980b. HMOs and the Medical Care Market. In *Socioeconomic Issues in Health,* 1980. Chicago: American Medical Association.

————. 1980c. *Health Maintenance Organizations: Dimensions of Performance.* New York: Wiley-Interscience. In press.

————, and Crane, S. 1980. Regionalization of Services within a Multi-Hospital Health Maintenance Organization. *Health Services Research.* In press.

————, Feder, J., Holahan, J., and Lennox, K.D. 1980. Health Maintenance Organizations. In Feder, J., Holahan, J., and Marmor, T., eds., *National Health Insurance: Conflicting Goals and Policy Choices.* Washington, D.C.: Urban Institute.

Lum, D. 1975. The Health Maintenance Organization Delivery System: A National Study of Attitudes of HMO Project Directors on HMO Issues. *American Journal of Public Health* 65:1192–1201.

McAuliffe, W.E. 1979. Measuring the Quality of Medical Care: Process versus Outcome. *Milbank Memorial Fund Quarterly/Health and Society* 57 (Winter):118–152.

McCaffree, K.M., Boscha, M.V., Drucker, W.L., Richardson, W.C., and Diehr, P.K. 1976. Comparative Costs of Services. In Richardson, W.C., ed., *The Seattle Prepaid Health Care Project: Comparison of Health Service Delivery,* Chapter 3. National Technical Information Service, PB No. 267488-SET.

McClure, W. 1978. On Broadening the Definition of and Removing Regulatory Barriers to a Competitive Health Care System. *Journal of Health Politics, Policy, and Law* 3 (Fall):303–327.

McElrath, D.C. 1961. Perspective and Participation in Prepaid Group Practice. *American Sociological Review* 26:596–607.

Mechanic, D. 1975. The Organization of Medical Practice and Practice Orientation among Physicians in Prepaid and Nonprepaid Primary Care Settings. *Medical Care* 13(3):189–204.

———. 1976. *The Growth of Bureaucratic Medicine.* New York: Wiley-Interscience.

Miller, J.L. (Vice president, Health Net, Blue Cross of Southern California). 1980. Oral interview, with J.B. Trauner, May 1.

Moore, S. 1979. Cost Containment through Risk-Sharing by Primary-Care Physicians. *New England Journal of Medicine* 300:1359–1362.

Newhouse, J.P. 1973. The Economics of Group Practice. *Journal of Human Resources* 8 (Winter):37–56.

Owens, A. 1977. What Doctors Want Most from Their Practices Now. *Medical Economics* 54 (1) (March 7):88–92.

———. 1978. What's Behind the Drop in Doctors' Productivity? *Medical Economics* 55 (3) (July 24):102–105.

Roghmann, K.J., Gavett, J.W., Sorensen, A.A., Wells, S., and Wersinger, R. 1975. Who Chooses Prepaid Medical Care? Survey Results from Two Marketings of Three New Prepayment Plans. *Public Health Reports* 90 (November/December):516–527.

———, Sorensen, A.A., and Wells, S. 1980. Hospitalizations in Three Competing HMOs during Their First Two Years: A Cohort Study of the Rochester Experience. *Group Health Journal* 1 (1):26–33.

Sagel, S.S., Evens, R.G., Forrest, J.C., and Bramson, R.T. 1974. Efficacy of Routine Screening and Lateral Chest Radiographs in a Hospital-Based Population. *New England Journal of Medicine* 291:1001–1004.

Saward, E.W., and Greenlick, M.R. 1972. Health Policy and the HMO. *Milbank Memorial Fund Quarterly* 50 (April, Part 1): 147–176.

Shapiro, S., Jacobziner, H., Densen, P., and Weiner, L. 1960. Further Observations on Prematurity and Perinatal Mortality in a General Population and in the Population of a Prepaid Group Practice Medical Care Plan. *American Journal of Public Health* 50:1304–1317.

———, Weiner, L., and Densen, P. 1958. Comparison of Prematurity and Perinatal Mortality in a General Population and in the Population of a Prepaid Group Practice Medical Care Plan. *American Journal of Public Health* 48:170–185.

———, Williams, J., Yerby, A., Densen, P., and Rosner, H. 1967. Patterns of Medical Use by the Indigent Aged under Two Systems of Medical Care. *American Journal of Public Health* 57:784–790.

Sloan, F.A. 1974. Effects of Incentives on Physician Performance. In

Rafferty, J., ed., *Health Manpower and Productivity.* Lexington, Mass.: D.C. Heath.

Smillie, J.G. 1976. Recruitment of Physicians: Large Prepaid Group Practice. In Dorsey, J.L., and Kane, J., eds., *Physician Recruitment, Performance Evaluation: The Role of the Medical Director.* Washington, D.C.: Group Health Association of America.

Social Security Administration, Office of Actuary-Office of Research and Statistics. 1971. *Medicare: Health Insurance for the Aged: Geographic Index of Reimbursement by State and County.* SHEW Publication (SSA) 74–11710. Washington, D.C.: Government Printing Office.

Somers, A.R., ed. 1971. *The Kaiser-Permanente Medical Care Program: A Symposium.* New York: Commonwealth Fund.

Sorensen, A., and Saward, E. 1978. An Alternative Approach to Hospital Cost Control: The Rochester Project. *Public Health Reports* 93(4):311–317.

Strumpf, G.B. 1979. Public Payor Participation in HMOs. Paper presented at conference on Health Maintenance Organizations, sponsored by ABT Associates in Boston, Mass., November 1–2.

Wersinger, R.P. 1975. *The Analysis of Three Prepaid Health Care Plans in Monroe County, New York, Part 3: Inpatient Utilization Statistics, January 1, 1974–December 31, 1974.* Rochester, N.Y.: University of Rochester School of Medicine and Dentistry, Department of Preventive Medicine and Community Health.

———. 1979. Personal communication, May 1.

———, and Sorensen, A. 1980. *An Analysis of the Health Status, Utilization and Cost Experience of an HMO Population Compared with a Blue Cross/Blue Shield Matched Control Group.* Rochester, N.Y.: University of Rochester School of Medicine and Dentistry, Department of Preventive, Family and Rehabilitation Medicine.

Zelten, R.A. 1979. *Alternative HMO Models.* University of Pennsylvania, National Health Care Management Center Issue Paper No. 3.

This paper is a summarization of six years of work on HMOs, presented in Luft (1978a, 1978b, 1980a, 1980b, 1980c) and Luft and Crane (1980). Research support has been provided by the Social Security Administration/Health Care Financing Administration Grant No. 10-P-90335/9-01 and the National Center for Health Services Research Grant No. HS02975-02. Preparation of this summary was supported by the National Center for Health Services Research under Contract 233-79-3016. I am grateful to various members of the Health Policy Program for their assistance and am particularly indebted to Joan B. Trauner for her help in preparing this paper.

Address correspondence to: Harold S. Luft, Ph.D., Health Policy Program, School of Medicine, University of California, 1326 Third Avenue, San Francisco, CA 94143.

The Performance of Health Maintenance Organizations: An Analytic Review

FREDRIC D. WOLINSKY

*Center for Health Services Research and Development,
American Medical Association*

E VER SINCE 1970 WHEN PAUL ELLWOOD (1971) FIRST
coined the phrase "health maintenance organizations" (HMOs)
and Richard Nixon (1971) quickly made them the official national policy goal, HMOs have been the most touted, discussed,
analyzed, and hotly debated alternative health care delivery system in
the United States. Coming into formal existence through the HMO
Act of 1973 (PL 93-222) and its subsequent amendments (Department of Health, Education, and Welfare, 1974, 1975; PL 94-460; PL
95-559), HMOs have been officially targeted as a national priority (PL
93-641) and as one of the potentially key components of a national
health insurance system. Accordingly, one would assume that by now
a common understanding of what HMOs are, what they are supposed
to do, and what and how well they actually do it would have emerged.
Unfortunately, this is not the case. In the present paper we seek to
resolve part of this problem by 1) reviewing the nine most often cited
reviews of the HMO performance literature; 2) identifying the incentive and disincentive structures operating in HMOs; 3) exposing the
methodological problems associated with evaluating the performance
of HMOs; and 4) analytically reviewing the recent literature evaluating the performance of HMOs.

Milbank Memorial Fund Quarterly/*Health and Society*, Vol. 58, No. 4, 1980
© 1980 Milbank Memorial Fund and Massachusetts Institute of Technology
0160/1997/5804/0537-52 $01.00/0

Fredric D. Wolinsky

Findings and Conclusions from
Previous HMO Performance Reviews

Although there has not yet been a definitive evaluation of HMO performance, the issue has been discussed in several hundred papers, articles, and books. In particular, there have been nine reviews of these evaluations (or, if you will, nine "state of the HMO field" papers), which are generally considered to be quite informative, if not authoritative. We shall begin by highlighting the findings and conclusions reached in these nine reviews, whose bibliographies, when taken collectively, form an extensive reference list.

The Klarman Review

In an early review, Klarman (1963) used data collected between 1950 and 1961 to assess the effects of prepaid group practice on hospital use (the term HMO had not yet been coined). A simple comparison of hospitalization days per 1,000 members per year showed that during 1950 the rate of use in prepaid plans ranged between 490 and 685 days, while in Blue Cross plans the rate was 888 days, and for the United States population as a whole the rate was 1,165 days. By the year 1960–1961 the rates in prepaid group practice plans had risen somewhat, ranging from 544 to 730 days, with Blue Cross rates rising markedly to 1,060 days, and the rate for the United States population rising to 1,265 days. Klarman considered nine theoretical explanations for the differences between hospitalization rates in prepaid group practice and in conventional health insurance plans. The explanations included differences in 1) the ranges of benefits; 2) the availability of ambulatory care services; 3) access to hospital beds; 4) the possibility of skimping on medical care in the prepaid plans (by failing either to diagnose or to treat existing medical conditions); 5) physician reimbursement; 6) physician control over hospitalization; 7) the role and use of specialists; 8) the willingness of primary care physicians to provide private home health care; and 9) the length of patient stays. After considering these explanations in turn, he concluded:

> Of increasing prominence today is the presence or absence of controls. Controls take various forms and may be carried out by

salaried physicians, by subscribers confronted with financial deterrents, or by self-insured plans in which the members actively cooperate; or controls may, in effect, be imposed by lack or inaccessibil-
ity of hospital beds. The organizational framework of group practice
may constitute a source of control over hospital use, as well as a
vehicle for providing ambulatory services. (Klarman, 1963:963–
964)

In essence, Klarman attributed the effect to the differences in the
controls that influence the organization, the physician, and the patient.

The Weinerman Review

Reviewing basically the same data as Klarman, Weinerman (1964:880)
focused on patients' perceptions of group medical care, arguing that
"the proof of group practice must lie, after all, in the satisfaction of
those who use its special type of service." He found that those enrolled in prepaid group practice were significantly more apt to express
complaints concerning "waiting times, inadequate explanations by
doctors, difficulty in getting house calls, and lack of interest in the
patient as a person" (Weinerman, 1964:885). From these data he
distilled the nature of the patient perception problem and cast it in
sociological terms: "The local practitioner is pictured as more ready to
accommodate the patients' wants . . . whereas the structure of group
practice is seen as bending the previously conditioned member to its
doctor-oriented rules of procedure" (Weinerman, 1964:886).
Weinerman (1964:887–888) went on to sketch the implications of the
problem: "Most importantly, the attitudes of patients—whether rational or not—profoundly affect the degree to which the program
succeeds in its function, that of protecting its members' health. . . .
The uneaten specialty on the dinner plate in the most excellent of
restaurants makes little contribution either to nutrition or appetite."
   In essence, Weinerman was offering a radically different explanation for the smaller number of hospitalization days in prepaid group
practice. He implied that it may not be the greater efficiency in
prepaid group practice, but the fact that such alternative health care
delivery systems were just so much less "acceptable" (i.e., in terms of
the expected and traditionally personal patient-practitioner relationship) that they resulted in a decline in health service utilization.

The Donabedian Review

Donabedian's (1969) review is more comprehensive than either Klarman's or Weinerman's, and was prepared without reference to them in order to maintain an independent view. Donabedian studied choice of plan, subscriber satisfaction, utilization of ambulatory and hospital services, and the quality of care. He concluded that the major reasons that individuals enroll in a prepaid group practice plan (PGP) (when given the choice through employee benefits) are geographic proximity, not having a private physician as a regular source of care, not being ideologically opposed to "socialized medicine," and the wider range of benefits. Once the employees had chosen membership in prepaid group plans, they were apt to complain about the impersonality of care, the clinic or charity medical care atmosphere, long waiting periods to see a physician, and the difficulty of obtaining house calls. On the other hand, the same subscribers felt that they received good quality medical care in the prepaid group practice, but credited the quality to the availability of technical, diagnostic, and consultative resources rather than to the quality of the physicians themselves. With regard to utilization, Donabedian (1969:11) argued that "the key question is not what is the level of utilization that is associated with any system of organizing care but what precisely happens to utilization and why." In other words, the utilization question should focus on whether the utilization rate is appropriate rather than on what the actual rate is. After an analysis stratified according to disease category (even though the data did not provide a clear answer to the question), Donabedian (1969:15) concluded that "the findings are consistent with the conclusion that [conventional insurance plans] overhospitalize for the common respiratory conditions and the more minor surgical conditions such as benign neoplasms, tonsillectomies and accidental injuries."

In addition to showing that the prepaid plans reduced costs (through lowered hospitalization rates) while maintaining appropriate levels of utilization, the data indicated further cost reductions from the substitution of cheaper ancillary services for the more expensive physician services (also where appropriate). Overall, Donabedian (1969:24–25) presented a very strong case for "the capability of prepaid group practices to achieve a more rational pattern in the use of medical resources, its ability to control costs, and the greater protection it generally offers against the unpredictable financial ravages of illness."

The Greenlick Review

Building on the earlier reviews, and making ample use of the massive data resources of the Kaiser Foundation Hospitals' Health Services Research Center, Greenlick (1972) assessed the impact of prepaid group practice on American medicine. As in the previous studies, he concluded that comprehensive coverage at a reasonable premium was the major attraction bringing subscribers into prepaid group practices. Greenlick (1972:110) also found that "the expenditures for providing medical care services for a total population covered by prepaid group practice programs are less than the expenditures for care to similar populations covered in the traditional individual fee-for-service system." The reduced cost, however, could not be attributed to efficiencies of scale, but rather arose from "system efficiencies," such that "by integrating the financing and the organization of medical care, PGP can reduce incentives for the physician or the population to prefer that equivalent services be provided on an in-patient rather than on an out-patient basis." In essence, Greenlick concluded that although all the data were not yet in, it was clear that prepaid group practices had several major advantages over conventional plans, the advantages stemming from the different incentives placed before physicians and patients alike.

The Roemer-Shonick Review

Building on Donabedian's, Klarman's, and Weinerman's reviews, and updating them with data from more recent studies, Roemer and Shonick (1973) prepared an extensive review of HMO performance. They focused their review on subscriber composition, participation of physicians, utilization rates, quality assessments, costs and productivity, health status outcomes, and patient attitudes. After reviewing the data, they concluded that

> the "prepaid group practice" (PGP) model of HMO continues to yield lower hospital use, relatively more ambulatory and preventive

service, and lower overall costs (counting both premiums and out-of-pocket expenditures) than conventional open-market fee-for-service systems. Economies of scale are still not proved. New data point to reduced disability from the PGP model of HMO, as well as to more favorable consumer attitudes (based mainly on the economic advantage, in spite of certain impersonalities of clinics) than exist toward conventionally insured private solo practice. The medical care foundation [individual practice association] . . . has yielded some evidence of economies in physician's care, but none in hospital use. (Greenlick, 1972:271)

Having built up HMOs as the answer to the crisis in health care, Roemer and Shonick go on to identify the two "principal hazards" that are inherent to the HMO concept: 1) the notion of inequitable "risk" selection, in which the HMO accepts as enrollees only the healthy, for whom the provision of health care is relatively inexpensive; and 2) the provision of poorer quality care through skimping. Moreover, these authors warn that once IIMOs move into the mainstream of American health care it will become even more important to maintain vigilance to detect these two hazards, because both the critical approach to a new idea and the self-regulation of a new industry will wear off.

The Gaus et al. Review

Gaus et al. (1976) examined enrollment selectivity, utilization of services, accessibility of care, and patient satisfaction in ten HMOs serving Medicaid patients as opposed to the fee-for-service Medicaid population. With respect to utilization, Gaus et al. found a significant difference in hospitalization only for staff and group models, not for individual practice associations (IPAs). Gaus et al. (1976:3) concluded "that capitation payment to an HMO alone is not significant enough to produce major changes in utilization and that organized multispecialty group-practice arrangements with largely salaried physicians may be more significant." This indicates that some incentives (those related to the organizational delivery of care) are more effective than others (those related to financing). Gaus et al. also found that original health status, use of ambulatory services (including preventive services), patient satisfaction, and access were remarkably similar in both the general Medicaid population and the HMOs.

The Luft Reviews

In three recent papers, Luft (1978a, 1978b, 1979, 1980a; see also his 1979 paper and his forthcoming book, 1980b) has presented the most detailed and critical reviews of the literature on HMO performance to date (even though he makes the serious mistake of assuming that the results of each study should be given equal weight in assessing HMO performance). In particular, from a comprehensive review of the primary literature he has focused on the performance issues of how HMOs actually save money, why they appear to provide more preventive services, and whether they lower the rate of growth of medical care costs. Demonstrating that total costs (both premiums and out-of-pocket expenditures) are from 10 to 40 percent lower in HMOs than in conventional health insurance plans, Luft (1978a:1336) notes that "most of the cost differences are attributable to hospitalization rates about 30 percent lower than those of conventionally insured populations . . . due almost entirely to lower admission rates. . . . There is no evidence that health maintenance organizations reduce admissions in discretionary or unnecessary categories; rather, the data suggest lower admission rates across the board."

According to Luft, there are three possible interpretations of these data: 1) given that discretionary care exists in all categories of hospitalization, an effective HMO may limit discretionary use across the board; 2) self-selection may have the effect that healthier people, who don't need as much hospitalization, come into HMOs; and 3) HMOs may be skimping at the same time that conventional insurance plans "overtreat" discretionary cases. With regard to the issue of whether or not HMOs provide more health maintenance than conventional insurance plans, Luft (1978b:163–164) concludes that "the greater use of preventive services by HMO enrollees appears to be attributable to their better financial coverage, not the preventive care ideology [purported to exist in HMOs]. When people have full coverage for 'preventive' ambulatory visits, they have at least as many, if not more, services under the F[ee] F[or] S[ervice] system than in an HMO. These results are entirely in accord with data for hospitalization— HMO enrollees seem to get fewer services if everything else is held constant."

Focusing on the ability of HMOs to reduce the growth rate of medical care costs, Luft (1980a:1) concludes that "since the early

1960s, total costs for HMO enrollees have grown at a slightly lower rate than for people with conventional insurance coverage. Hospitalization rates show substantial reductions within specific HMOs over a 20 year period." Some of the HMOs' long-term reductions in hospitalization, however, may merely reflect changes in the age-sex mix of their enrollment populations.

Summary

In general terms, these reviews seem to agree on five points: 1) Hospitalization rates in HMOs are up to 45 percent lower than those in conventional insurance systems (this is clearly the case for PGP models, although it is not so clear for IPA models) 2) Total costs are less in HMOs than in conventional insurance systems (again, largely because of lower hospitalization rates, and more pronounced in PGP than in IPA models). 3) Seemingly higher levels of preventive care utilization in HMOs may actually be a reflection of the more extensive coverage that they offer in comparison with conventional health insurance plans. 4) HMO enrollees tend to be more satisfied with the technical aspects of the medical care they receive than are those in conventional insurance plans, but the conventionally insured are more satisfied with their patient practitioner relationships. 5) Although the evidence on the quality of care received in HMOs is not complete, the quality appears to be at least equal to, if not better than, that received in the average conventional insurance plans. Nonetheless, the most important and agreed-upon point to emerge from these reviews is that *although reduced costs and lower hospitalization rates in HMOs are rather well documented, we still do not know how they are achieved.*

Defining HMOs and Their Incentive Structures

Although the nine reviews discussed above claim to have accurately assessed the performance of HMOs, there are two general sets of problems that they (and the studies on which they are based) have failed to consider in sufficient detail. That is, in order to accurately assess the performance of HMOs, and especially to determine their potential for a major role in any form of national health insurance (NHI), one must first be cognizant of the various problems that preclude their simple, direct assessment. Specifically, one must consider the definitional problems of what an HMO actually is, distinguish some of the basic types of HMOs from each other, and delineate the general and specific structural incentives and disincentives that affect HMO performance.

Definitional Problems With the HMO Concept

Like the confusion and controversy surrounding NHI (see Wolinsky, 1980), much of the debate and furor over HMOs may be traced to definitional problems, as a result of which different groups *talk by* rather than *talk to* each other. This confusion occurs because the historical conception of HMOs as Kaiser Health Plan (or Ross-Loos) groups, the legislative definition of HMOs provided by PL 93-222, and the contemporary definition of HMOs as any prepaid health care delivery system, do not agree. To be sure, the PL 93-222 (1973:2) definition, with the DHEW (1974) modifications in brackets, is the most specific: "For purposes of this title, the term 'health maintenance organization' means a legal entity which (1) provides [or arranges for the provision of] basic and supplemental services to its members in the manner prescribed by subsection (b), and (2) is organized and operated in the manner prescribed by subsection (c)." Subsection (b) contains four subsections and subsection (c) contains eleven, all in bureaucratese, and all followed by an entire section of definitions. Thus, although the PL 93-222 definition (as amended by PL 94-460) is the most specific, it is generally used only to distinguish between federally qualified and nonqualified (for feasibility grants and guaranteed start-up loans) HMOs, because it is so cumbersome.

The traditional Kaiser Health Plan definition of HMOs (cf. Greenlick, 1972), while somewhat easier to comprehend than PL 93-222's definition, is not without its own problems. In the main, this traditional definition suggests that all HMOs are closed-panel, hospital-based, group practice models, with enrollment restricted to members of the founding industrial groups (e.g., the Kaiser shipbuilding industries) and subsequent corporate sponsors. The proliferation of HMOs not sponsored by industry, of open-panel plans, and the enrollment of the unemployed and aged under Medicaid and Medicare contracts make this traditional Kaiser Plan imagery less than optimal.

Accordingly, a more general definition is necessary in order to include the numerous variations on the HMO theme that are currently in existence. Luft (1978a:1336) has used the following definition, which is also well suited to the present paper: "An organization will be considered an HMO if it assumes a contractual responsibility to provide or assure the delivery of health services to a voluntarily enrolled population that pays a fixed premium that is the HMO's major source of revenue." This definition allows us to focus on the larger issue of the performance of HMOs in general, and also allows us to compare and contrast the performances of the specific types of HMOs.

A Typology of HMOs

As we have already seen, there is a considerable amount of variation within the general category of HMOs. Nonetheless, it has become common for health services researchers, policy makers, and the public to delineate only two grossly distinct types in order to simplify comparisons (cf. Roemer and Shonick, 1973). These two types are generally referred to as "prepaid group practices" (PGPs) and "individual practice associations" (IPAs). In PGPs, all of the physicians are members of the same group practice and are reimbursed on the basis of a fixed salary or salary plus profit-sharing, with the group usually servicing the HMO exclusively, and either owning or contracting with the hospital(s) to which its patients are admitted.

On the other hand, the IPA is a loose federation of independent, individual physicians who agree to treat patients enrolled in a third party's HMO (frequently jointly sponsored by medical societies and insurance companies) in their own private offices, being reimbursed by the HMO on a fee-for-service basis (usually less an overhead discount rate of from 10 to 40 percent), and having less than 10 percent of their total patient load coming from the HMO. In essence, the difference is that, although both types of HMOs provide health care to their patients in a prepaid fashion, physicians in PGPs typically are salaried while physicians in IPAs are reimbursed on a fee-for-service basis, and health care is generally delivered from one central location (or satellites thereof) in PGPs, but is delivered out of the individual offices of the independent physicians in IPAs.

Such an arbitrary dichotomization of HMOs into PGPs and IPAs, however, is quite misleading in that there may well be more variation within each type than between types. Hester (1979:406) has argued that such an arbitrarily dichotomous conceptual model of HMOs is "greatly oversimplified. It neglects key characteristics of the internal structure of those institutions and uses aggregate measures of both inputs and outputs that often blur essential differences in performance." Empirical support for Hester's statement may be found in an analysis of the data reported in the *National HMO Census of Prepaid Plans, 1978* (Department of Health, Education, and Welfare, 1979). Regression analyses of those data reveal that, on the average, group model PGPs (essentially a group practice in which the physicians have a proprietary interest) experience 57.3 more days of hospitalization per 1,000 members than do staff model PGPs (where physicians' services are contracted on a straight salary basis, and where they have no proprietary interest). This difference is both statistically and substantively significant.

Even more compelling reasons than these differences in health outcomes are the theoretically significant structural input differences among HMOs. Table 1 briefly highlights this point by identifying only eight different HMO types according to their different structural configurations. As Table 1 indicates, not all HMOs are alike nor is it simply a case of PGPs versus IPAs. Although this point may seem obvious, it has been seriously overlooked in each of the most often cited reviews of HMO performance (cf. Luft, 1980a, 1978a, 1978b, 1979, 1980b; Gaus et al., 1976; Roemer and Shonick, 1973; Greenlick, 1972; Donabedian, 1969; Weinerman, 1964; Klarman, 1963). As a result, those reviews inevitably suffer from a considerable amount of "conceptual measurement error," because they (and the studies on which they are based) do not isolate the individual effects of the different structural incentives and disincentives of each HMO on its own performance. Accordingly, the five points on which the nine reviews do agree are rather difficult to accept, let alone interpret.

Structural Incentives and Disincentives for HMO Performance

The tandem goals of HMOs are to provide comprehensive health care of high quality to the members, and to provide that care as efficiently as possible. In other words, the *ideas* behind HMOs are *comprehensive health care* and *cost containment*. The principal design characteristic that

TABLE 1
Eight Different Types of HMOs

Structural Characteristics	HMO Models*							
	1	2	3	4	5	6	7	8
HMO owns the hospital, which serves only HMO subscribers	+	+	−	−	−	−	−	−
Physicians are:								
a) Salaried staff of HMO	+	−	−	−	−	−	−	−
b) Salaried group practice of HMO	−	−	+	−	−	−	−	−
c) Group practice legally separate from the HMO	−	+	−	+	−	−	−	−
d) One established group practice contracting their services to the HMO while maintaining their private group practice	−	−	−	−	+	−	−	−
e) Several established groups independently contracting their services to the HMO while maintaining their private group practices	−	−	−	−	−	+	−	−
f) Fee-for-service practitioners who contract individually to service HMO subscribers while maintaining their private practice for other patients	−	−	−	−	−	−	+	−
g) Fee-for-service practitioners who contract through a separate legal entity to serve HMO subscribers while maintaining their private practices for other patients	−	−	−	−	−	−	−	+

Source: Adapted from "A Report from the Pennsylvania Medical Care Foundation. Prepaid Health Care Primer for Practicing Physicians: Health Maintenance Organizations and Individual Practice Associations," 1978. *Pennsylvania Medicine* 81 (9):10–19.
*Examples of the eight models are: 1) Group Health Plan of Puget Sound (a classic "staff" model). 2) Kaiser Foundation Health Plan (a classic "group" model). 3) Harvard Community Health Plan. 4) Genesee Valley Group Health Association. 5) Med Center Health Plan. 6) Philadelphia Health Plan (a classic "network" model). 7) Employers Mutual of Wausau. 8) Forbes Health Maintenance Plan of Pittsburgh (a classic "IPA" model).

makes HMOs more likely than conventional health care delivery systems to deliver comprehensive health care is the fact that, in the HMO, health care is provided through virtually unlimited access to a complete health care system, with the consumer's cost for that unlimited access being fixed and prepaid. Similarly, the principal design characteristic that makes HMOs more likely to achieve cost containment is that the HMO is placed on a fixed budget, out of which it must meet all the expenses associated with providing the comprehensive health care. Underlying these two design characteristics is the premise that both goals of the HMOs (comprehensive health care and cost containment) can best be achieved by using a systems perspective in which all of the inputs are responsive to a centralized administration. In essence, in order to provide cost containment and comprehensive care, each health care delivery system (i.e., each HMO) must be well integrated in the structural sense. This is the case for all HMOs at the general level, but the extent of structural integration (i.e., structural incentives and disincentives that influence the delivery and consumption of health services) differs markedly from HMO to HMO.

For example, in HMO model 1 (from Table 1) the HMO assumes a supervisory and administrative role with the hospital and the physicians. As a part of this process various incentives (and disincentives) are brought into play, which ultimately affect the delivery and consumption of health services through their promotional or prohibitive nature. For physicians, these incentives may be external or internal. External incentives include a mandatory case review by colleagues to verify the need for a hospitalization recommended by the physician handling the case. Internal incentives include tying the physician's income to the HMO's profit and loss statement (e.g., when physicians are placed at risk for the fiscal health of the plan, after receiving a fixed basic salary). Under such conditions physicians may be more hesitant to hospitalize, especially in proprietary situations where skimping may be financially rewarding. As one physician remarked (see Enright, 1979:127), "Doctors are accustomed to hospitalizing people. When they're put at risk, they begin to examine what they're doing wrong."

A somewhat different picture illustrates HMO model 8 (from Table 1). In this IPA model the HMO does not assume a strict supervisory and administrative role over the hospital. In fact, it merely contracts with the hospital for the right to bring its patients there. Similarly, there are only very weak incentives for physicians to exercise cost containment, as they are not at risk for the financial success of the hospital, nor are their prospective hospital admissions so subject to their colleague's scrutiny. Accordingly, the IPA is not likely to be as successful at cost containment as is the PGP and, within categories of IPAs and PGPs, there will be a considerable variation in performance (e.g., hospitalization rates) because of different incentives and disincentives.

Specific Incentives and Disincentives

The general realm of incentives and disincentives operative in an HMO includes three categories based on who (or what) actually receives the impact of the incentive: 1) organizational incentives, 2) physician incentives, and 3) patient incentives. In theory, the principal *organizational incentive* is the capitation system of reimbursement. That is, for each of its members the HMO receives a fixed premium in return for providing all the health care the member may need. Accordingly, the HMO must stay within the budgetary constraints imposed by the capitation system, because it may not levy any additional charges. In practice, however, the principal organizational incentive is whether or not the HMO is at risk for hospitalization, and the extent to which it prepares for such risk. Although by definition all HMOs are at risk for hospitalization (as well as for all other expenses incurred while caring for their members under the capitation system), the true extent of an HMO's risk, and the manner in which it employs incentives to reduce hospitalization (and thus reduce costs), vary considerably. For example, the HMO may stress the increased use of preventive ambulatory or outpatient care in order to decrease hospitalization rates. The HMO may also try to reduce discretionary hospitalization by having all potential hospitalizations recommended by any individual physician reviewed for merit by a panel of other physicians. Finally, the HMO may reduce hospitalization by restricting the supply of hospital beds. The expected net effects of all of these organizational incentives is to reduce costly hospitalization while increasing relatively inexpensive preventive ambulatory or outpatient care.

There are two major types of *physician incentives* in HMOs: 1) the effect of their being placed at risk for the delivery of care; and 2) the effect of their being reimbursed on a salary system rather than on a fee-for-service basis. Being placed at risk for the provision of care essentially places physicians in a proprietary or profit-sharing situation. Under profit-sharing it is to the physician's advantage to decrease expenses, which can be most easily done by decreasing that very expensive item, hospitalization, especially since most hospitalization is initiated by the physician (cf. Andersen and Anderson, 1979; Fuchs, 1974; Wolinsky, 1980). Like the HMO organization itself, physicians have three major ways to reduce hospitalization. 1) They may increase the use of preventive care (reducing the need for hospitalization by early detection and treatment). 2) They may substitute outpatient care and procedures for inpatient care. Or 3) they may choose to reduce the discretionary use of hospital services, such as expensive but unnecessary laboratory tests, or to reduce discretionary hospitalization itself, for such operations as tonsillectomies, hysterectomies, appendectomies, and cholecystectomies (LoGerfo et al., 1979). Any of these approaches should have the net effect of reducing costs. The other major physician-oriented incentive (actually a disincentive) occurs when physicians are reimbursed through a salary (or salary plus profit-sharing) system rather than on a fee-for-service basis. Under the salary system (which is the physician's analogue to the organizational incentives of the capitation system), the physician receives the same income regardless of the number of times he or she sees a given patient, either in the office or in the hospital. As a result, under the salary system there should be a decrease in utilization of hospital and ambulatory care, since any discretionary service utilization represents a diseconomy for the physician. Accordingly, under a salary system the use of hospital and physician services should be less than in a fee-for-service system, all other things being equal.

The major *patient incentive* is the elimination of the out-of-pocket costs (either completely, or retaining only small coinsurance payments such as $2.00 per visit) usually associated with the consumption of health services. As a result of eliminating the financial barrier of out-of-pocket costs, patients tend to use more preventive and outpatient care (at least during their first association with the HMO), as well as to increase their demand for discretionary services. This should result in a considerable increase in overall ambulatory care, and a net long-term decrease in hospitalization (which, for those who had been conventionally insured, may have had relatively low out-of-pocket costs associated with it even before the HMO experience). Moreover, by eliminating out-of-pocket costs the potential for moral hazard is greater in HMOs than in conventional insurance plans. In other words, when the financial barrier of out-of-pocket expenses for physician utilization is removed, utilization of physicians' services should increase, all other things being equal.

As indicated above, we can directly assess the effect of any specific incentive only if the effects of the other incentives are held constant (or controlled). Unfortunately, it is difficult to study HMOs with the randomized experimental designs necessary to accomplish this task—the Seattle Prepaid Health Care Project (Diehr et al., 1976) notwithstanding. As a result, there have been few research situations (and few, if any, HMO performance reviews) in which clear and unambiguous tests of these incentives have been made. Therefore, future HMO performance studies and reviews will need to identify the different structural incentives operating, as well as the extent of their operations. Otherwise, combinations of countervailing incentives will continue to go undetected, obscuring the analysis and resulting in artificial evaluations of HMO performance. The results of several recent studies of health service utilization support this need to identify the structural characteristics of the specific health care delivery system, when health outcomes are being examined (Dutton, 1978, 1979; Kronenfeld, 1978; Shortell et al., 1977; Williams et al., 1978; Wolinsky, 1970).

Methodological Problems
in Evaluating HMO Performance

In addition to the general set of problems in defining HMOs and identifying their incentive structures, there is a second general set of problems of a more methodological nature, which the nine HMO performance reviews (and the studies on which they are based) have also failed to consider in sufficient detail. Specifically, there are three methodological issues that warrant further attention before any analytical review of the literature: 1) the effects of adverse self-selection and other population differences; 2) the development and selection of the health outcome measures used to assess HMO performance; and 3) the efficacy of survey versus plan-audit data collection techniques. Until these issues are carefully considered, summary statements concerning HMO performance will remain ambiguous, if not downright misleading.

Adverse Self-Selection and Other Population Differences

The first methodological issue to be considered is the two-sided question of adverse self-selection and other population differences. That is, if it is not possible to arbitrarily and randomly assign subjects to HMOs that represent the different combinations of incentives and disincentives, or to traditional health care delivery systems, the comparability of subjects in the different systems must be established. The possibility that voluntary HMO enrollees were significantly different from those not electing (volunteering) to enroll in HMOs was first suggested by Bashshur and Metzner (1970:106), and has come to be known as *the risk-vulnerability hypothesis:*

> Persons in the younger age groups, single persons and those with no dependents and those of lower socioeconomic status . . . may be viewed as having a lesser economic "stake" and therefore feeling themselves less vulnerable to serious economic loss in meeting health needs. Older persons, those with dependents, on the other hand, may be considered to run a greater economic risk or to be greater health risks (or both) and hence to be more vulnerable.

According to this hypothesis, the more vulnerable, either in the economic or the health sense, are more likely to enroll in HMOs than are the less vulnerable. If this is the case, HMOs might appear to be less cost efficient merely because they commence with a more morbid or potentially morbid population requiring more care (Berki et al., 1977a, 1977b, 1978; Ashcraft et al., 1978). For an excellent review of the relevant literature, see Berki and Ashcraft (1980).

The recent data on the effects of voluntary disenrollment from HMOs make the risk-vulnerability hypothesis even more important. Wollstadt et al. (1978) have shown that individuals without dependents voluntarily disenrolled from HMOs at a rate twice as fast as those with families. Moreover, among those with families, the larger the family size (i.e., the more economically vulnerable), the less likely was voluntary disenrollment. Those who voluntarily disenrolled also had a much higher rate of out-of-plan use (indicative of established patient-practitioner relationships) than those who remained in the HMO. Taken together, these data suggest that the voluntary disenrollment process may well be reinforcing the alleged effects of the risk-vulnerability hypothesis in creating noncomparable populations. That is, there may be not only an adverse self-selection process, but also a complementary adverse voluntary disenrollment process.

The other side of this problem is that even if perceived health risk and economic vulnerability are similar throughout the HMOs and the conventional comparison groups, measures of outcome (such as indicators of health service utilization) are not directly comparable unless they are first adjusted for other population characteristics (most notably age, sex, race, and socioeconomic status). Such adjustments are necessary because of the effects these predisposing and enabling factors have on the use of services (Andersen, 1968; Andersen and Newman, 1973; Aday et al., 1980). Thus, without adjustment for the differential distribution of these characteristics across the health care delivery systems to be compared, the effects of the HMO's incentives can not be accurately assessed, and may appear to be contradictory from study to study. This is evident in Table 2, which contains a summary of the unadjusted results of eighteen previous studies of HMO performance, made by calculating the ratio of utilization in the HMO to the utilization of the fee-for-service comparison system (Diehr et al., 1976). Ratios less than unity indicate better HMO performance, and ratios greater than unity indicate poorer HMO performance (relative to the fee-for-service comparison group). Considering the fact that "in 6 of the studies (4, 7, 9, 10, 11, and 12) sociodemographic correlates are either not provided or would suggest lower utilization in general by prepaid group practice patients" (Diehr et al., 1976:1), the ratios in Table 2 reflect how volatile unadjusted and otherwise noncomparable results may be.

Health Outcomes: The Comparison Measures

As we have already seen, performance studies of HMOs have focused, in the main, on hospital and physician utilization (Table 2). In fact, we limited our own explication of the incentives and disincentives that make up the various HMO types to a discussion of what the hypothesized effects of the various incentives would be on physician

TABLE 2

Ratios of Utilization and Cost Measures in Prepaid Groups to Those in Fee-for-Service Independent Practices, in Eighteen Studies*

Study	Hospital		Physician		Total Costs
	Admissions	Days	Visits	Surg. Proc.	
1. Densen et al. (1958)	.86	.91	—	.82	—
2. Anderson and Sheatsley (1959)	.57	.47	.92	.65	.90
3. Densen et al. (1960)	.80	.78	—	.79	—
4. Falk and Senturia (1960)	.85	.55	.77	.48	—
	.77	.40	1.61	.52	—
5. Densen et al. (1962)	1.01	1.00	—	—	.86
6. Williams et al. (1964)	1.04	1.05	1.32	1.05	.89
	1.11	1.00	1.13	1.61	—
7. Dozier et al. (1964)	.65	.81	1.06	—	.77
8. Shapiro et al. (1967)	—	.87	.98	—	—
9. Chamberlain (1967)	.60	.53	—	—	—
10. National Advisory Com. (1967)	.68	.69	.94	.42	.54
11. Perrott and Chase (1968)	.50	.47	—	.45	—
12. Perrott (1971)	.49	.49	—	.33	—
13. Robertson (1972)	.49	.40	2.13		—
14. Hastings et al. (1973)	.80	.76	1.48		—
15. Hetherington et al. (1975)	1.05	.42	1.07		.89
16. Broida (1975)	1.54	1.41	2.29		—
17. Reidel et al. (1975)	.57	.58	—		—
18. Wersinger et al. (1976)	.64	.63	—		—

*Based on material adapted by Thomas Dolan from an earlier compilation by Goldman and Steinwald (1973), and published in Diehr et al. (1976). Areas of Study in Table 2.

1. Health Insurance Plan of Greater New York (HIP) and Blue Shield (BS) of New York City.
2. HIP and Group Health Insurance, Inc. (GHI), of New York City.
3. HIP and GHI of New York City.
4. Steelworkers enrolled in three health care plans: Kaiser-Permanente (KP) Medical Care Program in California, Blue Cross (BC) plans in various locations, and commercial carrier plans in various locations.
5. HIP and union-administered fee-for-service plan in New York City.
6. KP-San Francisco Bay area, BC/BS New Jersey, and General Electric health plan in Utica, New York. A possible explanation for the comparable hospital utilization in the three plans is that the sample size was inadequate for reliable comparisons of hospital utilization. In addition, there were large geographical differences nationally among the three patent populations.
7. KP-California and BC/BS California. Patient discharge rate is shown in place of hospital admissions rate.
8. Old Age Assistance recipients in New York City served by HIP and fee-for-service practitioners.
9. Various unidentified prepaid group-practice plans nationwide, BC subscribers nationwide.
10. KP-California and population at large, California. Physician visits data compare KP-California with residents of the western U.S.
11. Federal employees enrolled in various prepaid plans and BC/BS plans nationwide.
12. Federal employees enrolled in Group Health Association (GHA) and in BC plan, Washington, D.C. Surgical procedures data compare federal employees in prepaid group practice plans and in BC plans nationwide.
13. Public school teachers enrolled in an unidentified prepaid group practice plan and an unidentified nonprofit plan.
14. Employees of Algoma Steel Corporation, Sault Ste. Marie, Ontario, enrolled in either the Sault Ste. Marie and District Group Health Association or an indemnification plan administered by the Prudential Insurance Company of America.
15. Subscribers to two prepaid group practice plans, two commercial carrier plans, and two "provider" plans (including BC/BS), in California. The authors attribute the relatively low admission rate of the commercial plans to their acceptance of fewer "high-risk" patients.
16. Prepaid enrollees compared with fee-for-service patients, Marshfield Clinic, Marshfield, Wisconsin.
17. Federal employees in the Washington, D.C., area enrolled under the high-option Blue Cross-Blue Shield Government-Wide Service Benefit Plan compared with those enrolled in Group Health Association, Inc.
18. Enrollees under a foundation-type plan, Health Watch, and a BS/BC-sponsored multispecialty prepaid group practice, Rochester, New York. Rates exclude maternity-related and psychiatric admissions.

and hospital utilization. Such traditionally limited approaches, however, pose two rather serious limitations for any subsequent analysis. *First*, by using only hospital and physician utilization as indicators of health outcomes, *a considerable part of the important conceptual domain of health services is omitted,* including nonphysician ambulatory visits, such as those by registered nurses, nurse practitioners, and physician assistants (which are often substituted for physician visits in HMOs), accessibility of care (time and distance to the physician's office as well as waiting time, both to schedule appointments and on arrival for scheduled appointments), patient satisfaction, the quality and continuity of care, the efficiency of care (economic issues), and the effectiveness of care (how well the delivery system is structurally integrated).

Second, by using only the gross summary measures of physician and hospital utilization, *a considerable amount of measurement error is introduced.* That is, when the only measure of ambulatory care is the gross per capita number of physician visits, or when the only measure of hospital care is either the gross admissions per 1,000 members or the per capita days of hospitalization, it becomes very difficult (if not impossible) to interpret (partition) the results accurately and ultimately evaluate the performance of HMOs. For example, knowing the gross per capita number of physician visits per year does not allow one to determine the effects of the various incentives, because although preventive and outpatient care may increase, the number of physician visits to hospitalized patients and the number of hospitalized patients themselves may decrease in a countervailing fashion. As a result, it would appear that physician visits were unaffected by the incentives operating in the HMO, when in fact the *mix* of physician visits had actually changed markedly. A similar example is provided by hospitalization rates. If the organizational and physician incentives operating in HMOs have the desired effects, those effects should be most prominent in terms of reduced surgical hospitalizations and surgery-induced hospitalization days. Using a gross hospitalization measure, however, might well mask the dramatic nature of the drop in surgical hospitalization. Accordingly, when health outcomes among different HMOs or conventional health care delivery systems are being compared and contrasted, it is necessary to determine the comparability and the degree of measurement error of the health outcome measures under examination.

Fredric D. Wolinsky

Data Collection Problems:
Patient Surveys versus Plan Audits

To collect data on health outcomes, either the patient survey or the plan-audits technique is used, each of which has its own methodological problems. In the plan-audits technique, data are collected by abstracting information from the record-keeping system of the health plan. In other words, an archival record search is made, and whatever utilization has been recorded by the plan for a given individual becomes that individual's utilization data for the HMO performance study. The single most important problem with the plan-audit technique is that only in-plan utilization is counted. Out-of-plan utilization (primarily ambulatory care services), which occurs to some extent in all plans and has been estimated to be as high as 53.9 percent of total utilization under extreme circumstances, goes unmeasured (Greenfield et al., 1978; Corbin and Krute, 1975; Bashshur et al., 1967, Freidson, 1961). Therefore, HMOs may appear to be more efficient (or not to be substituting more ambulatory care for less hospital care) because the plan auditing technique underreports the actual amount of health services used by plan members.

A second important problem with using plan-audit data occurs when data from different plans are to be compared. It is quite likely that each HMO institutes its own data collection and retrieval systems, each system being based on somewhat different definitions and having rather different degrees of completeness and accuracy. Accordingly, any observed differences in plan-audit data between HMOs may well be a function of the different ways in which records were kept or audited, rather than reflections of "true" differences in HMO performance.

On the other hand, the patient survey technique, while eliminating the problem of measuring the out-of-plan use of services (but not necessarily the problem of noncomparability), is much more expensive and time-consuming. In addition, patient surveys have their own special problems, including those in general recall, in the reporting of detailed specific information such as initial diagnosis, determining whether the services were used for preventive or for restorative care, and what specific treatment regimen was prescribed. In other words, while the patient survey technique captures out-of-plan utilization, it introduces general and specific recall problems (which, even though they occur in the form of intercoder reliability problems in plan-audits, are at least relatively constant across the smaller number of doctors and nurses, compared with the variance across the larger number of enrollees). Therefore, when the performances of HMOs are compared with each other or with those of conventional health care delivery systems (as control groups), the methods of data collection must be comparable.

A Review of HMO Performance

Having defined and identified the incentive structures and the methodological problems involved in studying HMOs, we now come to the analytic review of HMO performance itself. The most comprehensive and direct tack would be to collect the necessary and detailed information for all HMOs currently in operation. Such an approach, however, is clearly beyond the limits of the present paper. A more feasible approach is to briefly describe the current population of HMOs, by means of the most comprehensive census data available, and then to analytically review the recent primary literature on HMO performance in light of the issues described above.

A Brief Survey of Prepaid Group Practices

The most comprehensive and timely source currently available for data on all HMOs is the *National HMO Census of Prepaid Plans, 1978,* compiled by the Office of Health Maintenance Organizations (Department of Health, Education, and Welfare, 1979). The HMO census contains relevant data (albeit somewhat limited and not necessarily uniform) for each of the 203 HMOs in the United States as of November 30, 1978 (since that time the number of HMOs has grown by approximately 15 percent, with most of the newest HMOs being IPAs). These data indicate that total membership in HMOs has risen to 7,470,963 individuals, of which 1) more than two-thirds are in the larger HMOs (those with 100,000 or more members), 2) nearly three-fourths are in the older HMOs (those in operation for ten or more years), and 3) nearly half are in California. On the average, the monthly premium for families in all plans was $95.32 (covering the most comprehensive, high-option plan available).

In addition to these more general descriptive statements, Table 3 contains the means, medians, and standard deviations for the general membership, Medicare membership, Medicaid membership, federal employees membership, number of years in operation, hospitalization days per 1,000 members per year, and number of physician encounters per member per year by HMO type (loosely categorized as staff, group, or IPA models). The data in Table 3 show that these general characteristics of HMOs are as varied as the incentives that comprise their organizational structures. Moreover, comparing the relative sizes of the means, medians, and standard deviations clearly indicates that these distributions are quite skewed, providing more support for the argument that not all HMOs are alike and that they may not be directly compared without using the appropriate statistical controls.

Multivariate analyses of these data reveal that when HMO performance is defined as hospitalization days per 1,000 members per year, a significant prediction model can be obtained. That is, using dummy variables for group models, IPA models, and federal qualification as an HMO yields a regression equation having an explained variance of .11, in which the overall and individual effects of the dummy variables are all significant at the .05 level:

$$\text{Hospitalization days per 1,000 members per year} = 425.6 + 57.3 \text{ group} + 78.7 \text{ IPA} - 50.4 \text{ federal qualification} + \text{error.}$$

In other words, even though the HMO census data are far less than optimal, (i.e., the data are not adjusted for different age and sex distributions, nor is the classification of HMO types an exceedingly rigorous one), they indicate that HMO performance ranges from 375.2 days per 1,000 members per year in federally qualified staff models (where the greatest combination of incentives is in operation), to 504.3 days per 1,000 members per year in nonfederally qualified IPA models (where the least amount of incentives is in operation), with qualified and nonqualified group models in between at 432.5 and 482.9 days, respectively, per 1,000 members per year. These data provide additional support for the need to classify HMOs in terms of their combinations of incentives.

TABLE 3
Means, Medians, and Standard Deviations of HMO Characteristics by HMO Type in 1978*

HMO Types	Characteristic	Mean	Median	Standard Deviation
All HMOs (N = 203)	Enrollment:			
	General	37,923	9,061	159,759
	Medicare (N = 61)	6,170	497	16,743
	Medicaid (N = 35)	6,570	2,792	11,057
	Federal employee (N = 55)	10,608	1,188	28,529
	Number of years in operation	6.566	4.570	8.568
	Hospitalization days per 1,000 members per year	454.535	438.000	134.583
	Physician visits per member per year	3.282	3.287	0.951
Group Model HMOs (N = 78)	Enrollment:			
	General	69,963	3,463	248,192
	Medicare (N = 27)	10,678	1,035	23,824
	Medicaid (N = 9)	13,515	6,504	18,486
	Federal employee (N = 24)	18,336	2,754	39,753
	Number of years in operation	8.274	5.350	8.846
	Hospitalization days per 1,000 members per year	462.00	458.000	142.814
	Physician visits per member per year	3.202	3.250	0.9016

Staff Model HMOs (N = 52)			
Enrollment:			
General	19,186	9,851	37,716
Medicare (N = 19)	2,033	233	4,237
Medicaid (N = 14)	3,038	1,693	3,625
Federal employee (N = 18)	6,736	1,157	16,770
Number of years in operation	6.450	4.317	8.562
Hospitalization days per 1,000 members per year	410.710	394.500	112.281
Physician visits per member per year	3.319	3.350	0.827
IPA Model HMOs (N = 70)			
Enrollment:			
General	15,686	8,000	29,612
Medicare (N = 15)	3,299	185	7,278
Medicaid (N = 12)	5,484	2,107	7,561
Federal employee (N = 13)	1,703	922	2,712
Number of years in operation	4.919	3.550	8.122
Hospitalization days per 1,000 members per year	485.476	480.500	135.885
Physician visits per member per year	3.343	3.367	1.117

*Adapted from Department of Health, Education, and Welfare (1979).

An Analytic Review of the Recent HMO Performance Literature

We now proceed with the analytic review of the recent literature (1977 or later) on HMO performance, in light of the issues raised above. We focus on the recent literature for three reasons: 1) given the large volume of the extant literature, some limitations are necessary for practical reasons; 2) previous reviews have summarized the literature up to the last few years; and 3) the increased amount of information commonly provided in the more recent HMO performance studies permits a more thorough review of how certain conclusions have been reached, why they may be in error, and how they can be adjusted. To maximize continuity, these studies are reviewed in loosely defined groups based on the research project or institutional affiliation of the authors.

The Stanford Project. In an attempt to assess the effects of supply-side and demand-side incentives on the use of physician services, Scitovsky et al. (1979) conducted a twelve-month study of 4,200 individuals enrolled in two prepaid plans. All respondents were employees (or their dependents) of Stanford University, and were faced with a triple-choice situation (with a conventional Blue Cross-Blue Shield plan as the alternative). One prepaid plan was a Kaiser plan (a closed-panel, group model with completely integrated facilities), and the other was a fee-for-service group practice that was not at risk for hospital costs, with only 15 percent of its revenue coming from prepaid plans. The Kaiser plan had a token copayment for physician office visits ($1.00); the other prepaid plan had a 25 percent coinsurance charge for all physician visits. On the one hand, Scitovsky et al. hypothesized that the at-risk physician incentives in the Kaiser plan would result in lower physician utilization. On the other hand, it was expected that physician utilization would be lower in the fee-for-service group practice, because of the 25 percent patient coinsurance disincentive. Unfortunately, the design of the study does not allow these individual effects to be accurately partitioned, so that it is impossible to determine why whatever happened, happened. Nonetheless, Scitovsky et al. report that after allowance for age composition, socioeconomic status, health status, attitudes toward seeking care, length of membership in plan, family size, and plan satisfaction, the mean number of physician visits per person per year is about the same. After the data are adjusted for physician affiliation (having a plan physician as the regular source of care), however, Kaiser patients use .48 more physician and .79 more physician-plus-paramedic visits per person per year.

On the surface these data may seem to indicate that the Kaiser plan is less efficient, but there are at least three other plausible and competing interpretations that can not be rejected. First, the increase in the use of physician services may reflect a more aggressive substitution of ambulatory care for hospital care in the structurally well-integrated (plan-owned hospital facilities) Kaiser plan. Because hospitalization rates are not reported, such trade-offs can not be documented. Second, the relative effect of the coinsurance patient disincentive of the other prepaid plan may exceed the effect of the well-integrated Kaiser plan incentives, a possibility that can not be assessed with these data, either. Third, the differences in physician use may be a function of differential plan selection (cf. Wolinsky, 1976) based on the uncontrolled effects of social class characteristics (such as occupational prestige) as opposed to the controlled effects of socioeconomic status (such as income). That is, members of the Kaiser plan are predominantly support staff at Stanford, whereas members of the other plan are predominantly faculty. Therefore the different levels of the use of physician services may be a function of different lifestyles, which would not necessarily be reflected by income distributions. In an earlier paper assessing differences among those enrolling in the two plans, Scitovsky et al. (1978) simply declared that this was not the case, and proceeded to eliminate occupation and education from the analysis, concluding that family income and proximity to the health plan's medical center are the major factors affecting choice. Support for a rival lifestyle interpretation, however, comes from the fact that 45 percent more of the fee-for-service plan members (faculty) had a specific plan physician as their regular source of care than did Kaiser members, which may be interpreted as a basic function of their lifestyle. In sum, although the Scitovsky et al. study provides an interesting look at the use of physicians' services in two prepaid plans, methodological shortcomings prohibit any explicit tests of the structural incentives in operation.

The Seattle Project. As part of the Seattle Prepaid Health Care Project, Williams et al. (1979) examined the use of mental health services in a prepaid group practice and in an individual practice association (in which the physicians were not at risk). Although there were no out-of-pocket costs to enrollees in either plan, the IPA emphasized individual psychotherapy, and the PGP had a more diverse orientation, employing a variety of practitioner and therapeutic modalities. Although enrollees were not randomly assigned, and as a result there were some small (yet statistically significant) differences between the IPA and PGP enrollees, the resulting effects of adverse selection appear to be counterbalancing. Accordingly, these data invite a rather direct comparison. Williams et al. (1979:148) report: "The percent using any mental health services was twice as great in the PGP as in the IPP [IPA], although persons using any services tended to have more visits in the IPP as compared to the PGP. A significantly higher proportion of enrollees were hospitalized in the IPP than in the PGP."

These data support three hypotheses concerning HMOs: 1) In an HMO (especially in the PGP model), paramedical services will be actively substituted (where appropriate) for more costly physician services. 2) The better integrated the hospital services (PGP versus IPA), the lower the number of hospitalization days and admissions. And 3) the better integrated the HMO is overall (PGP versus IPA), the more likely it is to have a health maintenance orientation, as reflected in extending more preventive (e.g., counseling and paramedical mental health) services to its enrollees. Although they do not provide a direct test of Goldensohn and Fink's (1979) hypothesis (that psychiatric treatment reduces the use of other physician's services), the data given by Williams et al. (1979) appear at first to be consistent with it, as do those of Levin and Glasser (1979), in their survey of the use of mental health services.

On closer inspection, however, the data of Williams et al. more clearly support Mechanic's (1979, 1980) hypotheses that increased and internalized psychological or psychosocial bodily concerns result in high levels of symptom sensitivity and reporting, which should ultimately lead to the increased use of physician services. Using other data from the Seattle project, Diehr et al. (1979a:937) demonstrate this phenomenon, concluding that mental health utilizers "consumed more somatic services than other enrollees, even controlling for background variables." Patrick et al. (1978) have also demonstrated that patients with chronic emotional problems, and their families, use more physician services, and the authors question whether reduced costs can ever be the outcome of such increased emotionally induced physician utilization. Unfortunately, the Patrick et al. study does not provide any cost comparison data with which to evaluate the performance of its PGP.

In another aspect of the Seattle project, LoGerfo et al. (1979) studied the rates of surgical care in the PGP and the IPA. Specifically, they were interested in determining whether differences in the surgical rates existed and, if so, what accounted for them. Calculating exposure-adjusted ratios (IPA:PGP) resulted in gross ratios of 3.8:1 overall, 5.8:1 for tonsillectomies, 6.3:1 for hysterectomies, 1.7:1 for cholecystectomies, and 1.7:1 for appendectomies. These ratios indicate that much more surgery takes place in the IPA than in the PGP. To determine whether or not the differences are due solely to more appropriate discretion in the PGP, LoGerfo et al. (1979:1) used a variety of acceptable (but not definitive) algorithms to isolate only those surgeries that were "necessary, appropriate, or justified." After reviewing the data they found ratios of 2.8:1 overall, 2.8:1 for tonsillectomies, 6.8:1 for hysterectomies, 1.7:1 for cholecystectomies, and 1.4:1 for appendectomies. These ratios indicate that even when the analysis is restricted to justifiable surgery, the rates are significantly higher (for tonsillectomies and hysterectomies) in the IPA than in the PGP. Because the characteristics (including health status) of the enrollees in the IPA and the PGP are very similar, this points to the effect of organizational incentives as the reason for less surgery in the PGP. Because all of these surgical procedures were justified, LoGerfo et al. (1979:12) concluded that "there is substantial evidence to support the contention of underprovision of surgical care in prepaid group practices as an explanation for observed differences in surgical rates."

In short, the PGP appears to have been skimping on services. Although there are some measurement and sampling problems involved in this study (such as the determination of "justifiable" surgery, the rather small number of types of surgical procedures, and the fact that true estimates of the number of people at risk for each procedure are not available), they are not of sufficient magnitude to completely offset the serious implications of skimping. Therefore, these data suggest that although placing physicians at risk for hospitalization costs (as in the PGP, and not in the IPA) eliminates a significant amount of unnecessary surgery, the effects of the incentives are dysfunctional: they go beyond reducing unnecessary services, perhaps far enough to induce skimping on necessary and justifiable services. Moreover, a subsequent analysis (Diehr et al., 1979b) of the effects of the increased access to medical care (offered by both the IPA and the PGP) on health status produced poorer health status evaluations on four out of five self-report measures (after one year's experience in the HMO). In addition, after one year enrollees were less healthy on all five measures than those in a comparison group (in a limited access, or nonenrolled situation). Unfortunately, the subjective self-report nature of these data severely limits their reliability and validity, let alone their generalizability, as they are highly subjective and susceptible to the low levels of satisfaction with the patient-practitioner relationships typically found in HMOs (relationships that were neither examined nor described).

In a related paper, however, LoGerfo et al. (1978) reached a far more favorable conclusion concerning the quality (process) of care in the PGP—a conclusion consistent with Williamson et al.'s (1979) unpublished summary of the literature on the quality of care in HMOs. Focusing on the care associated with urinary tract infections, LoGerfo et al. (1978:494) found that the quality of care was significantly better in the PGP. Specifically, "there was a greater recording of pertinent history and physical exam items in the prepaid group practice; the prepaid group practice used markedly more urine cultures and slightly more urinalyses in the laboratory evaluation of these patients; and the prepaid group practice physicians tended to use a more uniform and appropriate set of antibiotics."

They also found better quality care processes in the PGP for common infections (LoGerfo et al., 1977) and hypertension management (LoGerfo, 1975). Merging these findings with their earlier study on the appropriateness of hospitalization leads one to conclude that although there may be more of a tendency to skimp (entirely) on the delivery of care in the PGP, once the decision to provide care has been made the quality of the delivered care is better than that of the IPA. An alternative explanation would be that PGPs skimp only on expensive services (i.e., surgery) and not on inexpensive ones (i.e., laboratory examinations). In either case, the implication of skimping remains, although the nature of the skimping (i.e., selective vs. across-the-board) is unclear. Unfortunately, the design of the Seattle project precludes any comparisons of either the PGP or the IPA with a conventionally insured control group (from the patient's perspective).

The Berki Papers. In four papers reporting on different aspects of a large study of a quadruple-choice health plan situation, Berki and his colleagues (Berki et al., 1977a, 1977b, 1978; Ashcraft et al., 1978) have presented the most detailed and sophisticated analyses of a field study to date. Focusing on enrollment choice and the expectation and actual use of services, they employed a variety of statistical controls and analytic approaches, and concluded that

> having a private physician as the source of care is the best single predictor, its absence predicting a higher probability of enrollment in the closed, and its presence in the open-panel HMO. Higher risk life state families, younger and with more children, are more likely to join the open-panel plan than the closed or retain BC/BS; higher incomes and larger numbers of chronic conditions appear to have the same effects. Higher levels of health concern, on the other hand, predict a greater probability of choosing the closed-panel plan. (Berki et al., 1978:682)

This indicates the occurrence of statistical interaction such that having or not having a private physician as a regular source of care specifies the effects of health concern and stage of family life cycle on enrollment choice. In the presence of a private family physician, health concern does not affect enrollment choice, whereas family life stage does (the open-panel HMO being chosen). The opposite holds true in the absence of a private family physician (the closed-panel HMO being chosen).

Perhaps more interesting than their actual analysis is the conceptual refinement that Berki et al. offer. Specifically, they divide the risk-vulnerability hypothesis into two parts, financial vulnerability and health risk. Focusing on financial vulnerability (uniquely operationalized as per capita income rather than family income, in order to focus on relative vulnerability), they argue that open-panel HMO selection (i.e., selecting IPAs) versus retention of Blue Cross and Blue Shield (the Blues) is the most clear-cut test, since the difference between these two plans involves only choosing among insurance plans (risk) and not among physicians (providers). Comparisons of per capita income of those retaining the Blues and those choosing the IPA, however, do not reveal significant differences. Comparisons of family incomes do reveal significant differences, although they are in the opposite direction (IPA families have approximately $2,800 more income and thus less financial vulnerability than Blues families). Unfortunately, Berki et al. ignore their own insights and focus on general comparisons of HMO versus Blues selection (rather than on specific comparisons of IPAs versus Blues), which show that enrollees in any type of HMO have significantly lower per capita incomes than their Blues counterparts. Nonetheless, following their own conceptual breakthrough (comparisons of IPA versus Blues enrollees), they find no support for the financial vulnerability hypothesis. Similarly, Berki et al. (1977b:112) conclude that in terms of illness conditions there is also "no evidence of adverse health risk self-selection in an employed population."

After the enrollees had had one year's experience in the HMO, Berki and his colleagues (Ashcraft et al., 1978) refocused their analysis on satisfaction, utilization, and costs. Following an insightful panel analysis of HMO enrollees who remained in the HMO throughout the study, as well as those who had retained the Blues throughout, they concluded:

> Lack of access to and dissatisfaction with previous sources of care distinguished the preenrollment experience of those who selected the closed-panel plans; their postenrollment experience produced increased satisfaction reflecting that their expectations in these areas were met. Continuing enrollees in closed-panel plans were somewhat less satisfied after a year of experience than they were earlier. Those who joined the open-panel did so because of the expanded benefits and financial advantages which, their postenrollment experience showed, were accurately perceived. . . . [C]ontinuing enrollees in both types of plans made fewer illness but more preventive visits; new enrollees used greater numbers of both types of services after enrolling than before. (Ashcraft et al., 1978:14)

These data support three hypotheses concerning HMOs: 1) that the use of preventive care will be increased, which may ultimately result in reduced overall costs (although beyond the diagnosis and treatment of hypertension and diabetes, the data are not very clear on this point); 2) that the overall use of ambulatory services increases (at least during the first year), apparently concomitant with a decrease in hospitalization (although these data are not presented); and 3) that HMO enrollees are more satisfied overall (as a function of increased general access), but their level of satisfaction declines somewhat over time (probably as a function of less than optimal patient-practitioner relationships in the closed-panel plans).

Kaiser Plan Studies. Focusing on consumer satisfaction, Pope (1978) used multivariate analytic techniques on data from samples of currently active and recently terminated subscribers to the Kaiser-Permanente Medical Care program. He found that, among current subscribers, satisfaction is the highest for those who have a regular plan physician, are older, and live in families who rate their own health as excellent. Pope found that those who terminated their enrollment, as a result of dissatisfaction with Kaiser, are more likely to rate their own families' health as less than excellent, do not have a regular plan physician, and have been local residents for quite some time. Although Pope carefully points out that these results may be a function more of expectations than of the delivery (or nondelivery) of medical care in HMOs (a problem that the data can not resolve), there are two other serious limitations on these data. First, the response rate is rather low among the active subscribers (65 percent) and extremely low (29 percent) among those terminating their membership; only 6 and 16 percent, respectively, did not respond because they could not be reached. Therefore the satisfaction expressed by the terminating sample is likely to be biased, overrepresenting outlier values. Second, because satisfaction data are not presented for a comparable group from the conventionally insured population, the effects of HMOs on satisfaction can not be determined.

Using data on enrollees in Kaiser-Permanente's Oregon region, Freeborn et al. (1977:115) assessed the relative effects of health and of socioeconomic status on the use of ambulatory services. Controlling for the effects of age and sex, they found "health status to correlate more highly than socioeconomic factors with the utilization of services.... An exception was the use of preventive services, which was not significantly related to health status measures but rather, for women, to education, and to a lesser extent, income."

Unfortunately, an overreliance on zero-order correlations casts doubt on the results of this attempt to explicate the relative causal effects of health and socioeconomic status on ambulatory care use. The data do, however, suggest that enrollment in an HMO does not bring about equity in the use of preventive services, especially when predisposing characteristics such as education are considered. In effect, these data indicate that even in the absence of financial barriers, health services (at least preventive ones) will not be used unless there is a concomitant predisposition (or preventive health orientation).

Using data on 3,892 individuals enrolled in the Kaiser Foundation Health Plan of Portland, Lairson and Swint (1978, 1979) focused on the determinants of preventive and nonpreventive utilization of medical care service. Employing a modified version of Aday and Andersen's (1975) framework for the study of access to medical care, Lairson and Swint obtained results from a series of regression analyses (both ordinary least-squares and logistic) indicating that, for nonpreventive services, utilization is a function of health status, age, and sex; for preventive services, utilization is a function of education (positive), income (positive for dependents' utilization only), and age (positive for the young and the old). These data support the interpretation suggested earlier, that although enrollment in HMOs may remove the economic disincentives that serve to restrict the use of preventive services, enrollment in the HMO alone does not produce equity in preventive health behavior. Rather, preventive health service utilization is closely related to lifestyle and the ability to successfully negotiate with the HMO's bureaucratic system, both of which may be proxy-measured by education. In short, once enabling barriers are removed, one has to be predisposed in order to use services. In the preventive services case (when health status is controlled), this reduces to the preventive health orientation, which is directly related to education. Because Lairson and Swint do not control for the effects of different lengths of plan membership, it is impossible to determine whether or not the effect of education on preventive service utilization decreases with continued exposure to the HMO and its alleged preventive health or health maintenance orientation.

Using data collected from three samples of low-income individuals (a group enrolled in the Kaiser Health Plan of Oregon, a matched group of Medicaid recipients, and a group enrolled in the Kaiser plan who also retained their Medicaid eligibility), Johnson and Azevedo (1979b) sought to assess two general hypotheses: 1) that the use of services and the resultant costs of low-income enrollees in a PGP model HMO would be lower than those for a matched Medicaid group; and 2) that the use of services and resultant costs of the low-income PGP enrollees would also be less than those for a matched group of Medicaid recipients who were concurrently enrolled in the

PGP. Their intent was to assess the cost-containment strategy of enrolling Medicaid recipients in PGPs, as opposed to the traditional fee-for-service system, and to assess the added costs (if any) of allowing the PGP-enrolled Medicaid recipients to retain their Medicaid privileges. Both of the general hypotheses were supported, implying that medical care expenditures for the Medicaid population (where the cost was $151 per capita per female under 65) can be reduced by enrolling them in PGPs (where the cost was $124 per capita for females under 65), as long as the PGP-enrolled Medicaid population is not concurrently allowed to retain its Medicaid eligibility (where the cost was $167 per capita per female under 65). Unfortunately, these data do not allow for any controls in terms of differential health status or the appropriateness of the care received, nor do they consider the out-of-plan use of the PGP sample. Accordingly, Johnson and Azevedo's conclusions are somewhat suspect, although the $27 to $43 cost reductions per capita per female under 65 may be of sufficient magnitude to weather any subsequent adjustments for such measurement error.

Other Studies.   Christianson and McClure (1979) have examined the competitive effects of HMOs on the delivery of care throughout their geographic area. Specifically focusing on the growth of HMOs in Hawaii (Christianson, 1978) and in the Minneapolis-St. Paul area, where there has been an explosion of HMO growth, Christianson and McClure (1979:812) found that "competition has helped to reduce hospitalization, contain costs and improve access to medical services. At the same time it has focused attention on consumer satisfaction with medical services, increased the range of consumer choice and given consumers better information about providers." Much of this advantageous effect of HMOs on competition (an effect based largely on anecdotal information), however, may be the result of circumstances unique to the Minneapolis-St. Paul situation. Other studies, however, have also demonstrated (to varying degrees) the competitive impact of HMOs on the larger geographic health care system (Lavin, 1978; Goldberg and Greenberg, 1977, 1979; Greenberg, 1977). In addition, Enthoven (1978a, 1978b) has theoretically assessed the potential of HMOs for systematic cost containment, and has reached a favorable conclusion for certain market situations. Accordingly, Christianson and McClure have tempered their earlier statements on the competitive effects of HMOs by noting that such effective competition is *most likely* to develop in communities meeting three conditions: 1) at least two reputable HMOs are available to the public; 2) employers contribute the same fixed amount for an employee, regardless of the plan the employee chooses, and the selection of cheaper plans brings a rebate to the employee (for the difference); and 3) efficient plans are allowed to increase their membership by offering better coverage at lower premiums.

Greenfield et al. (1978) set out to assess the extent of out-of-plan use of services by Medicare members enrolled in the Health Insurance Plan (HIP). Using data from HIP records and Social Security Administration files, they drew a 10 percent sample (N = 5,202) of HIP Medicare enrollees and a 0.5 percent sample (N = 4,548) of non-HIP Medicare beneficiaries living in the same area. They found that almost one-third of the HIP Medicare enrollees used out-of-plan services, which accounted for the bulk of the $47 per capita extra that it cost the Medicare system for their care as opposed to the general Medicare population. Thus, enrollment in an HMO (HIP) did not reduce, but actually increased the overall per capita cost of medical care. These results, however, may not be generalized because under Medicare the HIP enrollees were not at risk, even if they used out-of-plan services (because all bills were paid by Medicare anyway). Therefore, patient incentives for using only in-plan services did not exist, nor did HIP exert much pressure to minimize out-of-plan service utilization.

In comparing the hospital cost experience of three competing HMOs, Gavett and Smith (1978:328) focused on elaborating measures of hospital cost experiences. They argued that five factors affect these experiences: "1) the hospital service mix used, 2) the admissions rate, 3) the hospital mix used, 4) the length of stay, and 5) the intensity of resources used within a particular hospital service." Therefore each of these five factors must be taken into consideration when hospitalization costs are examined. Using data from an IPA, a centralized and fully integrated PGP, and a decentralized loosely integrated PGP (and controlling for these five factors), Gavett and Smith (1978:334) concluded that "the difference in risks selected into each of these plans, rather than the structure and controls within these plans and their financial incentives appear to explain most of the differences in hospitalization rates. Those faced with the likelihood of more serious health problems tended to elect the foundation plan, and those less likely to face serious problems elected one of the closed panel plans."

These data indicate that a modified version of the adverse selection problem is in effect, in which the most vulnerable enrollees choose IPAs in order to continue their existing patient-practitioner relationships, whereas the less vulnerable (who are less likely to have an ongoing patient-practitioner relationship to maintain) choose a PGP for purely economic reasons. This supports the Berki et al. (1977b) data presented earlier. Moreover, Gavett and Smith report that although HMOs reduce hospital costs, the *degree* of cost reduction (after controlling for the five factors) is not as high as the level generally attributed to HMOs. They are quick to point out, however, that the low level of hospital cost savings in their HMOs is probably the result of serious adverse selection, a substantially lower ratio of hospital beds to population in the community, compared with the national average, and the fact that the plan physicians were not effectively at risk for hospitalization costs. These data, then, suggest that traditionally successful HMO performances *may* be artifacts both of measurement error (not controlling for the five factors influencing hospital costs) and of adverse self-selection (comparison group problems), although they do not provide a definitive test of the plan's incentive structure.

As part of a larger demonstration project, Fuller et al. (1977) evaluated the utilization, cost, and satisfaction experiences of 834 Medicaid recipients experimentally enrolled in a PGP. Data were collected on the experimental group for the 22 months preceding, and the 22 months following their enrollment in the PGP. Data were collected on the Medicaid control group for the first 12 months after the enrollment of the experimental group in the PGP. The compositions of the two groups are strikingly similar. Analysis of the data (Fuller et al., 1977:705) indicates that for those enrolled in the PGP "ambulatory physician encounter rates decreased 15 percent, drug utilization was down 18 percent, hospital admissions decreased 30 percent, and hospital days declined 32 percent after enrollment."

When overall cost comparisons are made for a comparable benefit configuration (a dental rider was added to the PGP coverage to attract Medicaid enrollees), a 37 percent savings was realized over three years in the PGP compared with the Medicaid population. Unlike other Medicaid studies, that by Fuller et al. reported a voluntary dropout rate of only 2.5 percent, which they cite as indicating increased satisfaction and good acceptance of the care provided in the PGP. The low dropout rate, however, is more likely a function of the attractiveness of the dental rider in the PGP, which would not be available to the traditional Medicaid population. Unfortunately, Fuller et al. were *not* able to partition the reductions in health services utilization across even the broad categories of appropriate versus nonappropriate care. Accordingly, it is not clear exactly what occurred: Did the PGP skimp? Did the control group overserve? Or some of both?

Pett (1979:42), in a seemingly "well-contained, experimental opportunity," examined the differences in hospitalization rates between government enrollees in a staff model HMO and in an IPA. Because the enrollees in both plans were nearly identical (except for ethnic status), and because the cost and range of benefits in both plans were identical, Pett argued that the only explanation for the marked differences in hospitalization rates was the differences in organizational incentives and physician personnel. He found the admissions per year per 1,000 enrollees to be 56.8 in the staff model and 83.2 in the IPA; hospitalization days per year per 1,000 enrollees were 246.3 in the staff model and 381.7 in the IPA. Unfortunately, Pett was not able to accurately partition the extent of the differences due to each of five incentives that differed in the two HMOs: 1) the IPA physicians were motivated to increase admissions, as their incomes were directly related to their level of activity through their fee-for-service reimbursement system; 2) the staff model physicians were subject to organized peer review, but the IPA physicians were not (throughout most of the study); 3) the IPA physicians expressed considerably more resentment at the notion of control through peer review than did the staff model physicians; 4) the IPA delivered its care through a very loose federation of independent practices, and the staff model delivered all of its care at the well-integrated group practice site; and 5) 80.8 percent of the IPA physicians were foreign medical graduates, whereas 75.7 percent of the staff model physicians were trained in the United States. As a result, although Pett was able to show rather conclusively that the IPA had higher hospital utilization, he could not determine which incentives were responsible. Moreover, because he did not control for the appropriateness of hospitalizations, he could not determine whether the difference was due to skimping in the staff model or to overuse in the IPA. Finally, because he did not report any data on ambulatory care use, he could not determine whether the staff model was substituting outpatient care for inpatient care.

To determine why individuals and families disenroll from HMOs, Wollstadt et al. (1978) analyzed enrollment and disenrollment data (both voluntary and mandatory) for Medicaid enrollees in the East Baltimore Medical Plan. They found that voluntary disenrollment peaked 3.6 months after the plan had opened, while mandatory disenrollment remained relatively constant throughout the study, suggesting that initial enrollees had higher rates of disenrollment than later enrollees. This may indicate start-up difficulties in establishing patient-practitioner relationships en masse, a hypothesis supported by Forthofer and Glasser (1979). They have shown that the use of physician services by new enrollees in a PGP is significantly lower during their first quarter of enrollment, but their use of diagnostic procedures (laboratory and radiological) is rather high, presumably as a function of the need to establish baseline data. On the other hand, Johnson and Azevedo (1979b) have shown that, over four years of continuous enrollment in a Kaiser Plan, a study of 828 low-income enrollees did not reveal any changes in the annual rate of office visits or drug utilization. Similarly, Mullooly and Freeborn (1979) report that in their six-year (with quarterly data points) retrospective cohort study of Kaiser-Permanente of Oregon, not only were there no start-up costs (either to patients or the HMO) for ambulatory care utilization during a cohort's enrollment, but also the utilization rates for high users, nonusers, and average users all remained relatively constant throughout the study period.

Taken together, these data seem to indicate that although there may not be any start-up costs for the HMO (in terms of a first enrollment quarter utilization surge), there may be some start-up costs for the enrollee (in terms of obtaining a personalized patient-practitioner relationship). When enrollment and utilization are considered at the same time, the potential start-up costs for the enrollees appear to be higher than those for HMOs. Wollstadt et al. (1978:148) found that "of those in the plan for six months, three-quarters of the continuously enrolled had used plan facilities, while less than one in five of the voluntarily disenrolled sought care from the plan. . . . When comparing those enrollees who used the plan facility at least once, differences in facility use between these three groups [enrolled, voluntarily disenrolled, and mandatorily disenrolled] disappeared." Thus, it would appear that disenrollment is a function of poor or nonexistent patient-practitioner relationships of the traditionally personal style, problems that would be at a peak during the start-up period. This interpretation, however, is somewhat clouded by the fact that these Medicaid recipients are not faced with the same incentive structure as the normally employed HMO population. That is, there is no cost-saving incentive for the Medicaid enrollee to "suffer through" the HMO and its initial poor patient-practitioner relationship. Medicaid enrollees who disenrolled were given back their Medicaid cards, entitling them to comprehensive health care also without cost.

Using data on the use of ambulatory services in five delivery systems, Dutton (1979) focused on the effects of the gross organizational differences in solo practice, fee-for-service group practice, prepaid group practice, public clinics, and hospital outpatient emergency room departments. Multiple regression analyses of her data (Dutton, 1979:221) showed that "sources used primarily by the poor—hospital outpatient departments, emergency rooms, and public clinics—contained important structural and financial barriers, and had the lowest rates of patient-initiated use. The prepaid system in contrast, maximized patients' access to both preventive and symptomatic care and did not seem to inhibit physician-controlled follow-up care."

As a result, the poor, who are not likely to be HMO enrollees because they are generally not members of the employed groups to whom HMO benefits are offered (except through relatively rare Medicare and Medicaid contracts), are deterred from seeking both preventive and somatic care. At the same time, the fee-for-service system encourages physicians to expand their follow-up services, which is quite an expensive process (relatively speaking) for the poor who must use it.

Summary and Conclusions

Two Common Themes

Although the data and conclusions reviewed in this paper were quite varied and often contradicted each other, two common themes can be identified, which future HMO performance studies should take into consideration. *First,* the research designs employed have not been framed clearly enough, in varying degrees, to provide conclusive evidence to support or reject the hypothesized effects of the incentive and disincentive structures. That is, even in the more sophisticated designs, some complications exist, either because they were not anticipated, or because adjusting the research design to compensate for them was impractical. *Second,* the orientation of these studies has been far more descriptive than analytic (in the deductive, hypothesis-testing sense). Although this tendency is typical for a developing substantive area, a continuation of this trend would be wasteful. Unfortunately, just such a pursuit has recently been suggested for future research on HMOs (see Hester, 1979).

What We Can Say About HMOs

As a result of these two common themes, very little can be conclusively stated about the performance of HMOs. We can, however, make four statements: 1) The total cost for the delivery of health care in an HMO is less than that in a conventionally insured delivery system. 2) The total cost for the delivery of health care in a PGP appears to be less than that in an IPA. 3) The major factor involved in reducing the costs reflected in statements 1 and 2 is the lower level of hospitalization usually found in the HMO (especially in the PGP) 4) *We do not know how or why* statements 1, 2, and 3 are true.

Methodological Deficiencies in the HMO Literature

In addition to these four statements on HMO performance, we may also identify the three most serious deficiencies in the literature of HMO performance. *First,* there is *the design or biased comparisons problem.* That is, in addition to the absence of randomized controlled experimental designs, unadjusted and/or partial comparisons between PGPs, IPAs, and control (conventionally insured) groups are tenuous, at best. This problem may be either blatant (as in the total absence of a control group), or subtle (as in adverse selection). *Second,* there is *the problem of reciprocal causation.* That is, while a study may, for example, focus and report performance data on physician utilization, it may neglect to consider the effects of that physician utilization on hospitalization experiences, and vice versa. In short, the performance of

HMOs on one aspect of the use of services is statistically considered in isolation from the other aspects of service utilization, although they are considered to be related in the conceptual model. *Third,* there is *the problem of reliability and validity of measurement.* For example, when hospitalization is the performance indicator under examination, only the gross rate is measured, rather than the five factors that comprise gross hospitalization experiences.

Emergent Hypotheses

Finally, although the data do not permit us to make any more definite statements about the performance of HMOs, four additional hypotheses have emerged that warrant future study. *First,* those who are already ill apparently pick the IPA (in multiple-choice situations) because they already have a private physician as their regular source of care, as a result of their being ill. That is, if you are already ill, the chances of your having seen a physician on a regular basis (concerning your illness) are higher than if you are not ill. When presented with a multiple-choice situation, it would be more reasonable for you to choose the IPA so that you could continue your patient-practitioner relationship. *Second,* there may well be an anomaly concerning the quality of care received in HMOs. Although PGPs may be more likely to skimp on surgical care than IPAs (or, it would be assumed, than conventional health care systems), the quality of care actually received in the PGP is better. This may reflect the difficulty of simultaneously attaining the HMO's tandem goals of comprehensive health care and cost containment. *Third,* disenrollment from the HMO, among non-Medicaid and non-Medicare enrollees in PGPs, may be a function of the lower quality and quantity of the traditionally personal patient-practitioner relationship to which they have been accustomed. This would be especially critical during initial enrollment periods when patients' demand for personal relationships may considerably exceed the providers' potential supply. *Finally,* enrollment in the HMO may not produce equity in the use of preventive health services; rather, the use of preventive health services may continue to be a function of social class characteristics (especially education and occupational prestige). That is, if, as Luft (1978b) has argued, HMOs do not provide a more preventive orientation than the fee-for-service system, then the effects of education and occupational prestige on preventive service utilization will not be diluted simply by exposing individuals to HMOs. On the other hand, if HMOs really do have more of a health maintenance orientation (i.e., if Luft is wrong), then the effects of education and occupational prestige on preventive service utilization should be diluted with increased and continued exposure to HMOs.

References

Aday, L.A., and Andersen, R. 1975. *Access to Medical Care.* Ann Arbor: Health Administration Press.

———, Andersen, R., and Fleming, G., 1980. *Health Care in the United States: Equitable for Whom?* Beverly Hills: Sage Publications.

Andersen, R. 1968. *A Behavioral Model of Families' Use of Health Services.* Chicago: Center for Health Administration Studies.

———, and Anderson, O. 1979. Trends in the Use of Health Services. In Freeman, H.E., Levine, S., and Reeder, L., eds., *Handbook of Medical Sociology,* 3d edition. Englewood Cliffs: Prentice-Hall.

———, and Newman, J. 1973. Societal and Individual Determinants of Medical Care Utilization in the United States. *Milbank Memorial Fund Quarterly/Health and Society* 51 (Winter):95–124.

Anderson, O.W., and Sheatsley, P.B. 1959. *Comprehensive Medical Insurance: A Study of Costs, Use and Attitudes Under Two Plans.* New York: Health Information Fund.

Ashcraft, M., Penchansky, R., Berki, S.E., Fortus, R., and Gray, J. 1978. Expectations and Experience of HMO Enrollees after One Year: An Analysis of Satisfaction, Utilization, and Costs. *Medical Care* 16:14–32.

Bashshur, R.L., and Metzner, C.A. 1970. Vulnerability to Risk and Awareness of Dual Choice of Health Insurance Plan. *Health Services Research* 5:106–113.

Bashshur, R., Metzner, C., and Warden, C. 1967. Consumer Satisfaction with Group Practice: The CHA Case. *American Journal of Public Health* 57:1991–1999.

Berki, S.E. and Ashcraft, M.L.F. 1980. HMO Enrollment: Who Joins What and Why: A Review of the Literature. *Milbank Memorial Fund Quarterly/Health and Society* 58 (Fall):588–632.

———, Ashcraft, M., Penchansky, R., and Fortus, R. 1977a. Health Concern, HMO Enrollment, and Preventive Care Use. *Journal of Community Health* 3:3–31.

————, Ashcraft, M., Penchansky, R., and Fortus, R. 1977b. Enrollment Choice in a Multi-HMO Setting: The Roles of Health Risk, Financial Vulnerability, and Access to Care. *Medical Care* 15:95–114.

————, Penchansky, R., Fortus, R., and Ashcraft, M. 1978. Enrollment Choices in Different Types of HMOs: A Multivariate Analysis. *Medical Care* 16:682–697.

Broida, J.H., Lerner, M., and Lohrenz, F.N. 1975. Impact of Membership in an Enrolled, Prepaid Population on Utilization of Health Services in Group Practice. *New England Journal of Medicine* 292:780–783.

Chamberlain, J. 1967. Selected Data on Group Practice Prepayment Plan Services. *Group Health and Welfare News* 8, special supplement: i–viii.

Christianson, J.B. 1978. *Do HMOs Stimulate Beneficial Competition?* Excelsior, Minn.: InterStudy.

————, and McClure, W. 1979. Competition in the Delivery of Medical Care. *New England Journal of Medicine* 296:812–818.

Corbin, M., and Krute, A. 1975. Some Aspects of Medicare Experience with Group Practice Prepayment Plans. *Social Security Bulletin* 38:3–11.

Densen, P.M., Balamuth, E., and Shapiro, S. 1958. *Prepaid Medical Care and Hospital Utilization.* Chicago: American Hospital Association.

————, Jones, E., Balamuth, E., and Shapiro, S. 1960. Prepaid Medical Care and Hospital Utilization in a Dual Choice Situation. *American Journal of Public Health* 50:1710–1726.

————, Shapiro, S., Jones, E.W., and Baldinger, I. 1962. Prepaid Medical Care and Hospital Utilization. *Hospitals* 36:62–68, 138.

Department of Health, Education, and Welfare. 1974. *Federal Register,* Vol. 38, No. 203. Washington, D.C.: Government Printing Office.

————. 1975. *Health Maintenance Organizations: Guidelines for Subparts B, C, D, E, and G.* Washington, D.C.: Government Printing Office.

————. 1979. *National HMO Census of Prepaid Plans, 1978.* Washington, D.C.: Government Printing Office.

Diehr, P.K., Richardson, W.C., Drucker, W.L., Shortell, S.M., and LoGerfo, J.P. 1976. *The Seattle Prepaid Health Care Project: Comparison of Health Services Delivery. Chapter 2: Utilization: Ambulatory and Hospital.* Seattle: School of Public Health and Community Medicine, University of Washington.

————, Williams, S.J., Shortell, S.M., Richardson, W.C., and

Drucker, W.L. 1979a. The Relationship between Utilization of Mental and Somatic Health Services among Low Income Enrollees in Two Provider Plans. *Medical Care* 17:937–952.

———, Richardson, W.C., Shortell, S.M., and LoGerfo, J.P. 1979b. Increased Access to Medical Care: The Impact on Health. *Medical Care* 17:989–999.

Donabedian, A. 1969. An Evaluation of Prepaid Group Practice. *Inquiry* 6:3–27.

Dozier, D., Krupp, M., Melinkoff, S., Shwarberg, C., and Watts, M. 1964. *Report of the Medical and Hospital Advisory Council to the Board of Administration of the California State Employees Retirement System.* Sacramento: The State of California.

Dutton, D.B. 1978. Explaining the Low Use of Health Services by the Poor: Costs, Attitudes, or Delivery Systems. *American Sociological Review* 43:348–368.

——— 1979. Patterns of Ambulatory Health Care in Five Different Delivery Systems. *Medical Care* 17:221–243.

Ellwood, P. 1971. Health Maintenance Organizations, Concept and Strategy. *Hospitals* 45:53–56.

Enright, S.B. 1979. I.P.A.: The Initials That May Mean Your Future. *Medical Economics,* February 19, 124–137.

Enthoven, A.C. 1978a. Competition of Alternative Health Care Delivery Systems. In Greenburg, W., ed., *Competition in the Health Care Sector: Past, Present, and Future.* Washington, D.C.: Federal Trade Commission, Bureau of Economics.

———. 1978b. Consumer-Choice Health Plan. *New England Journal of Medicine* 298:650–658 and 298:709–720.

Falk, I.S., and Senturia, J. 1960. *Medical Care Program for Steelworkers and Their Families.* Pittsburgh: United Steelworkers of America.

Forthofer, R.N., and Glasser, J.H. 1979. Utilization of Services of an HMO by New Enrollees. *American Journal of Public Health* 69:1127–1131.

Freeborn, D.K., Pope, C.R., Davis, M.A., and Mullooly, J.P. 1977. Health Status, Socioeconomic Status, and Utilization of Outpatient Services for Members of a Prepaid Group Practice. *Medical Care* 15:115–128.

Freidson, E. 1961. *Patients' Views of Medical Practice.* New York: Russell Sage Foundation.

Fuchs, V. 1974. *Who Shall Live? Health, Economics, and Social Change.* New York: Basic Books.

Fuller, N.A., Patera, M.W., and Koziol, K. 1977. Medicaid Utilization of Services in a Prepaid Group Practice Health Plan. *Medical Care* 15:705–740.

Gaus, C.R., Cooper, B.S., and Hirschman, C.G. 1976. Contrasts in HMO and Fee-for-Service Performance. *Social Security Bulletin* 39:3–14.

Gavett, J.W., and Smith, D.B. 1978. A Comparison of the Hospital Cost Experience of Three Competing HMOs. *Inquiry* 15:327–335.

Goldberg, L., and Greenburg, W. 1977. *The Health Maintenance Organization and Its Effects on Competition.* Washington, D.C.: Federal Trade Commission, Bureau of Economics.

———. 1979. The Competitive Response of Blue Cross and Blue Shield to the Health Maintenance Organization in Northern California and Hawaii. *Medical Care* 17:1019–1028.

Goldensohn, S.S., and Fink, R. 1979. Mental Health Services for Medicaid Enrollees in a Prepaid Group Practice Plan. *American Journal of Psychiatry* 136:160–164.

Goldman, M., and Steinwald, B. 1973. Prepaid Medical Care and Health Services Utilization: A Reexamination of the Evidence. Unpublished.

Greenburg, W. 1977. HMOs Stimulate Competition, FTC Concludes. *Hospital Progress* 58:10–11.

Greenfield, C., Densen, P., Jones, E., Kleinman, J., and Miller, J. 1978. Use of Out-of-Plan Services by Medicaid Members of HIP. *Health Services Research* 13:243–260.

Greenlick, M.R. 1972. The Impact of Prepaid Group Practice on American Medical Care: A Critical Evaluation. *Annals of the American Academy of Political and Social Science* 399:100–113.

Hastings, J., Mott, F., Barclay, A., and Hewitt, D. 1973. Prepaid Group Practice in Sault Ste. Marie, Ontario. Part 1, *Medical Care* 11:91–103; Part 2, *Medical Care* 11:173–188.

Hester, J.A. 1979. Research in Resource Allocation in a Prepaid Group Practice. *Milbank Memorial Fund Quarterly/Health and Society* 57 (Summer):388–411.

Hetherington, R., Hopkins, C., and Roemer, M. 1975. *Health Insurance Plans: Promise and Performance.* New York: Wiley.

Johnson, R.E., and Azevedo, D.J. 1979a. Examining the Annual Drug Utilization of a Cohort of Low Income Health Care Plan Members. *Medical Care* 17:578–591.

———. 1979b. Comparing the Medical Utilization and Expenditures of Low Income Health Plan Enrollees with Medicaid Recipients and Low Income Enrollees Having Medicaid Eligibility. *Medical Care* 17:953–966.

Klarman, H.E. 1963. Effect of Prepaid Group Practice on Hospital Use. *Public Health Reports* 78:955–965.

Kronenfeld, J.J. 1978. Provider Variables and the Utilization of Ambulatory Care Services. *Journal of Health and Social Behavior* 19:68–76.

Lairson, D.R., and Swint, J.M. 1978. A Multivariate Analysis of the Likelihood and Volume of Preventive Visit Demand in a Prepaid Group Practice. *Medical Care* 16:730–739.

———. 1979. Estimates of Preventive versus Nonpreventive Medical Care in an HMO. *Health Services Research* 14:33–43.

Lavin, J.B. 1978. The Town That's Squeezing Out Private Practice. *Medical Economics:* July 24, 27–44.

Levin, B.L., and Glasser, J.H. 1979. A Survey of Mental Health Service Coverage within Health Maintenance Organizations. *American Journal of Public Health* 69:1120–1125.

LoGerfo, J.P., 1975. Hypertension: Management in a Prepaid Health Care Project. *Journal of the American Medical Association* 233:245–248.

———, Lawson, E., Okamoto, G., Diehr, P.K., and Richardson, W. 1977. Quality of Care for Common Infections: Comparisons of Prepaid Group Practice and Independent Practice. Paper presented at the meeting of the American Federation for Clinical Research.

———, Lawson, E., and Richardson, W.C. 1978. Assessing the Quality of Care for Urinary Tract Infection in Office Practice: A Comparative Organizational Study. *Medical Care* 16:488–495.

———, Efird, R.A., Diehr, P.K., and Richardson, W.C. 1979. Rates of Surgical Care in Prepaid Group Practices and the Independent Setting: What Are the Reasons for the Differences? *Medical Care* 17:1–11.

Luft, H.S. 1978a. How Do Health Maintenance Organizations Achieve Their Savings? Rhetoric and Evidence. *New England Journal of Medicine* 298:1336–1343.

———. 1978b. Why Do HMOs Seem to Provide More Health Maintenance Services? *Milbank Memorial Fund Quarterly/Health and Society* 56 (Spring):140–168.

———. 1979. HMOs, Competition, Cost Containment, and NHI. Paper presented at the meetings of the American Enterprise Institute, Washington, D.C. October.

———. 1980a. Trends in Medical Care Costs: Do HMOs Lower the Rate of Growth? *Medical Care* 18:1–16.

———. 1980b. *Health Maintenance Organizations: Dimensions of Performance.* New York: Wiley.

Mechanic, D. 1979. Correlates of Psychological Distress among Young Adults: A Theoretical Hypothesis and Results from a

16-Year Follow-up Study. *Archives of General Psychiatry* 36:1233–1239.

———. 1980. The Experience and Reporting of Common Physical Complaints. *Journal of Health and Social Behavior* 21:146–156.

Mullooly, J.P., and Freeborn, D.K. 1979. The Effect of Length of Membership upon the Utilization of Ambulatory Care Services: A Comparison of Disadvantaged and General Membership Populations in a Prepaid Group Practice. *Medical Care* 17:922–936.

National Advisory Commission. 1967. *Report of the National Advisory Commission on Health Manpower.* Volume 11:197–228. Washington, D.C.: Government Printing Office.

Nixon, Richard. 1971. *Health Message of the President of the United States.* Washington, D.C.: Government Printing Office.

Patrick, D.L., Coleman, J.V., Eagle, J., and Nelson, E. 1978. Chronic Emotional Problem Patients and Their Families in an HMO. *Inquiry* 15:166–180.

Perrott, G. 1971. *The Federal Employees Health Benefits Program: Utilization Study.* Washington, D.C.: Health Services and Mental Health Administration.

———, and Chase, J.C. 1968. The Federal Employees Health Benefits Program: Sixth Term Coverage and Utilization. *Group Health and Welfare News,* special 8-page supplement, October.

Pett, L.J. 1979. Utilization of Hospital Services in the Individual Practice Association on Guam: A Comparative Analysis. *Medical Care* 17:420–429.

PL 93-222. 1973. *The Health Maintenance Organization Act of 1973.* Washington, D.C.: Government Printing Office.

PL 93-641. 1974. *The National Health Planning and Resources Development Act of 1974.* Washington, D.C.: Government Printing Office.

PL 94-460. 1976. *Health Maintenance Organization Amendments of 1976.* Washington, D.C.: Government Printing Office.

PL 95-559. 1978. *Health Maintenance Organization Amendments of 1978.* Washington, D.C.: Government Printing Office.

Pope, C.R. 1978. Consumer Satisfaction in a Health Maintenance Organization. *Journal of Health and Social Behavior* 19:291–303.

Riedel, D., Walden, D., Singsen, A., et al. 1975. *Federal Employees Health Benefits Program: Utilization Study.* Washington, D.C.: National Center for Health Services Research.

Robertson, R.L. 1972. Comparative Medical Care Use Under Prepaid Group Practice and Free Choice Plans: A Case Study. *Inquiry* 9:70–76.

Roemer, M.J., and Shonick, W. 1973. HMO Performance: The Recent Evidence. *Milbank Memorial Fund Quarterly/Health and Society* 51 (Spring):271–317.

Scitovsky, A.A., Benham, L., and McCall, N. 1979. Use of Physician Services under Two Prepaid Plans. *Medical Care* 17:441–460.

———, McCall, N., and Benham, L. 1978. Factors Affecting the Choice between Two Prepaid Plans. *Medical Care* 16:660–681.

Shapiro, S., Williams, J., Yerby, A., Densen, P., and Rosner, H. 1967. Patterns of Medical Use by the Indigent Aged under Two Systems of Medical Care. *American Journal of Public Health* 57:784–790.

Shortell, S., Richardson, W., LoGerfo, J., Diehr, P.K., Weaver, B., and Green, K. 1977. The Relationships among Dimensions of Health Services in Two Provider Systems: A Causal Model Approach. *Journal of Health and Social Behavior* 18:139–159.

Weinerman, E.R. 1964. Patients' Perceptions of Group Medical Care: A Review and Analysis of Studies of Choice and Utilization of Prepaid Group Practice Plans. *American Journal of Public Health* 54:880–899.

Wersinger, R., Roghmann, K.J., and Gavett, J.W. 1976. Inpatient Hospital Utilization in Three Prepaid Comprehensive Health Care Plans Compared with a Regular Blue Cross Plan. *Medical Care* 14:721–732.

Williams, J.J., Trussell, R.E., and Elinson, J. 1964. A Survey of Family Medical Care under Three Types of Health Insurance. *Journal of Chronic Diseases* 17:879–884.

Williams, S.J., Shortell, S.M., LoGerfo, J.P., and Richardson, W.C. 1978. A Causal Model of Health Services for Diabetic Patients. *Medical Care* 16:313–326.

———, Diehr, P.K., Drucker, W.L., and Richardson, W.C. 1979. Mental Health Services: Utilization by Low Income Enrollees in a Prepaid Group Practice Plan. *Medical Care* 17:139–151.

Williamson, J.W., Cunningham, F.C., and Ward, D.J. 1979. Quality of Health Care in HMOs as Compared to Other Health Settings: A Literature Review and Policy Analysis. Paper prepared for the Office of Health Maintenance Organizations, Department of Health, Education, and Welfare, Rockville, Md.

Wolinsky, F.D. 1976. Health Service Utilization and Attitudes toward Health Maintenance Organizations: A Theoretical and Methodological Discussion. *Journal of Health and Social Behavior* 17:221–236.

———. 1978. Assessing the Effects of Predisposing, Enabling, and Illness-Morbidity Characteristics on Health Service Utilization. *Journal of Health and Social Behavior* 19:384–396.

———. 1980. *The Sociology of Health: Principles, Professions, and Issues.* Boston: Little, Brown.

Wollstadt, L.J., Shapiro, S., and Bice, T.W. 1978. Disenrollment from a Prepaid Group Practice: An Actuarial and Demographic Description. *Inquiry* 15:142–149.

297

The Effects of Prepayment on Access to Medical Care: The PACC Experience

EMIL BERKANOVIC
LEO G. REEDER
ALFRED C. MARCUS
SUSAN SCHWARTZ

The data reported herein are taken from a larger study in which a prepaid medical foundation was compared with a non-prepaid free-for-service system on a number of factors pertaining to how health care is perceived by both Medicaid recipients and physicians. The data to be presented are confined to the issue of the impact of prepayment on Medicaid recipients' perceptions of their access to health care. Two sets of questions are explored. The first set bears directly on the issue of gaining access to care. The second set addresses the issue of the acceptability of the services received. Few differences were observed between the systems in either accessibility or acceptability. Thus, the fears of some critics of the HMO concept with respect to prepayment creating incentives for the denial of services are not supported by the data. It is concluded that the organizational features of medical practice which affect access are actually quite similar in the two systems.

An important concept in the present debate over the organization of health care is that of the Health Maintenance Organization (HMO). Although there are many organizational forms which have been included under this term, all have in common the delivery of prepaid health care to a defined population group. Advocates of HMOs contend that prepayment creates a financial incentive for the prevention and early detection of disease, thus avoiding the larger costs of treatment and, especially, hospitalization. Critics of this concept, on the other hand, argue that prepayment merely creates incentives to deny needed services (Klarman, 1971).

At present, there are a number of prepaid health care delivery systems throughout the United States. Although there are many differences among them, one of the major divisions into which these proto-HMOs can be divided is between prepaid, closed-panel group practice, and prepaid fee-for-service foundation practice (Ellwood, 1971). In the former, the population which is served is required to seek care only from the group, or panel, of physicians to whom they have made prepayment. In the latter, the population is

M M F Q / Health and Society / *Spring 1975*

free to choose any physician they wish, who then bills the foundation for the services he has rendered, and is reimbursed according to the foundation's fee schedule. Prepaid practices of both types are currently of great interest as sources of evidence bearing on the HMO concept.

Unfortunately, there is little evidence which can be brought to bear on the effectiveness and efficiency of each system. Indeed, the criteria by which effectiveness and efficiency should be judged are by no means clear. Thus, although the research which has been done within either mode of organizing care has addressed a number of interesting variables, the data are unclear with respect to the claims of the advocates of each system (Klarman, 1971). Further, from a policy perspective, it is essential that each system be shown to be superior to the present system of delivering care before the funds required for an extensive conversion of that system are committed.

The Present Study

The data reported herein are taken from a larger study in which a prepaid medical foundation was compared with a nonprepaid fee-for-service system on a number of factors pertaining to how health care is perceived by both Medicaid recipients and physicians. The importance of comparing prepaid foundations with non-prepaid fee-for-service systems lies in the fact that such foundations are likely to become the predominant form of HMO. Thus, the vast majority of physicians practicing in both systems said that they would be unwilling to practice in a closed-panel group, although 80 percent of those currently practicing under fee for service said they would be willing to participate in a prepaid foundation aimed at providing care for the poor. The data to be presented in this paper are confined to the issue of the impact of prepayment on access to medical care.

The foundation which was studied is the Physicians' Association of Clackamas County (PACC). PACC is a non-profit, physician-sponsored, prepaid medical service plan in Clackamas County, Oregon. The plan was established in 1938 and is sponsored by the Clackamas County Medical Society. All physicians practicing in Clackamas County who were active members of the medical society at the time of the study, with two exceptions, were members of PACC, as were all osteopathic physicians practicing in the county.

In 1967, the Clackamas County Medical Society proposed to the state of Oregon that the society, through the agency of PACC, administer and underwrite on a prepaid basis the physician, hospital, and prescription-drug portions of Medicaid for all welfare recipients residing in Clackamas County. In addition to the regular PACC members, there were fifty-three physicians practicing outside of Clackamas County who volunteered to participate in this program. Under the terms of the contract, Medicaid recipients may choose any physician they wish, whether participating or not. Physicians who are not participating, but who treat Clackamas County welfare patients are reimbursed by PACC according to the same fee schedule used by the Public Welfare Department.

Method of Study

Since no absolute standards exist against which to compare the experiences which are reported by persons seeking medical care in a particular setting, it was deemed essential that this study be comparative. Accordingly, the problems of gaining access to care reported by the Clackamas County Medicaid recipients are compared with those reported by Medicaid recipients in Washington County, where Medicaid is administered on a non-prepaid fee-for-service basis. Washington County was chosen both because it shares a number of characteristics in common with Clackamas County, and because the two counties are adjacent.

Simple random samples of welfare cases which had been eligible for Medicaid for a continuous period of at least one year were drawn in each county. There were 296 interviews completed in Clackamas County and 297 in Washington County. These numbers represent roughly 89 percent of original sample size after it had been adjusted for cases which were found to be ineligible for inclusion in the study. The interviews were conducted with the female head-of-house whenever there was one present.

Some differences were found between the two samples in the distributions of age, sex, race, and number of children in the family. These factors were routinely taken into account in all analyses. Tables including these factors are presented only when they alter an observed relationship between county and an outcome of interest.

No differences were observed between the samples in the distributions of education, recent illness experience, chronic illness experience, perceived health status, or self-reported utilization of either physician or hospital services. These factors, therefore, cannot explain any differences observed between these samples.

The interviews ranged over a wide number of topics pertaining to these respondents' perceptions, attitudes, and experiences of the medical services available to them. The data which follow, however, are taken from those questions which reflect the problems which the respondents experienced in attempting to make use of medical services.

Two sets of questions are explored for differences between Clackamas County and Washington County Medicaid recipients' responses. First, there are several questions which bear directly on the issue of gaining access to care. Second, there are some questions which address the issue of the acceptability of the services which these Medicaid recipients have used. Taken together, these questions are conceived as a set of indicators bearing on the extent to which the providers of medical care discourage the use of their services. Further, these perceptions are conceived as being more important in determing consumer behavior than are the "facts" as they might be determined by an impartial observer.

TABLE 1

"In the past 12 months, how much trouble have you had in getting
an appointment with a doctor in (. . . .) County? Would you say:
a lot, some, not very much, no trouble at all?"

	Clackamas County		*Washington County*	
A lot	9.8	(21)	3.8	(9)
Some	12.1	(26)	13.5	(32)
Not very much	14.9	(32)	13.1	(31)
None	63.3	(136)	69.6	(165)
	100.1	(215)	100.0	(237)

$X^2 = 7.18$, *d.f.* = 3, P/X^2 = NS, *g* = .14

TABLE 2

"In the past 12 months, how much trouble have you had in getting
an appointment for your children to see a doctor in (. . . .) County?
Would you say: a lot, some, not very much, no trouble at all?"

	Clackamas County		Washington County	
A lot	8.7	(18)	6.9	(17)
Some	9.6	(20)	6.9	(17)
Not very much	14.4	(30)	12.1	(30)
None	67.3	(140)	74.1	(183)
	100.0	(208)	100.0	(247)

$X^2 = 2.67$, *d.f.* = 3. P/X^2 = NS. *g* = .15

Results

The respondents were asked how much trouble they have had in attempting to obtain a doctor's appointment both for themselves and
for their children. Although the Clackamas County sample was
slightly more likely to say that they have had a lot of trouble to both
questions, the differences are quite small, chi square does not
achieve significance at the usual .05 criterion level, and the gamma
measure of association is low. It appears, therefore, that there was
no difference between the prepaid and the non-prepaid systems in
the ease with which Medicaid recipients were able to obtain physicians' appointments.

 Another indicator of the accessibility of medical care is the
ease with which a physician may be seen when one does not have
an appointment. The data bearing on this issue indicate that it was
somewhat more difficult to obtain an unscheduled doctor's visit in
Clackamas County than it was in Washington County. Yet,
although chi square achieves significance at below the .05 level,
gamma is low. Further, there is a reversal of linearity within this relationship. Thus, although Washington County respondents were
more likely to respond "no trouble at all," and Clackamas County
respondents were more likely to respond "a lot," the relationship
was reversed in the two intermediate categories. These findings
suggest that the relationship between prepayment and difficulty in
seeing a doctor without an appointment is weak at best.

TABLE 3

"Now, when you don't have an appointment, how much trouble is it to get to see a doctor in (. . . .) County? Would you say: a lot, some, not very much, no trouble at all?"

	Clackamas County		Washington County	
A lot	29.3	(79)	20.8	(56)
Some	16.7	(45)	18.2	(49)
Not very much	31.9	(86)	26.4	(71)
No trouble at all	22.2	(60)	34.6	(93)
	100.1	(270)	100.0	(269)

$X^2 = 12.64$, d.f. = 3, $P/X^2 = .006$, $g = .18$

The respondents were also asked how long they had to wait to see a physician with whom they had an appointment. The response categories for this question were stated as subjective appraisals, rather than as estimates of amount of time. The reason for this procedure was to obtain the respondent's feelings about the length of wait. It was assumed that a person who reports having to wait "a very long time" finds the service less acceptable, and, hence, is less likely to make use of it, than a person who reports waiting "not

TABLE 4

"When you have an appointment for yourself, how long do you usually have to wait in the doctor's office before he sees you? Would you say: very long, fairly long, not too long, not long at all?"

	Clackamas County		Washington County	
Very long	13.1	(38)	9.9	(29)
Fairly long	24.4	(71)	17.7	(52)
Not too long	40.5	(118)	43.5	(128)
Not long at all	22.0	(64)	28.9	(85)
	100.0	(291)	100.0	(294)

$X^2 = 7.49$, d.f. = 3, $P/X^2 = $ NS, $g = .17$

long at all." Further, it was assumed that a 30-minute wait could be appraised quite differently by different respondents.

Again, although Clackamas County respondents were slightly more likely to report waiting "very long" or "fairly long," the percentage differences are quite small, chi square fails to achieve statistical significance, and gamma is low. These data indicate, therefore, that there was essentially no difference between the pre-paid and the non-prepaid systems in the subjective length of time which patients must wait to see a physician.

In addition to difficulty in gaining access to medical services, the acceptability of the services which an individual receives will have an impact on his willingness to make further use of those services. Accordingly, the respondents were asked whether they had seen a physician in the past year whose competence they doubted, and whether they had been treated rudely or dis-courteously by a physician or a member of his staff.

Washington County respondents were somewhat more likely to report having questioned the ability of a physician they had vis-ited during the past year. Although the percentage difference is not large, chi square is significant at less than .05 level and gamma for this relationship is moderate. Further, a difference of approximate-ly this magnitude was found for all subgroups of the samples. It ap-pears, therefore, that Medicaid recipients are somewhat more critical of the care they receive in a non-prepaid system. An ex-amination of the verbatim reasons these respondents gave for hav-ing been critical failed to provide an explanation for this difference.

TABLE 5

"In the past 12 months, have you or any members of your family gone to a doctor whose medical ability you questioned?"

	Clackamas County		Washington County	
Yes	11.2	(31)	20.8	(60)
No	88.8	(246)	79.2	(228)
	100.0	(277)	100.0	(288)

$X^2 = 9.01$, $d.f. = 1$, $P/X^2 = .003$, $g = -.35$

TABLE 6

"In the past 12 months, can you recall any experiences when you or a member
of your family was treated rudely or discourteously by a doctor
or some member of his office or clinic staff?

	Clackamas County	Washington County
Yes	20.1 (56)	22.0 (64)
No	79.9 (223)	78.0 (227)
	100.0 (279)	100.0 (291)

$X^2 = .21$, $d.f. = 1$, $P/X^2 = $ NS, $g = -.06$

No differences were observed between the samples in the
percentage of respondents who reported having been treated
rudely or discourteously. Interestingly, however, about one in five
of these Medicaid recipients reported such experiences.

The respondents were also asked if the quality of care they or
their children had received over the past year was as good as that
received by other people. There were no differences between the
samples on either of these items, and well over 90 percent of the
respondents in each county answered "yes" to both. Further,

TABLE 7

"Considering the visits you and your family have made to the doctors
in this county over the last 12 months, how satisfied are you
with the care you have received?"

	Clackamas County	Washington County
Very dissatisfied	6.5 (17)	6.9 (19)
Somewhat dissatisfied	3.0 (8)	8.7 (24)
Somewhat satisfied	26.2 (69)	25.1 (69)
Very satisfied	64.3 (169)	59.3 (163)
	100.0 (263)	100.0 (275)

$X^2 = 7.96$, $d.f. = 3$, $P/X^2 = .047$, $g = -.12$

although over 80 percent of the respondents in each county indicated that they were satisfied with the health care they had received, the Washington County respondents were slightly more likely to report being dissatisfied.

It appears, therefore, that prepayment creates no disadvantages in the acceptability of the medical services available to these Medicaid recipients. Thus, from the patient's point of view, at least, prepayment has little adverse effect on the physicians' treatment of welfare patients. If prepayment leads to the creation of barriers to utilization, therefore, these data suggest that such barriers are encountered by the individual prior to his achieving patient status and do not extend to the treatment he receives as a patient.

Up to this point, the analysis has focused on indicators of the accessibility of medical services which are postulated to affect the use of such services. An alternative approach to the question of the impact of prepayment on access to medical care lies in assessing whether there is a difference between the prepaid and the non-prepaid respondents in their use of services at times when they recognized the need. These data indicate that the Clackamas County sample is slightly more likely to say that, during the past year, they or a member of their family did not go to the doctor when they thought they should. Again, however, chi square does not achieve significance and gamma is low. It appears, therefore, that there is little difference between the prepaid and the non-prepaid samples in their failure to seek care when the need is recognized.

TABLE 8

"In the past 12 months, have there been any times you felt that you or a member of your family needed to see a doctor but didn't go?"

	Clackamas County		Washington County	
Yes	33.4	(99)	26.9	(80)
No	66.6	(197)	73.1	(217)
	100.0	(296)	100.0	(297)

$X_2 = 2.68$, $d.f. = 1$, $P/X^2 = NS$, $g = .15$

There are two general trends which may be observed in the data which have been presented. First, prepayment does not adversely affect the acceptability of the medical care which these welfare recipients have received. Second, the effect of prepayment on a series of indicators of the accessibility of medical care is small and, in every case except one, not statistically significant. Yet there relationships are consistent in showing that the prepaid respondents are slightly disadvantaged with respect to access to care. Because of the consistency of this pattern, the possibility that prepayment in fact has an adverse effect on the accessibility of medical care could not be ruled out.

In order to explore this possibility, the relationships which have been presented were examined within categories of sex, age, race, and number of children in the family. It will be recalled that these were the background variables on which the distributions of the two samples were found to differ. In every case it was found that the differences between the samples were confined to respondents with three or more children living at home, and that the size of these differences was enhanced within this group. These respondents represented about a third of the Clackamas County sample.

Although there appeared to be no a priori reason why respondents with large families should be singled out for discriminatory treatment in attempting to gain access to medical care under prepayment, two attempts were made to explore this possibility. First, the samples were compared on the reasons which Medicaid recipients with three or more children gave for not seeking care for which they recognized the need. These data indicate virtually no substantive differences between the prepaid and the non-prepaid subsamples. If Medicaid recipients with large families are more likely to encounter problems in seeking access to medical care under prepayment, they are no more likely to cite any particular reason for not seeking needed care than are their less disadvantaged counterparts in a non-prepaid system.

Second, comparisons were also made between these subsamples on the suggestions which they offered regarding how the health care in their county could be improved. Again, there are virtually no substantive differences between these subsamples. Thus, those respondents who expressed the greatest access problems were not any more likely to call for a particular improvement in the care available to them.

TABLE 9

"In the past 12 months, have there been any times when you felt that you
or a member of your family needed to see a doctor, but didn't go?"

Three or More Children	Clackamas County		Washington County	
Yes	37.3	(41)	20.8	(27)
No	62.7	(69)	79.2	(103)
	100.0	(110)	100.0	(130)

$X^2 = 7.20$, $d.f. = 1$, $P/X^2 = .007$, $g = .39$

Taken together, then, these data indicate that, although
Medicaid recipients receiving medical care in a prepaid system
were slightly disadvantaged with respect to gaining access to care,
this finding was confined to those respondents with large families,

TABLE 10

Reasons why "In the past 12 months have there been times when you or a member
of your family needed to see a doctor, but didn't go?"

Three or More Children	Clackamas County		Washington County	
Financial considerations	9.0	(7)	7.3	(3)
Doctor or facility would not accept welfare	1.3	(1)	0.0	(0)
Didn't think doctor would adequately deal with the situation	2.6	(2)	12.2	(5)
Dislikes physician	15.3	(12)	21.9	(9)
Problem with access into system such as transportation	5.1	(4)	4.9	(2)
Problem of time or convenience	13.0	(10)	12.2	(5)
Recurring condition or just waited to see	26.9	(21)	31.8	(13)
Miscellaneous	26.9	(21)	9.8	(4)
	100.1	(78)	100.1	(41)

TABLE 11

Reasons for Agreeing That Health Care in (. . .) County
Could Be Improved

Three or More Children	Clackamas County		Washington County	
Quality of care should be better	5.2	(5)	5.3	(5)
Need to improve financing of care	7.3	(7)	7.4	(7)
Need more doctors or facilities	40.6	(39)	35.8	(34)
Doctors should take more interest in their patients	13.6	(13)	15.8	(15)
Need better information about where to go	2.1	(2)	3.1	(3)
Doctors should keep more convenient hours	5.2	(5)	1.0	(1)
Miscellaneous	26.0	(25)	31.6	(30)
	100.0	(96)	100.0	(95)

and was probably not attributable to the prepayment mechanism.
Thus, there was little in either the reason why these respondents
did not seek needed care or in the improvements they suggested for
their medical care which could be attributed to PACC's administration of Medicaid on a prepaid basis. This conclusion is reinforced by the data which indicated that prepayment does not adversely affect the acceptability of the care which these respondents
have received.

Discussion

The fact that little difference was observed between the counties in
the accessibility and acceptability of medical services for Medicaid
recipients has important implications for the Health Maintenance
Organization concept. The fears which some critics of this concept
have expressed with respect to prepayment creating incentives for
denying needed services are not supported by these data. Rather,
the data suggest that the organizational features of medical practice
which affect access are quite similar in the two systems studied.

This conclusion is supported by the fact that there were few differences between the counties in rates of self-reported utilization of either physician or hospital services. Although these self-reported rates are subject to considerable inaccuracy, there is evidence that such data are useful in providing relative approximations of utilization patterns for comparative purposes (Richardson and Freeman, 1972). Thus, the fact that these rates were approximately the same for the two counties reinforces the conclusion that there was no important difference between Clackamas and Washington counties in the accessibility or acceptability of medical care for Medicaid recipients.

One obvious implication of this conclusion is that the foundation-type HMO is unlikely to differ significantly in those organizational features of medical practice which the consumer must confront in order to obtain care. Hence, although these data do not bear on the issue of the technical quality of care under prepayment, it appears that the experience of seeking and receiving medical care is not much different in a prepaid foundation than it is in a non-prepaid fee-for-service system.

Indeed, it could be argued that there is little reason to expect that Medicaid recipients' perceptions of the care they receive would be much different in these two systems. From the recipients' point of view a fixed portion of his felt need for health care is paid in full in both systems. The process of seeking care is similar in both, as are the bureaucratic procedures which must be endured in order to make use of Medicaid. Further, only part of the recipient's health needs are provided for. Other needs, which may be of some urgency to him, must either be paid for out-of-pocket, or must be foregone. The fact that this care is prepaid in one county and non-prepaid in another is of little consequence from the recipient's point of view, unless this difference were to eventuate in gross inadequacies in the provision of the care requested by the recipient in one system of the other. One would not expect this to be the case, and the data indicate that it is not.

Emil Berkanovic, P.H.D.
School of Public Health
University of California, Los Angeles
Los Angeles, California 90024

Support for this study was received under SRS Project #97-P-00029/9-01.

References

Ellwood, P.M.
1971   "Health Maintenance Organization: concept and strategy." Hospitals
        45 (March): 53–56.

Klarman, H.E.
1971   "An analysis of the HMO proposal—its assumptions, implications,
        and prospects." In Health Maintenance Organizations: A Recon-
        figuration of the Health Services System. Proceedings of the 13th An-
        nual Symposium on Hospital Affairs, Center for Health Administra-
        tion Studies, Graduate School of Business, University of Chicago.

Richardson, A.H., and H.E. Freeman
1972   "Evaluation of medical care utilization by interview surveys."
        Medical Care 10: 357–362.

Health Status and Health Care Use by Type of Private Health Coverage

MARK S. BLUMBERG

Kaiser Foundation Health Plan, Inc.,
Oakland, California

THE HEALTH STATUS AND THE HEALTH CARE utilization of members of prepaid group practices relative to members of other health maintenance organizations is a subject of continuing interest and some controversy. The interest is raised by the fact that almost all studies have shown a lower volume of inpatient hospital use among members of prepaid group practices than among other populations, a situation recently reviewed by Luft (1980). The controversy relates to the reasons why this difference exists.

In an attempt to obtain pertinent information on this problem we sought data on the health status and health care utilization of populations under age 65 enrolled in prepaid group practices and in other types of private health coverage.

Source of Data

Each year the National Center for Health Statistics obtains extensive information through the Health Interview Survey (HIS) on health status and health care utilization, based on a sample of about 116,000 people in the civilian noninstitutional population of the United States.

Milbank Memorial Fund Quarterly/*Health and Society,* Vol. 58, No. 4, 1980
© 1980 Milbank Memorial Fund and Massachusetts Institute of Technology
0160/1997/5804/0633-24 $01.00/0

The HIS for 1975 contained detailed questions regarding the types of
private health coverage of the respondents. Particular emphasis was
placed on defining the population with private plans who were members of prepaid group practices (Choi and Ries, 1978). In the HIS
study (p. 1) "members of prepaid group plans were defined as including both those who belonged to plans classified as health maintenance
organizations (HMO) and those who belonged to other prepaid group
practice plans."

Thus the major distinction in the HIS survey, and in this paper, is
between those in prepaid group practice plans (PGPs) and those with
all other forms of private health care coverage. The latter category
includes those who were members of individual practice associations
(IPAs). In many recent studies, including some in this issue of the
Milbank *Quarterly,* the term "health maintenance organization"
(HMO) is used to encompass a variety of arrangements that include
both prepaid group practices (PGPs) and individual practice associations (IPAs).

This paper compares those in PGPs with those in all other forms of
private health care coverage, including IPAs.

The questions used in the HIS to obtain the respondents' type of
health coverage were complex. The major exclusions from private
health coverage were:

Government Plans
— Medicare
— Crippled Children's Services
— Medicaid
— Civilian Health and Medical Program of the Uniformed Services
(CHAMPUS)
— Veterans' benefits
Limited Plans
— Accidents only (e.g., school)
— Dread diseases only (e.g., polio, cancer)
— Liability insurance (e.g., automobile)
— Income maintenance (i.e., whether or not in hospital)
— Work loss benefits
— Dental only

The plans included are defined as those "specifically designed to pay all or part of the hospital, doctor, surgeon or other medical expense of the insured individual." There is some ambiguity as to whether a major medical plan that supplemented basic coverage would be considered as one or as two plans by a respondent. Indemnity plans, which pay a fixed number of dollars per hospital day, were included, regardless of the percentage of actual hospital charges these dollars might pay for.

The names of all plans reported by the respondents were listed by the surveyors. The classification into "PGP" and "all other" was based on decisions by the survey staff and not on the respondents' opinion of whether they or other household members were in an HMO. As noted above, individual practice associations (IPAs) were classified as other private coverage.

The HIS realized that respondents may not have been familiar with the terms health maintenance organization or prepaid group practice. In fact, only about one-half of the sample in a prepaid group practice—as determined by their plan name—knew that they were in an "HMO."

In summary, the HIS was unlikely to result in errors of omission on private health coverage. However, there was some chance that sophisticated respondents could have overstated their overlapping or duplicate coverage and all respondents probably included individual hospital indemnity plans as coverage, regardless of how little these plans paid per day. For our purposes, the major limitation of the data source was the inability to distinguish respondents who had been offered an HMO choice from those who had not.

Selection of the Subsample for Analysis

A published report from the National Center for Health Statistics provides considerable information about the characteristics of those with PGP coverage, as contrasted with those having other private coverage or no private coverage (Choi and Ries, 1978). The data showed that the population enrolled in a prepaid group practice plan, when compared with those with other private coverage, had a greater percent of persons with limitation of activity, a higher number of restricted-activity days per person per year, and a greater number of bed-disability days per person per year. They also showed that those in the PGP population had fewer short-stay hospital discharges per hundred persons per year but somewhat more doctor visits per person per year than those with fee-for-service coverage only.

We reviewed many unpublished tables from the 1975 HIS provided by the National Center for Health Statistics. The percent of respondents who claimed to have both PGP and other private coverage seemed high. In fact, some prepaid group plans that were not hospital-based provided hospital coverage through another private carrier such as Blue Cross. This is much more characteristic of PGPs in the East than of those in the West, which are more likely to have their own hospitals. This situation favored the use of data from western areas. In the present study, those with both PGP and other private coverage are classed with the PGP members.

We analyzed data on the health care coverage of the population under age 65 from HIS tapes for each of the western standard metropolitan statistical areas (SMSAs). Because of possible differences in health status and in patterns of health care utilization even within the West, we sought a more homogeneous area and selected those California SMSAs with sizable PGP enrollments for further study.

The study sample is shown in Table 1. As of July 1975, the eight metropolitan areas listed had a total population of 16.97 million of the state total of 19.68 million. It is probable that over 95 percent of the PGP members in California resided within one of these eight metropolitan areas. About one-third of the sample were in northern California and two-thirds were in southern California. Each of these areas was designated as "self-representing" by the HIS. In effect, the sample size in each of these SMSAs was proportional to its population, a fact that permitted pooling the samples without concern for sampling ratios.

These eight metropolitan areas provided a sample of 8,449 persons under age 65, of whom 1,278 were in prepaid group practices. Another 4,900 had other forms of private coverage, and 2,271 had no private coverage. Thus, 26.9 percent of the population under age 65 in these areas had no private health care coverage. This figure was higher than expected and may relate to adverse economic conditions in 1975.

The column to the right in Table 1 gives PGP members as a percent

TABLE 1

HIS Sample, under Age 65, by Private Health Coverage Status in Selected California Metropolitan Areas (1975)

Metropolitan Area*	Number of People in Sample by Type of Health Coverage			No Private Coverage as a Percent of All	PGP as a Percent of All with Any Private Coverage
	PGP	Other Private Coverage	No Private Coverage		
Northern California					
San Francisco-Oakland SMSA	322	779	387	26.0	29.2
Vallejo-Napa SMSA	24	53	54	41.2	31.2
Santa Clara County	76	451	140	21.0	14.4
Sacramento SMSA	89	248	130	27.8	26.4
Subtotal	511	1,531	711	25.8	25.0
Southern California					
Los Angeles City	254	674	343	27.0	26.8
Other L. A. County	322	1,273	559	26.0	20.2
San Bernardino-Riverside Counties	66	300	234	39.0	18.0
San Diego SMSA	73	364	221	33.6	16.7
Orange County	52	738	203	20.4	6.6
Subtotal	767	3,369	1,560	27.4	18.3
Total People	1,278	4,900	2,271	26.9	20.7

*Each of these areas is a standard metropolitan statistical area (SMSA), although the county names have been used for some areas. Los Angeles City and other L.A. County together comprise Los Angeles County, which is the Los Angeles-Long Beach SMSA.

of all those with private coverage in each of these study areas. The PGP market share was 20.2 percent of those with any private coverage.

The percent of the sample population who had no private health care coverage for each age under 65 is shown in Figure 1. Some of the variation by age is caused by the relatively small samples in the 1-year age intervals. There were nevertheless important and real differences by age. Over 40 percent of persons aged 22 and 23 had no private health coverage, and the figure was well over 30 percent for each age between 19 and 25. Many of these young adults could have had problems in obtaining private health care coverage since many were too old to continue coverage on their parents' health plans and had no suitable opportunity for joining a group to replace this lost coverage. People in this age group frequently have temporary work or work in industries where group health coverage is not common. Although they could obtain individual coverage, limited incomes and good health may discourage its purchase.

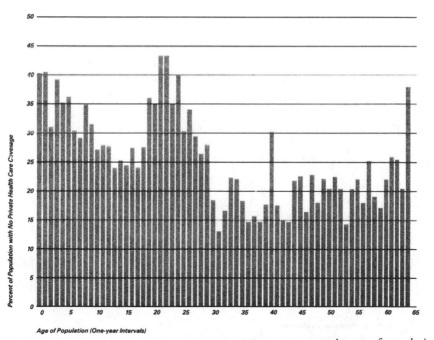

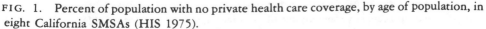

FIG. 1.   Percent of population with no private health care coverage, by age of population, in eight California SMSAs (HIS 1975).

Over 40 percent of those under age 2 had no private health care coverage. Their mothers were concentrated among those in their early twenties because age-specific birthrates peak for women in this age category. This gap in private coverage for young mothers and their infants contributes to the substantial Medicaid involvement with childbirth. As children get older, fewer are without private health care coverage. The percent was a minimum for those of high-school age.

Among adults, absence of private health coverage was lowest among those aged 30 to 40, and rose gradually after that. (The peaks in Fig. 1 at ages 40 and 64 were probably due to chance.)

Figure 2 shows the percent of those with private health care coverage who were enrolled in prepaid group practices. Apart from the variation caused by sampling, there are no major peaks and valleys. There is a slight decline in the PGP market share with increasing age from birth through 43 and a somewhat lower market share among those aged 44 through 64. The average PGP market share is higher among those under 18 than the average for all age groups (i.e., 20.7

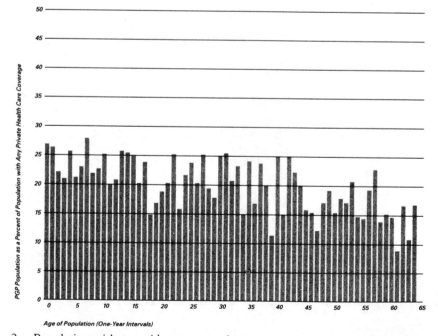

FIG. 2. Population with prepaid group practice coverage as a percent of population with any private health care coverage, by age of population, in eight California SMSAs (HIS 1975).

percent), which suggests that the PGP had more attraction for families with dependent children than did the alternative carriers.

This information on PGP market share by age cannot be used to determine the relative health status of those in PGPs and those with other private health care coverage. For example, one might believe that those in the PGP had fewer chronic conditions because the PGP share of those in the older age groups was less. But this conclusion depends on the assumption that the age-specific prevalence of chronic conditions in the PGP population is the same as or less than for those with other private plans. Direct measures of health status of populations by type of health care coverage are needed to determine their relative health status.

Health Status Findings

Information on the percent of persons in the sample with limitation of activity due to one or more chronic conditions is given in Table 2. Among those under age 65, heart conditions were the leading cause of such limitations, with hypertension and asthma also important. However, various conditions or impairments of the musculoskeletal system formed the largest group of those with such limitations (National Center for Health Statistics, 1977). The percent of persons

TABLE 2

Limitation of Activity Due to Chronic Conditions; Percent of People under Age 65, by Type of Health Coverage, in Selected California SMAs (1975)

Limitation of Activity Due to Chronic Conditions	Type of Health Coverage		
	PGP	Other Private Coverage	No Private Coverage
Percent unable to carry on major activity	1.0%	1.1%	4.6%
Percent limited in amount or kind of major activity	6.0	5.4	6.5
Percent otherwise limited in activity	4.1	4.3	4.1
Total percent limited in activity	11.1%	10.8%	15.2%
Average number of chronic conditions causing limitation in activity per person with limited activity	1.30	1.29	1.43

having any limitation in activity due to a chronic condition was slightly higher (11.1 percent) in the PGP sample than in other forms of private coverage (10.8). The highest percent (15.2) occurred among those who had no private coverage.

Table 2 also gives the average number of chronic conditions causing limitation per person with limited activity. The average for both categories of those with private coverage is similar but is somewhat higher for those with no private coverage.

Self-appraised health status is an important explanatory variable for respondents' use of hospital services. The multiple regression models of Newhouse and Phelps (1976) illustrate the empirical use of the variable. Although the health status question is subjective, the respondents' replies may be a combination of their actual health status and their opinion regarding it. Both aspects can contribute to respondents' use of health services. The self-appraised health status by health care coverage is shown in Table 3. The responses of the PGP sample and of the sample with other private coverage are almost identical in distribution. In contrast, the health status of those with no private coverage is somewhat worse than for those with private coverage.

The restricted-activity day is another measure of health status used by HIS and is defined (Bureau of the Census, 1975) as "one on which a person cuts down on his usual activity for the whole of that day because of an illness or an injury." Table 4 gives annual restricted-activity days per person (based on a 2-week sample period) by type of

TABLE 3

Self-Appraised Health Status of HIS Sample under Age 65, by Type of Health Coverage, in Selected California SMAs (1975)

| Self-Appraised Health Status | Type of Health Coverage | | |
	PGP	Other Private Coverage	No Private Coverage
Excellent	57.4%	56.9%	43.3%
Good	33.4	34.5	42.0
Fair	7.7	6.7	9.8
Poor	1.4	1.6	3.6
Not reported	0.2	0.3	1.3
Total	100.0%	100.0%	100.0%

TABLE 4

Annual Restricted-Activity Days per Person* for HIS Sample under Age 65
by Type of Health Coverage in Selected California Sites (1975)

Type of Restricted-Activity Days	Type of Health Coverage		
	PGP	Other Private Coverage	No Private Coverage
Number of bed-disability days	6.3	5.9	9.4
Number of other restricted-activity days	14.9	12.0	14.1
All restricted-activity days	21.2	17.9	23.5

*Based on a 2-week recall period.

health coverage. Note that these restricted-activity days include those due to either acute or chronic conditions. The number of days for PGP members was slightly higher than for those with other private coverage, and highest for those with no private coverage. These data show that total restricted-activity days resulting from chronic or acute conditions are somewhat higher among those in prepaid group practices than among those with other private coverage.

Physician Visits

A physician visit is defined by HIS as "consultation with a physician in person or by telephone, for examination, diagnosis, treatment or advice. The visit is considered to be a physician visit if the service is provided directly by the physician or by a nurse or other person acting under a physician's supervision."

Data on physician visits by type of health care coverage are given in Table 5. The number of physician visits per person per year was slightly higher for those with no private coverage and lowest for those with other private coverage, with an intermediate figure for those in PGPs, but the differences were small. The percent of those who had made at least one physician visit in the previous 12 months was highest for those in a PGP. The number of physician visits per person per year for those who had made at least one visit in the past 12 months was highest for those with no private coverage and lowest for those in a

TABLE 5

Physician Visit Measures for HIS Sample under Age 65 by Type of Health
Coverage in Selected California SMSAs (1975)

Physician Visit Measures*	Type of Health Coverage		
	PGP	Other Private Coverage	No Private Coverage
Number of visits per person per year	4.15	4.05	4.33
Percent with one or more visits in past 12 months	65.7%	60.0%	57.9%
Number of visits per person per year for those with at least one visit in past 12 months	6.32	6.75	7.48

*Based on 1-year recall period.

PGP. Note that the data for physician visits (and those for hospital
episodes) included all such services whether or not paid by the PGP.

Both doctor visits and hospital episodes were based on a recall
period of 1 year. In contrast, the question on HMO coverage per-
tained to the time of the survey. There was no way to determine the
health coverage status of the sample at the time of each doctor visit (or
for each hospital episode). This should not result in bias if health care
use does not differ substantially for those who changed coverage
within the study year. A paper on ambulatory services used by Kaiser
Foundation Health Plan members in Oregon (Mullooly and Freeborn,
1979) stated that, in general, these findings suggest that length of time
in plan does not affect ambulatory care use.

Hospital Use

The portion of the survey relating to hospital use was based on
respondent recall for the 12 months preceding the interview and thus
depends on the accuracy of recall for this period. (Most reports of HIS
data use a 6-month recall period for hospital utilization.) All short-
term episodes were included regardless of their location. The study
includes stays in federal hospitals and in hospitals outside the

respondents' areas of residence. For the prepaid group practice members, the hospital stays include those in facilities belonging to or associated with the PGP as well as other hospital stays, whether or not authorized and paid for by the PGP. Thus the utilization data include all services, even those not included in a PGP's utilization data. This is a potential improvement over data derived only from the records of PGPs and other third parties.

It is important to keep in mind that the survey was limited to the civilian, noninstitutional population (e.g., excluding residents of penal institutions and nursing homes). Active military personnel are excluded but their dependents are included, provided they did not live in group quarters.

Obviously, decedents could not be interviewed nor were their survivors interviewed about health use of decedents. This causes an understatement of health care use, particularly hospital services among the aged with high death rates. But this leads to little error in reported hospital use for the under-65 population studied here because their death rate is very low.

There was some concern that the sample size might not be adequate to provide comparative data on short-term hospital use, since such care is relatively uncommon among those under age 65. However, the sample provided a total of 919 stays and 5,585 short-term hospital days. The greatest length of stay observed for any hospital episode in this sample was 90 days, and there were a number of other observations between 60 and 90 days. Thus these aggregate data are not skewed by a few cases with excessively long stays.

The data on hospital use rates by type of health coverage are shown in Table 6. The lowest rate of hospital use in days per 1,000 persons per year occurred for the PGP members, and the highest for those with no private coverage. Despite the fact that those in the PGP are similar to those with other private coverage in their general health status, limitations of activity, and chronic conditions, the days per 1,000 were 22 percent lower for those in PGPs. Just over half of this reduction was due to shorter lengths of stay; the remainder was due to fewer episodes per 1,000 persons per year.

These hospital utilization figures follow the conventional approach of omitting well newborns but including sick newborns and obstetric cases. The Health Interview Survey determined the reasons for each hospitalization, but these data are on a separate tape that has not yet

TABLE 6

Annual Short-Term Hospital Use* per 1,000 in HIS Sample under Age 65,
by Type of Health Coverage

Hospital Use	Type of Health Coverage			
	PGP	Other Private Coverage	No Private Coverage	All Persons in Sample
Days per 1,000 persons per year	469.5	604.1	891.7	661.0
Episodes per 1,000 persons per year	93.1	104.6	126.4	108.8
Average length of stay (days)	5.04	5.78	7.05	6.08
Estimated nonobstetric episodes per 1,000 persons per year	75.1	91.7	100.9	91.8

*Excludes well newborns.

been analyzed. The sample under age 1 has been used as a proxy for obstetric deliveries in the preceding 12 months, since almost all deliveries occur in hospitals. The number of deliveries is not exactly equal to the number of children under the age of 1. The small number of stillborns and infant deaths tends to offset the small number of multiple births. Thus the annual volume of obstetric deliveries should be very close to the number of children under the age of 1.

The estimated nonobstetric episodes per 1,000, shown at the bottom of Table 6, were derived by subtracting the obstetric deliveries (Table 7) from all hospital episodes.

TABLE 7

HIS Sample under Age 65 and under Age 1, by Type of Health Coverage,
in Selected California SMSAs (1975)

HIS Sample	Type of Health Coverage			
	PGP	Other Private Coverage	No Private Coverage	All Persons in Sample
A. Number under age 1	23	63	58	144
B. Number under age 65	1,278	4,900	2,271	8,449
C. Crude birthrate per 1,000 under age 65 (A/B) × 1,000	18.0	12.9	25.5	17.0

Estimated obstetric delivery data by type of coverage are presented in Table 7. The figures in line C are simply obtained from the relation (A/B) × 1,000 and are estimates of crude birthrates for the samples of members with different types of health care coverage. The estimated crude birthrate of those with PGP coverage was almost 50 percent higher than for those with other private coverage (18.0 vs. 12.9). The highest rate was found for those with no private coverage, 25.5 per 1,000. About 40.3 percent of all those under age 1 in the selected California SMSAs had no private coverage.

Adjustments for obstetric hospital care are important since the admission rate per obstetric delivery is not likely to be changed by the mother's health care coverage. Furthermore, the number of nonobstetric admissions associated with pregnancy or sterilization can equal those for obstetric deliveries—e.g., tubal ligations, some hysterectomies, abortions, pre- and postpartum complications (National Center for Health Statistics, 1980). Hence, the magnitude of the difference between hospital admission rates for PGP and for other types of private health coverage, exclusive of all pregnancy and related conditions, was greater than shown.

Government Workers

In the State of California, all workers with Federal Employee Health Benefits in the study area were offered Kaiser Foundation Health Plan and some other PGPs under a plural- or dual-choice system. In addition, all State of California employees were offered similar plural choices if they resided in the study areas. The situation for local government employees including school districts was not as uniform but the great majority of these were also offered a PGP choice in the metropolitan areas included in the study. Hence government workers were an identifiable large pool of eligibles with a PGP choice through their work. For this reason, they were studied separately.

There were 697 government workers under the age of 65 in the sample. Of these, 220 or 31.6 percent were in a PGP, 56.4 percent had other private coverage, and 12.1 percent had no private coverage (some of the latter may have had veterans' benefits, CHAMPUS, or other government coverage). A major proportion of these plans for government workers required an employee contribution, which could explain why some had no private coverage. In addition, there were a few workers who were not eligible for coverage because of the nature of their work or other conditions of employment.

The data in Table 8 summarize the findings for this sample of government workers under age 65. (Note that these data are for workers only and do not include the workers' dependents.) The data on line a indicate that a higher percent of those in the PGP were

TABLE 8

Summary of Health Status and Measures of Health Care Use by Type of Health Coverage for Government Workers* under Age 65 in Eight California SMSAs† (1975)

Health Status and Measures of Health Care Use	Type of Health Coverage		
	PGP	Other Private Coverage	No Private Coverage
Sample size: number of workers	220	393	84
Limitation of activity due to chronic conditions			
a. Percent with a limitation	13.6%	10.2%	9.5%
b. Number of chronic conditions causing limitations per person with limitations	1.37	1.20	1.00
Self-assessed health status			
c. Percent "fair" or "poor"	11.4%	10.7%	7.1%
Restricted-activity days per year‡			
d. Bed-disability days	3.4	6.9	5.3
e. Other restricted-activity days	12.1	15.8	10.5
f. Total restricted-activity days	15.5	22.7	15.8
Physician visits§			
g. Per person per year	4.47	4.07	3.60
h. Percent of persons with one or more in past year	70.9%	65.9%	58.3%
Hospital Care§//			
i. Episodes per 1,000 person-years	82	109	95
j. Average stay in days	4.44	5.34	5.77
k. Days per 1,000 person-years	364	582	548

*Includes federal, state, and local government workers; excludes their dependents.
†San Francisco-Oakland; Los Angeles-Long Beach; Riverside-Ontario-San Bernardino; Vallejo-Napa; San Jose; Sacramento; San Diego; Orange County.
‡Based on 2-week recall.
§Based on 1-year recall.
//Excludes well newborns.

limited in activity because of a chronic condition than were those with other private coverage (13.6 vs. 10.2 percent). Those in the PGP were a little more likely to have a "fair" or "poor" health status (line c). However, those in PGPs had fewer restricted-activity days per year than those with other private coverage (lines d, e, and f). Average numbers of physician visits per person per year were higher among those in the PGP, as was the percent of persons with one or more physician visits in the past year (lines h and i).

Total hospital days per 1,000 person-years were only 364 in prepaid group practices, whereas they were 582 for those with other private coverage. This difference was due largely to a lower number of episodes per 1,000 person-years but due also to a shorter average stay for those in the PGPs.

Discussion

The present analysis provides objective information on a representative sample of the California metropolitan area population, which included prepaid group practice members who comprised about half of all such members under the age of 65 in the United States in 1975. Those in PGPs were 15 percent of the entire sample but were 21 percent of those with any private health coverage, because 27 percent of the sample had no private coverage.

Most government workers in California are offered an HMO choice. About 36 percent of government workers with private health care coverage in the study areas were in a PGP. These market share data are more pertinent to the issue of competition between private third parties than those that simply take PGP members as a percent of the general population. Persons with no private coverage are not part of the market for such coverage. A substantial portion of those in the private sector with "other private coverage" are not offered an HMO choice.

The study shows that those with no private coverage were less healthy and used more health care services than those with private coverage. A surprisingly high 27 percent of the entire sample under age 65 had no private health care coverage. Preschool children and adults in their early twenties were least likely to have private coverage. About 40 percent of the entire sample under age 1 had no private health care coverage. Many young adults had no private coverage in the period between losing their dependent status on their parents' plans and obtaining stable employment with health care coverage as a fringe benefit. In the United States, birthrate peaks for women at age 23. Thus, many young mothers and their infants are part of the significant population without private health care coverage.

Individual members of a prepaid group practice are self-selected since all have voluntarily enrolled. Those PGP members in groups that have dual or plural choice have also voluntarily enrolled. Thus the great majority of PGP members are self-selected. The real issue is the effect of this self-selection process on the health characteristics of those in the PGP.

On an a priori basis, most investigators believe that there are important offsetting factors that could influence the health characteristics of those who join PGPs under a dual-choice system or enroll as individuals (Donabedian, 1969). On the one hand, the generally broader benefits in the PGP might attract those who have more health problems. But, on the other hand, the necessity of selecting a new physician when joining a PGP may serve as a barrier to those in poorer health who are most likely to have active physician ties.

Direct measures of health status of a cross-section of those enrolled in PGPs and other private coverage are provided by this study. It is clear from the foregoing analysis of the California sample, summarized in Table 9, that the percents of those with limitations on activity due to chronic conditions, and of those whose self-appraised health status was "fair" or "poor," were slightly higher among PGP members than among those with other private coverage. The PGP population had somewhat more restricted-activity days and bed-disability days per person (due to both acute and chronic conditions) than those with other private coverage. The rate of physician visits for PGP members was about the same as for those with other private coverage, but those in PGPs were more likely to have made at least one visit to a physician during the preceding year.

The population sample in this study resided in eight different metropolitan areas of a large state. Although the health status of the PGP members was similar to that of those with other private coverage, on the average, it is possible that this relation could have varied from area to area. But the present analysis indicates that PGPs are not favored with a healthier population in California. The results of the present

TABLE 9

Summary of Health Status and Measures of Health Care Use by Type of
Health Coverage for Population under Age 65 in Eight California
SMSAs* (1975)

Health Status and Measures of Health Care Use	Type of Health Coverage		
	PGP	Other Private Coverage	No Private Coverage
Sample size: number of people	1,278	4,900	2,271
Chronic conditions			
a. Percent of sample with chronic conditions causing limitation in activity	11.1%	10.8%	15.2%
b. Average number of chronic conditions causing limitations per person with limitation in activity	1.30	1.29	1.43
Self-assessed health status			
c. Percent "fair" or "poor"	9.2%	8.3%	13.4%
Restricted-activity days per year†			
d. Bed-disability days	6.3	5.9	9.4
e. Other restricted-activity days	14.9	12.0	14.1
f. Total	21.2	17.9	23.5
Physician visits‡			
g. Per person per year	4.15	4.05	4.33
h. Percent of persons with one or more in past year	65.7%	60.0%	57.9%
Hospital care,†§ episodes per 1,000 person-years			
i. Obstetric delivery	18.0	12.9	25.5
j. All other	75.1	91.8	100.9
k. Total episodes	93.1	104.7	126.4
l. Average stay in days	5.04	5.78	7.05
m. Days per 1,000 person-years	469.5	604.1	891.7

*San Francisco-Oakland; Los Angeles-Long Beach; Riverside-Ontario-San Bernardino;
Vallejo-Napa; San Jose; Sacramento; San Diego; Orange County.
†Based on 2-week recall.
‡Based on 1-year recall.
§Excludes well newborns.

study were similar to those of the more limited 1968 study (Roemer et al., 1972) conducted in Los Angeles County.

Despite morbidity equal to or greater than that of persons with other private coverage, the PGP population did use substantially fewer short-term hospital days per year because of lower admission rates and shorter lengths of hospital stay. (Note that the present study included *all* hospital use, including any that might not have been covered by the PGPs.)

Because the PGP members have a much higher crude annual birthrate than those with other private health coverage (18.0 vs. 12.9 per 1,000 under age 65), the disparity in use of nonobstetric hospital services was even greater than that in total hospital use. And for every obstetric delivery admission, there is usually at least one other conception-related admission. The high obstetric delivery rate of those in the PGP was consistent with a rational decision by those offered a choice of plans, because PGPs have generally offered far more complete maternity benefits than alternative plans.

During any given year, there are many factors that influence the relative health status of those enrolled in a PGP (or any other form of health care coverage). These factors include the characteristics of all those who join and those who terminate (including births and deaths), as well as changes in the continuing members caused by the passage of time. Each year, each continuing member becomes a year older, and net changes in the PGP due to gaining or losing members may or may not offset the risk effects of this aging process of the majority of members who continue. It is impossible to determine the health status of those in PGPs relative to that of any other population except by direct questions or observations regarding the health status of all (or a sample) of the populations being compared.

For these reasons, it is not possible to draw conclusions about the health status of PGP members in general solely on the basis of the health status of those who joined recently. (It is equally fallacious to impute the health status of those in the PGP from the characteristics of those who terminate).

Luft (1980) has raised the question of whether PGP members are more averse to hospital care than nonmembers. The physician visit rates of PGP members are at least as high as for those with other health care coverage. As the patient controls the visit rate to a considerable degree, those in PGPs do not appear averse to seeking physician services. Nor is any evidence offered to support the hypothesis that PGP members simply dislike hospital care. A review of many unpublished and published surveys on reasons for selecting a PGP plan under a dual-choice system has failed to show that the reputation of the PGP regarding per member hospital use was ever mentioned by the respondents, either pro or con. Health economists understandably are interested in the differences in hospital use for various forms of health care coverage. But this interest may not be shared by the average person.

Alternative Hypotheses

Most of the published speculation on what contributes to the lower hospital use by PGP members concerns some process within the PGP, and the predominant fee-for-service (FFS) sector is tacitly considered the norm. The fee-for-service sector is predominant in the volume of services provided but its position as the norm can be challenged. A number of alternative hypotheses occur if the PGP is considered the norm and FFS is considered aberrant in its behavior.

We offer an alternative set of speculative hypotheses on the observed differences in hospital use between the PGP and FFS. These hypotheses are based on the different economic incentives faced by providers and enrollees of these two types of private health care coverage and their corresponding delivery modes.

1. With fee-for-service, patients are often willing and able to shop for nonemergency office care since their third-party coverage of office services is still limited by deductibles, copayments, and exclusions. As a result, prices for many office services reflect a somewhat competitive market.

2. In contrast, FFS patients are less able or willing to shop for hospital services. In addition, the physician fees and other cost components of hospital care are more completely covered by third parties than those for office (or home) services. This makes FFS patients less sensitive to prices for inpatient care than for office care.

3. The considerable practice expenses of FFS physicians are largely for office services. Physician services in the hospital result in little

practice expense to physicians, particularly at the margin. Hence, compared with office services, a much higher proportion of physician fees for hospital services is net revenue.

4. As a consequence, physician net income per hour for hospital services substantially exceeds their net income per hour for office services. This disparity has widened over time, in part because of the substitution of usual and customary fees for fees based on fixed relative values. This system permits fees for hospital services to increase more rapidly than those for office services.

5. These circumstances provide FFS physicians with a growing economic incentive to hospitalize, particularly for some medical and surgical care that could be performed effectively without admission to a hospital. This incentive is reinforced by some noneconomic benefits to the physician for hospital care (e.g., house officer services).

6. The FFS patient also has economic incentives favoring hospitalization, since the out-of-pocket costs to the patient are likely to be less for the hospital care than for extensive office (or home) care.

7. The individual physicians comprising the prepaid group practice have little or no personal economic incentive affecting the place where appropriate care is given since their individual incomes do not depend on the location of the care they provide. Physicians in prepaid group practice and physicians in FFS practice probably share many of the same noneconomic incentives to hospitalize.

8. The PGP patients are likely to have negligible out-of-pocket costs, regardless of where their care is provided. Consequently, their economic concern is limited to the indirect costs (e.g., family convenience) of hospital care compared with those of office care.

Conclusion

Luft et al. (1980) have summarized the relative hospital utilization of those in HMOs, as follows:

> Total medical care costs are substantially lower for HMO enrollees than for the general population and these lower costs are attributable to lower hospitalization rates. The reasons for this lower hospitalization are less clear. . . . Two major alternative explanations remain: (1) that HMOs provide the appropriate level of care, and the conventional system too much; and (2) that utilization differ-

ences are attributable to the self-selection of different types of people into HMOs and into the conventional system. (Luft et al., 1980:178–179)

We believe that, for those with private health care coverage, the findings presented in this analysis greatly increase the likelihood that the first explanation is correct and that the second is not. The PGP will be understood better when more is known about the alternative forms of health care coverage and delivery with which it is compared.

References

Bureau of the Census, 1975. *Health Interview Survey, Interviewer's Manual.* Washington, D.C.: Government Printing Office.

Choi, J., and Ries, P. 1978. Sociodemographic and Health Characteristics of Persons by Private Health Insurance Coverage and Type of Plan: United States, 1975. *Advancedata* 32. National Center for Health Statistics, Department of Health, Education, and Welfare. Washington, D.C.: Government Printing Office.

Donabedian, A. 1969. An Evaluation of Prepaid Group Practice. *Inquiry* 6(3):3–27.

Luft, H.S. 1978. How Do Health Maintenance Organizations Achieve Their Savings? Rhetoric and Evidence. *New England Journal of Medicine* 298:1336–1343.

———. 1980. HMO Performance: Current Knowledge and Questions for the 1980s. *Group Health Journal* 1(1):34–40.

———, Feder, J., Holahan, J., and Lennox, K. 1980. Health Maintenance Organizations. In Feder, J., Holahan, J., and Marmor, T., eds., *National Health Insurance: Conflicting Goals and Policy Choices.* Washington, D.C.: Urban Institute.

Mullooly, J.P., and Freeborn, D.K. 1979. The Effect of Length of Membership upon Utilization of Ambulatory Care Services. *Medical Care* 17(9):922–936.

National Center for Health Statistics. 1977. Limitation of Activity Due to Chronic Conditions. *Vital and Health Statistics.* DHEW Publication No. (HRA) 77-1537-Series 10, No. 111. Public Health Service. Washington, D.C.: Government Printing Office.

———. 1980. Utilization of Short-Stay Hospitals: Annual Summary of the United States, 1978. *Vital and Health Statistics.* PHS Publication No. 80-1797-Series 13, No. 46. Public Health Service. Washington, D.C.: Government Printing Office.

Newhouse, J.P., and Phelps, C.E. 1976. New Estimates of Price and Income Elasticities of Medical Care Services. In Rossett, R.N., ed., *The Role of Health Insurance in the Health Services Sector*. New York: National Bureau of Economic Research.

Roemer, M.I., Hetherington, R.W., Hopkins, C.E., Gerst, A.E., Parsons, E., and Long, D.M. 1972. *Health Insurance Effects, Services, Expenditures, and Attitudes under Three Types of Plans*. Ann Arbor: Bureau of Public Health Economics, Research Series No. 16, University of Michigan.

Acknowledgments: The author appreciates the prompt review given to an earlier draft by several readers, particularly Harold S. Luft and Peter Ries. Many subsequent comments by others were also of value. D. Taya Dunn of the Kaiser Foundation Health Plan, Inc., Central Office performed all of the computer analyses used in this study, at the Computer Center of the University of California at Berkeley.

Address correspondence to: Dr. Mark S. Blumberg, Kaiser Foundation Health Plan, Inc., One Kaiser Plaza, Oakland, CA 94612.

IV Other Issues

Milbank Memorial Fund Quarterly/*Health and Society, Vol. 57, No. 3, 1979*

Research in Resource Allocation in a Prepaid Group Practice

JAMES A. HESTER

Massachusetts Institute of Technology

HEALTH MAINTENANCE ORGANIZATIONS (HMOs) have long been proposed as one mechanism for controlling health care costs and encouraging a more rational allocation of resources to health care needs. Although a wealth of literature has been published on the concepts of HMOs, the theory of their operation, and their performance in gross terms, very little information has been available on the details of how they function, and especially on the analytic tools used to make internal decisions on how to allocate staff and capital. The Southern California Region of the Kaiser-Permanente Medical Care Program (K-P) has made a major commitment over the last four years to a program of applied research directed toward improving the analytic capabilities available for short-term staffing, budgeting and rate setting decisions, and for long-term member and facility expansion policies. This paper provides an overview of the types of projects undertaken, and includes brief summaries of some of the more significant findings.

The paper's intent is twofold. First, it supplies some specific insights into the surprising diversity that exists among local areas of a large-scale HMO. This diversity makes simplistic approaches to resource allocation questions infeasible in the long term. Second, the paper offers a perspective on the prospects and problems in health services research somewhat different from that recently presented by Mechanic (1978). He has argued for an isolation of health services research for immediate policy implementation, in tones reminiscent of the supporters of basic research in the hard sciences:

> The most serious problem affecting the future of health services research is the expectation that a modest research investment will provide solutions to the political dilemmas of health care. It is both naive and counterproductive to anticipate any direct relationship between such research and policy implementation. The demand that health services research questions be formulated in terms of immediate political issues, moreover, debases the processes of problem formulation, compromises adequate data acquisition, and inevitably leads to disappointment and frustration. (Mechanic, 1978: 129–130)

Yet in an era of increasing scarcity of health resources neither society, through its government, nor operational organizations through their internal staffs, can afford the luxury of long-term commitments to researchers who, as a whole, have not inspired much confidence in their ability to select or carry out research projects that will lay strong foundations for later practical applications. Perhaps one approach to building this confidence is to redirect some attention away from the ever-changing and faceless policy makers and toward the managers of major large-scale delivery systems.

As has been illustrated by the work described in this paper, the issues surrounding the ongoing allocation of resources within such institutions provide a rich set of opportunities for research that challenges the researcher, advances the state of the profession, and results in significant organizational change. Although institutional settings are by no means insulated from the political pressures and constraints that Mechanic describes, they are reduced enough to make unnecessarily pessimistic his assessment that "health services research will (and, indeed, should) always be in the background in the formulation of important policy decisions unless the decisions are purely technical ones. But few important health services issues are simply matters of knowledge or technical expertise" (Mechanic, 1978: 130).

The institutional setting for the work described in this paper was the Kaiser-Permanente Medical Care Program, which provides high-quality, comprehensive medical services to over 1.4 million members in southern California. The medical care is delivered through seven relatively autonomous medical centers distributed over a 20,000-square-mile service area. The resources available to the program include 1,400 full-time salaried physicians, 140 nurse practitioners, and 1,826 staffed acute-care beds. The operating costs for these resources, which are primarily supported by revenue from the dues paid by the program's membership, were $540 million for fiscal 1978. Because of the autonomy that has evolved for each of the seven medical centers, K-P presents an unparalleled natural experiment in which seven sets of group practices are functioning with identical benefits for members and incentives to providers. The decisions that determine what resources will be available, and when and where, are made at many levels throughout the organization, including senior regional management, the area administrators responsible for each medical center, and the department heads, chiefs of service, and supervisors responsible for the day-to-day delivery of care (Somers, 1971). Each medical center uses administrative structures and staffing patterns that are unique, influenced only by broad regional guidelines on either total dollars spent, or total staffing levels per thousand members. But the principal actors who shape these structures and patterns are the physicians in each medical center, especially the chiefs of service and local medical directors.

One indication of the great diversity among the areas is shown by their different approaches to providing primary care services. Some areas have developed independent departments of family practice, utilizing a combination of family practitioners and nurse practitioners, supported by a carefully structured network of linkages to specialists in the departments of internal medicine, pediatrics, and obstetrics and gynecology. Other medical centers rely, instead, on a single department of internal medicine, using primarily physicians as the provider, with a small number of nurse specialists who function in restricted roles. A similar diversity is evident in the behavior of the medical centers over time. K-P has been in existence for more than twenty-five years, and significant differences in the long-term trends in key parameters such as inpatient utilization rates remain unexplained. For example, two medical centers that ten years ago had essentially the same inpatient utilization, as measured by patient days per thousand members, have experienced opposite long-term trends, one increasing while the other has decreased, so that today the inpatient utilization rates, adjusted for age and sex, differ by 55 percent.

A key question for management in such a setting is how to determine what changes in resource allocations would result in better performance, and how to provide incentives to the area directors for making such changes. Formal analysis of alternatives can play a role in some issues. However, given the nature of the management of medicine, there are major constraints on the impact that analysis can have in such decisions. K-P provides an almost ideal setting for analysis: a large-scale prepaid health program in which the decision makers have direct control over and responsibility for all major resources, and the managers have demonstrated an enlightened attitude toward supporting the analytic staffs and the data collection required to conduct meaningful studies. During the last four years, a large number of applied research projects have been completed, which provide good insight into the limitations of analysis even in such a favorable environment. The next section of this paper will review a selected set of cases from the work completed in four subject areas and the final section will summarize some of the lessons to be learned from our experience. It should be emphasized that not all the points made in this paper can be generalized to all HMOs. The opportunities, needs, and constraints faced by prepaid health care vary with each setting.

Applied Research in Resource Allocation

The analyses described below were carried out in an unusual setting, and it is important to understand some of the characteristics of the environment before the substance of the work is reviewed. During the four-year period under review (1974–1978), the staff directly involved in the projects originally envisioned for the Applied Research Unit expanded approximately tenfold, from four analysts to slightly over forty. Even a program the size of K-P could not make a commitment of this magnitude to "research." The principal reason for such growth was the steady expansion of the ongoing responsibilities, primarily staff support to both regional management and the area administrators in the twice-a-year operating and capital budget cycles. Approximately three-fourths of the applied research efforts during the four years were spent on developing the forecasting and analysis tools necessary for the short-range and long-range planning cycles described elsewhere (Richter, 1978; Rubenstein, Hester, and Brannin, 1978), and on producing those forecasts twice a year. The research projects have encompassed all aspects of the analysis, including membership forecasting, inpatient and outpatient utilization, and selection of sites for new facilities. As both the tools and the institutional framework for the planning analysis have stabilized, the character of these projects has shifted from applied research to a greater emphasis on routine production and continuing development. The formalization of these responsibilities has resulted in the spin-off of two operating groups, one for short-range planning support, the other for long-range planning support, with the result that the regional applied research staff is again at the original size of four analysts.

A twice-a-year budgeting cycle implies that the staff responsible is continuously in production of a major set of operating forecasts: data collection and preparation, analysis of initial projections, review with administrators, and a seemingly never-ending cycle of updates and modifications. Because of the way in which staff were assigned, almost every individual involved in the applied research projects outlined below was also responsible for some aspect of this routine planning support. The continuing exposure to the blunt pragmatic probing by seasoned line administrators and regional managers inevitably shaped both the scope and the execution of the applied research projects. Much of the work represents attempts to apply simple quantitative tools to large, previously unanalyzed data bases in order to answer fundamental questions about the characteristics of K-P's membership and their use of medical care services. There has been no pretense of generating either highly refined causal models or finely tuned optimizations, for reasons discussed in the concluding section. Instead, the theme of the work has been twofold: first, the development of simple new tools for budgeting staff and facilities, and second, descriptive analyses in support of specific major issues of management.

The originators of the topics chosen included the research staff itself, line managers in the K-P facilities, regional managers in the southern California central office, and corporate staff for the K-P program as a whole in Oakland. The realities of organizational dynamics shaped both the topics selected (e.g., note the absence of a major evaluation of nurse practitioners) and the pace of completing the work. Some indication of the interaction between organizational dynamics and research issues will be given, but a full discussion of this theme is beyond the scope of this paper.

The efforts described here divide naturally into four categories of analysis: 1) membership, 2) ambulatory care, 3) inpatient utilization, and 4) special projects. Selected major projects in each category are discussed in order to give an indication of the nature of the projects and their consequences. Each piece of work summarized is substantial enough to merit a separate paper to do full justice to the analysis; each analysis has been documented in internal K-P reports. Formal papers on several of the projects are now being prepared for publication.

Membership Studies

Outpatient Membership Project. In a prepaid group practice with multiple locations, a precise understanding of the size and composition of the membership being served at each location is essential to the functioning of the program. In the short term, the allocation of staff and total operating budget to each location must be based upon the membership served by each location. Even errors as small as 3 to 5 percent in this allocation can result in significant inequities in the physician staffing and other resources available at each location to service the needs of its members. In addition, long-range (three to ten years) planning for the allocation of capital for facility expansion must be based upon forecasts of the geographic distribution of the total growth in membership, and the draw-off of membership from existing facilities that is caused by the addition of new medical centers. This is not a simple problem, since the location of new facilities in an area can, and usually does, stimulate additional growth in membership. However, the effects of this stimulus can be analyzed separately. Finally, both cross-sectional and longitudinal analyses of utilization rates at each location require a consistent definition of the population at risk at each location.

Since the allocation of resources based on the size of the membership is such an important issue, K-P initiated a major review of its allocation methodology. The outpatient membership project examined the extent to which the members of each of the seven medical centers identified with that center and used it to obtain most of their medical care. Given a network of facilities located close enough to each other to offer each member a choice among two or more possible service locations within a reasonable driving time, it is not obvious that a well-defined membership exists for each medical center. It is quite conceivable that members might switch back and forth among several facilities, according to the availability of services, so that no meaningful distinct membership could be identified. The project analyzed the utilization records of a 1 percent sample (13,000 members) of the program's membership over a one-year period. The results demonstrated that a well-defined membership does in fact exist for each area, and that a member-oriented allocation was feasible. The key findings were:

1. Almost 90 percent of the members who used outpatient services in the eleven-month period obtained 100 percent of their care from a single medical center; i.e., they did not split *any* of their utilization with another source of care (Table 1).

TABLE 1
Use of One of Six Medical Centers by a 1-Percent
Sample (13,000) of the Members (1976)

	Number of Centers Used					
	1	2	3	4	5	6
*Percent of sample using center	89.20	9.90	0.74	0.14	0.02	0

*Based on records of visits to doctors' offices.

2. Consequently, each medical center in the region was found to be providing the overwhelming majority (typically 95 percent) of its outpatient services to health plan members affiliated principally with that medical center.

3. The age sex profiles of the membership for the several medical centers did vary significantly (Table 2) and needed to be accounted for in analyzing utilization, especially of inpatient services.

TABLE 2
Age Composition of Members of Seven Medical Centers (1978)

Age (years)	Medical Center							Entire Region
	A	B	C	D	E	F	G	
0-14	23%	27%	23%	25%	22%	24%	24%	24%
15-44	49	49	51	49	49	51	52	50
45-64	21	20	20	19	23	19	19	20
65+	7	4	6	7	6	6	5	6
Total	100%	100%	100%	100%	100%	100%	100%	100%

These findings imply that it is possible to identify the membership served by each medical center, and to compare the differences in characteristics that should significantly influence the amount and composition of the utilization of medical care.

On the basis of these results, a proposal was made to the regional medical group management to use these data to produce a new member-based allocation. Even though the initial response to the proposal was favorable, almost eighteen months passed before the change was implemented. Since the proposed change implied significant shifts in the official allocation of members and thus of resources among the seven medical centers, a number of detailed studies were made to explain exactly why the changes occurred. The departure of the key managers who had approved the change required starting almost from scratch with a new review committee. Finally, the desire to produce more reliable estimates of the size of the over-65 population required waiting for the expansion of the sampling fraction in the data system that supported the allocation.

Membership Termination Study. This study documented for the first time the turnover of membership that results both from involuntary disenrollment due to job change, moving, etc., and from voluntary disenrollment. Because of the myriad possibilities for change in the status of membership, for example, those due to changes in benefit coverage, conversions to individual coverage, and transfers between different employer groups, it had previously been impossible to determine the true level of membership terminations. A precise set of definitions was used, along with a 10 percent sample (140,000 members) drawn from a special membership file that linked enrollment histories, to analyze both the overall termination rate and how it is affected by such matters as age, geographic location, and coverage.

The results of the study had a major effect on the conceptual framework underlying the analysis of membership growth in the program. In the past, attention had focused exclusively on the net increase in membership, which tended to be in the range of 5 to 7 percent per year. With a turnover rate of approximately 17 percent per year, it became clear that the net growth was the residual of two major gross flows: an inflow of 23 percent new members and an outflow of 17 percent due to terminations, both voluntary and involuntary. Since small shifts in either of the gross flows could have a major impact upon their difference, i.e., the net growth, it was easier to understand the volatility of the fluctuations in net growth of members experienced during the 1970s. In addition, concern over the effect of the large volume of new members identified here, approximately 260,000 in 1978, led to the special project on new member entry described below.

Ambulatory Care Analysis

Early in the development of our research priorities, the decision was made to have an ongoing series of projects exploring the delivery of outpatient services. The consensus among both the support staff and the administrators was that ambulatory care offered long-term potential for changes that would result in greater satisfaction to members and providers, and greater efficiency.

Urgent Care Study. The largest single study in this group was a 2.5-year analysis of the delivery of urgent care services to a sample of 7,000 adults (over 14 years of age) at a medical center and its affiliated satellite clinics. Patients were supplied with questionnaires and their written answers used to develop a profile of the members who visited outpatient clinics and requested general medical and surgical care on an urgent basis, i.e., within forty-eight hours of initial contact. Two surveys were conducted approximately nine months apart in order 1) to develop a broad-based description of the magnitude of the demand for urgent care, the characteristics of the members who asked for urgent care, and the respective roles of different departments in handling these patients; and 2) to assess the impacts of several significant operational changes in key outpatient clinic areas. Specifically, the surveys sought to answer the following questions:

1. What are the characteristics of the members who utilize these clinics? In particular, what proportion of them perceive themselves as having "regular physicians"?

2. Are characteristics such as the member's age, sex, and length of time in the health plan significant determinants of the likelihood that users of medical short-appointment clinics will have a regular physician?

3. What are the characteristics of the physicians identified as being the members' regular physicians? For example, where are they located, and what is their specialty?

4. Why do patients with regular physicians visit short-appointment or walk-in clinics, instead of their own physicians?

5. Do patients come to these clinics with new or with old medical problems? Have they seen a physician previously for the same complaint?

The second survey, which included 5,000 patients, showed that those adults who used urgent care represented all age groups (Fig. 1), were relatively long-time members of the health plan, and tended to be habitual users of same-day or walk-in clinics. In addition, approximately one-half of the patients surveyed reported having a regular or family physician. The findings indicated that members who had regular physicians were in fact "splitting" their utilization of outpatient services. This was confirmed by the patients' response to the question on why they were using the medical short-appointment clinic and walk-in clinics instead of their regular physicians. Although many patients mentioned the difficulty in getting to see their physicians, almost one-quarter (23.8%) of the

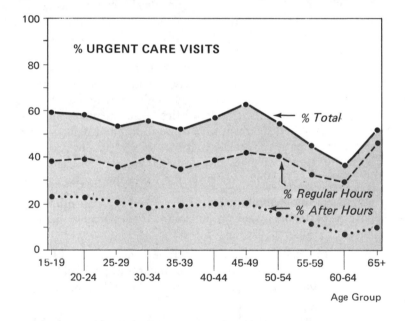

FIG. 1. Estimated proportion of 5,000 outpatient visits for urgent care to the departments of internal medicine, family practice, obstetrics and gynecology, and surgery, plotted by age groups.

respondents said that they didn't generally go to their physicians for the type of problem they were having. These members apparently tended to see their regular physicians for specific ongoing or chronic problems. For complaints such as colds, flu, etc., they perceived the medical short-appointment clinic as the more appropriate site for care. This finding is also supported by the results of asking for the patients' descriptions of their medical complaint: 42.2 percent were described as new illnesses.

Changes in clinic staffing and scheduling policies, both across departments, and in one case in the same two departments over time, were shown to influence the member's choice in predictable ways. For example, a simple change was made in scheduling procedures, which had the appointment clerk inquire whether the member had a regular physician, and referred the patient to his doctor when he had one. This change reduced the number of members who had been using walk-in clinics for urgent care, even though they had a regular physician. Given that the demand for urgent care was found to be 40 to 60 percent of the total demand for primary outpatient care (Fig. 1), how each department handles urgent care requests has implications for developing effective resources for urgent care. A second medical center has already made use of the results of this project in planning an urgent care center for its members.

Primary-Care Module Evaluation. At the medical center, a multiobjective evaluation was conducted of an experimental primary-care module that tested the expanded use of nurse practitioners, as well as a carefully structured network of referral linkages to the principal specialty departments, internal medicine, pediatrics, and obstetrics and gynecology. Some objectives of the primary-care module were improving the continuity of care through consistent use of the patient's primary-care physician for all nonemergency ailments; better use of resources through the use of nurse practitioners; improved access to care through better telephone communication from physician to patient, closer patient-physician relations, and overall better organization within the module; improved quality of care through closer specialist relations with the family-practice primary-care module; and increased satisfaction to patient and provider.

The evaluation compared the performance of this module with that of a traditional family practice department, along the dimensions of cost, accessibility, member satisfaction, provider satisfaction, and quality of care. Such a broad-based evaluation necessitated collaboration among several regional support departments and the facility personnel. It supplemented routine data obtained from encounter forms and accounting sources with special patient surveys at the time a service was provided. The overall results of the evaluation were quite favorable, and have resulted in the adoption of this model as the approach for providing primary care in the area. The second module has already been placed in operation.

Both studies met the formal objectives established when they began, but in many ways they were the most disappointing projects attempted. While the research staff believed that most of the general findings were the result of region-wide structural characteristics and thus applicable to the six other medical centers in the program, for the most part medical group management perceived the analyses as not being transferable outside the one center where they were conducted. These reactions crystallized our appreciation of the degree to which each medical center viewed both its problems and their solutions as being unique.

We also gained more understanding of the limitations of the existing routine data on outpatient services, and the recognition that special surveys or other techniques of collecting primary data could not fill this gap on a routine basis. The problems with the existing outpatient data were not atypical for a large multilocation system. Basic definitions of departments, type of service, etc., had not been updated and existing definitions were applied inconsistently from department to department. This situation has been partially remedied through a major two-year effort, which was part of the implementation of an improved performance budgeting system within the medical group.

However, one difficulty remains in employing data from routine sources to conduct meaningful analyses: the absence of information on the presenting medical problem and diagnosis. In the urgent-care study and other similar efforts, it became clear that an episode-based analysis is needed (Solon, 1967), to be able to analyze the interaction between the group member and the system of delivering health care. If analysis focuses on the single encounter between patient and system, a false profile of how the system functions can be obtained. Almost two-thirds of initial visits result in follow-up care, so that the patient must usually be seen for more than one visit. Also, the multiple entry points in the health care system generate special problems. False economies in one department, for example in the evening after-hours clinics, can result in lack of definitive care, so that the patient soon reappears at some other point in the system.

Dealing with this issue requires accurate, reproducible coding of medical problem and diagnosis. This has been achieved in research and smaller operational settings (Barnett, 1973; Greenfield et al., 1978), but not at the scale (six million provider contacts per year) involved in K-P. Since research applications by themselves cannot justify the costs involved, the program is currently reviewing whether its management analyses will require such data.

Inpatient Utilization

Estimates of inpatient utilization rates at specific medical centers are an essential component of both long- and short-range planning in the program. In the short term, forecasts of patient days are the measure of workload volume, which drives the budgets for hospital staffing. In the long-range analyses, the timing and size of major additions to the number of beds are linked directly to projected utilization by members. The use of inpatient services within the program shows a degree of variation that has yet to be explained. If we compare utilization rates in the seven medical centers, we find a 55 percent variation even after adjusting for age and sex differences (Table 3). If we look at region-wide trends over time, we find that raw utilization (not adjusted for age/sex changes in membership) has declined an average of 1 percent per year over the last eight years, and age-specific utilization has decreased almost twice that fast.

TABLE 3

Comparison of Annual Inpatient Utilization Rates at Seven Medical Centers (1976)

Inpatient Utilization (Days/1000 Members)	Medical Center							Entire Region
	A	B	C	D	E	F	G	
Actual	480	399	426	528	430	493	309	441
Age/sex adjusted	448	437	424	519	411	504	333	441

Inpatient Utilization Study. This study utilizes the computerized 100 percent sample of discharge abstracts, which has been maintained in the program since 1969, as a resource in explaining the behavior described above. The utilization data have been combined with age- and sex-specific membership data to allow a population-based analysis. The analysis first computes the utilization rate expected for each area if it followed regional average patterns. The variation from expected is then explained by three types of factors: age-sex composition of membership, admission rates, and lengths of stay. Case mix is adjusted by using either the diagnosis categories of the Professional Activity Study (PAS) or the diagnosis-related groups (DRGs) developed by Fetter and Mills (1976). The analysis is carried out for each of the five major services (obstetrics, gynecology, pediatrics, medicine, general surgery) at each medical center, as well as for the medical center as a whole.

The study has not been completed as yet, so that its final results and impact cannot be described. First indications are that variations in morbidity patterns from area to area, as well as differences in physician patterns of practice, will be important in explaining the data in Table 3. Preliminary results of the analysis by service have already been incorporated into the short-term forecasts prepared for setting hospital budgets.

Inpatient Case-Mix Analysis. In a related effort, the case mix of each of the K-P hospitals has been compared both with each other and with a sample from community hospitals. This study is not population-based like the previous one. It looks only at the patient load admitted to each hospital and estimates the relative complexity of the case mix it represents and the impact of that case mix on the average length of stay and average cost.

The K-P data for one year (1976) were obtained from the 100 percent sample of discharges already described. Data on clusters of community hospitals, for the same year, were purchased from a discharge abstract service. The first step was to construct the detailed profile of the case mix served by each institution by allocating each discharge into one of 383 DRGs. The DRGs are more appropriate than the traditional categories of the International Classification of Diseases, Adapted (ICDA) or the PAS categories for analyzing the impact of case mix on resource use, because they take into account the effect of secondary diagnoses, operations, and complications (Fetter and Thompson, 1975). The distributions were consolidated into case-mix indices by using total length of stay by DRG as a weighting factor. The analysis separated out the relative importance of two types of effects—differences in the mix of patients hospitalized, i.e., case mix, versus differences in the manner in which patients with the same medical problem were managed, i.e., performance.

Interpretation of the distributions and indices is now under way. However, preliminary results agree with the early findings of the inpatient utilization study and reveal a significant variation in case mix among the K-P medical centers. Both of these studies began because of a concern over how differences in inpatient utilization affect resource allocation. Inpatient days are a fair measure of resource use in planning future facilities, but they are a poor measure of costs per case in estimating the impact of case mix on operating costs. Carrying out the case-mix analysis disclosed one of the disadvantages of prepaid medical care. since no hospital bill is prepared for each patient, there was no record on a case-by-case basis of the services used. This meant that it was impossible to determine the average cost per case for the different types of cases. Surrogate cost data from fee-for-service hospitals can be, and have been, used to make approximate calculations. However, a full analysis of the effects of case mix on *costs* will not be possible until the equivalent of a patient billing system is installed. As was the situation in the problem of missing data on medical problems for outpatient services, such a data system could not be justified if they were to be used only in an analysis. It appears that an automated admit, discharge, and transfer system, combined with portions of automated order-entry systems, can be justified by their impact on hospital operations. If so, they will provide the core of the required cost data system. In summary, although prepaid health plans do not require detailed resource-tracking systems for external billing, such systems may be quite useful for the internal management of medical center budgets and rates.

Special Projects

The project described here is representative of the short-term interdepartmental efforts requested by senior regional management to resolve pressing, immediate questions. Since the analysis phase typically lasts only two to three months, any new efforts to collect significant source data are precluded.

New Member Entry Project. The manner in which approximately 260,000 new members each year enter the Southern California Region of the Kaiser-Permanente Medical Care Program was reviewed by a special regional committee. The objective was to develop recommendations that would improve the entry system in three ways:

1. More appropriate matching of services to the needs of new adult members, especially for those with immediate medical problems.

2. Improved control over entry, to reduce the peaked workload that now results from the concentration of new enrollments effective in the first month of the year.

3. Improved orientation of new members, to make them more familiar with proper utilization of services, and to encourage them routinely to use one particular medical center and provider as a source of care.

The committee's findings and recommendations covered all aspects of the region's response to new members: processing of applications and issuing of membership cards, providing initial acute and routine medical services, orienting and educating the members, and linking new members to a particular location of care and a regular provider. It was not possible to single out one or a few functions that could be concentrated on, to the exclusion of the rest.

The report relied heavily upon the experience of the committee members and of other individuals in the program who were interviewed during the course of its work. This expertise was supplemented by statistical analysis, which usually confirmed the first impressions of the committee but from time to time provided some surprising insights. The data for this analysis came from a combination of the special files of membership status developed from the termination study described previously, the 1 percent member-oriented sample of outpatient utilization based upon encounter data, and special surveys conducted at two medical centers. Such statistics were useful; however, the most important information came from the lengthy candid exchanges among the committee members during their working sessions. After distribution of the preliminary report of the committee, these discussions were expanded to include all senior managers.

Two of the principal findings that shaped the recommendations were:

1. The number of new members entering the program each year is substantial in all medical centers, but varies widely from area to area. Even with the closing of new group enrollment in 1978, 260,000 new members should be added, representing 103,000 new families. For a typical medical center (200,000 members), this represents 160 new members each working day, 110 being adults over 15. The percentage of members who were new in 1976 averaged 18 percent region-wide, but varied from 31 percent in one medical center to 14 percent in two other medical centers (Table 4).

TABLE 4

Number and Age Distribution of New Members
in Seven Medical Centers (1976)

Members	Medical Center							Entire Region
	A	B	C	D	E	F	G	
Number new members	43,700	45,200	19,600	27,400	50,600	28,200	19,500	234,200
Percent new members	17%	20%	14%	15%	31%	14%	17%	18%
Total members	257,000	220,000	138,000	185,000	164,000	199,000	116,000	1,279,000

2. New members seek and obtain their first medical services much more quickly than was anticipated. They account for a significant fraction of outpatient services. In 1976, approximately 45 percent of new members had an initial contact for care within their first three months of membership. This rate is comparable to that of the health plan membership as a whole, and appears to represent needs for specific acute or chronic care as opposed to physical examinations. Overall, new members account for about one-fifth of the outpatient services provided.

The recommendations are expected to be incorporated as specific objectives for each department involved. They encompass a broad scope of program operations, including the first health assessments after the member joins the roll of the regular physician, the distribution and content of membership cards and orientation literature, and the timing of new admissions to membership.

Some Observations

In assembling the above summary of applied research projects, it has been impossible to resist the temptation to reflect on the current limitations to the effective application of analysis to questions of resource allocation faced by providers in general and by health maintenance organizations in particular. This is admittedly a significantly restricted subset of possible applications, yet the topics involved are essential ones for the translation of broader policy analyses into changes in how people actually obtain medical care. These particular applications also face the most demanding requirements from the decision makers involved. If these analyses turn out to be in error, to have neglected a key factor or misestimated a response, the manager involved has to live with the consequences of those mistakes, often for a long time. Also, since resource reallocations usually imply that some medical centers will get a smaller staff and fewer facilities, the intensity of the probing of staff analysts by the "losing" manager is something that must be experienced to be appreciated. This interaction over time, in fact, represented an ultimate quality-control system upon much of the work presented here. As such, it had some obvious limitations; for example, emotions occasionally overruled logic, and the critic's lack of formal analytic background sometimes hindered the unraveling of the critical comments and using them to make adjustments in the methodology. However, in comparing these experiences with the more traditional reference system for papers, I believe that the sustained interaction over time with an interested group of critics was more effective in revealing flaws in logic, alternative approaches, and basic inconsistencies or errors in source data. For the reasons detailed below, much of the extensive body of analytical work published to date is not very helpful in such a setting. This is not meant as a condemnation of the work, but rather to emphasize that the requirements are different.

Health Maintenance Organizations: Uniform Concept, Diverse Reality

Health maintenance organizations have received steadily increasing attention as an alternative form of organizing, providing, and reimbursing health care services. For the most part, HMOs are classified into two primary types, prepaid group practices with physicians organized into multispecialty groups and paid an annual salary, and groups of independent practitioners, which are looser affiliations of physicians who are reimbursed on a fee-for-service basis. Although some awareness appears to be developing of the great diversity that exists among existing HMOs, even among those that fall into the prepaid group practice model, this understanding is not widely shared. The prepaid group practice form of HMOs is an extremely complex organization involving numerous formal contractual arrangements among health plan administrators, medical care providers, and the administrators of clinic and inpatient facilities. The resulting institutional relations, financial incentives, and administrative practices vary widely and often influence the performance of the HMO as measured by any number of key standards: cost, accessibility, quality of services, member satisfaction, etc. In addition, as was emphasized in the introduction to this paper, multiple service locations, even when restricted to just a single HMO, usually imply the likelihood of significant variations in administrative practices and the local organization of care, which can readily confound analyses that do not take them into account.

In short, the conceptual model of an HMO that is often employed in comparative analyses between the prepaid and fee-for-service sectors, or is used in analyzing policy options for HMOs in general, is usually greatly oversimplified. It neglects key characteristics of the internal structure of those institutions, and uses aggregate measures of both inputs and outputs that often blur essential differences in performance. Some of the difficulties include the following:

1. The importance of the dynamic nature of both the membership and provider staffing is often underestimated. In our work we have found numerous examples were the 15–20 percent turnover in membership per year, and the slightly lower rates of turnover of physicians per year, affect the development of member-physician relations, member behavior in seeking care, and demands upon marketing and enrollment staff.

2. The incentives felt by individual salaried physicians on the staff are complex, and the role of economic incentives, such as the bonus offered by the Southern California Region of the Kaiser-Permanente program, may be greatly overestimated. Similarly, the economic benefits of the practice of preventive medicine are questionable in the eyes of the average staff physician (Luft, 1978).

3. The per capita amount and mix of both inpatient and outpatient services utilized by HMO members varies widely and cannot be explained by simple age-sex adjustments. Utilization rates appear to be influenced not only by internal factors such as member characteristics, provider attitudes, accessibility to care, and out-of-pocket costs, but also by external factors such as geographic setting and community provider standards.

Tools for Analysis

One of the principal reasons for the confusion outlined above and for the major limitations on analysis at the current time is the lack of adequate tools for describing the behavior of a HMO at a detailed, as opposed to gross, level. In order to make valid cross-sectional comparisons, or to anticipate "what happens if . . . ," the following tools are needed:

1. Reasonable models of behavior of members and providers, to predict the impact of differences in structural variables and other changes.

2. Accurate, reproducible measures of key inputs and outputs for both inpatient and outpatient services.

3. Routine collection of key data on mix of services, costs, and accessibility as part of an ongoing management information system that provides both summary reports to regional management and regular operating reports to line supervisors.

4. Techniques for combining impacts when the organization has multiple objectives.

In spite of the extensive research in health care delivery during the last three decades, the tools available in these areas fall short of the need. The understanding of key incentives and the factors motivating behavior, which is incorporated in many of the formal models that attempt to explain the behavior of users and providers, is often somewhat naive and idealistic. For example, models are needed that can estimate outpatient utilization while taking into account the effect of member characteristics, economic incentives, and characteristics of the delivery system within an HMO framework. Does a more definitive handling of a medical problem during the patient's first visit reduce the need for follow-up visits and thus result in lower total cost per episode? What is the impact of significant improvements in access upon utilization in a setting where out-of-pocket costs are negligible? How does the time required for a task change when a more skilled (or less skilled) provider is used?

The measures of output for inpatient utilization that allow analysis of case complexity have steadily improved during the past several years. We have been satisfied with the preliminary results of such classification systems as the diagnosis-related groupings (DRGs) mentioned before. This is unfortunately not true for outpatient utilization. The difficulties of obtaining reproducible coding of outpatient utilization are substantial because of the need to combine the formal diagnoses with the more general presenting symptoms in order to capture the full range of cases. The revised classification scheme developed for the National Ambulatory Care Survey is currently being assessed. Also, it is highly desirable to be able to describe outpatient utilization in terms of the total services associated with the episode of care for a given medical problem. Even within a prepaid group practice, which theoretically provides all outpatient services, the difficulty of linking discrete services spread out over a period of many months, and provided at multiple locations, is great.

A final difficulty has been the basic one of obtaining a consistent interpretation of even simple sets of definitions and complete reporting on services in a system where literally hundreds of persons are involved in collecting the source data. Even within the same organization, ensuring consistent reporting of outpatient utilization by discrete categories turned into a major one year project. As for measures of input, although measuring total costs and the amount of mix of staff time would seem to be relatively straightforward, stubbornly persistent problems have been encountered in obtaining sets of cost centers that reflect the actual structure of the delivery system, accurate accounting of direct costs to those cost centers, and meaningful allocations of indirect costs.

Many of the data used in these analyses came from a set of special computerized reporting systems, which collected data on an ongoing basis. These included a 100 percent sample of hospital discharge abstracts, a 1 percent sample of all outpatient utilization, and a 10 percent sample of members and their membership transactions. A substantial support staff (twelve clerks and five analysts) was assigned to these systems to enter the source data, ensure data quality, and program both routine and special reports. While many new HMOs have comparable or even better systems of collecting source data, very few of them have reached the stage of organizational maturity where they have the resources required to collate and interpret these data in special studies of the type described here. An additional problem for many of the new HMOs is their size; for example, with 30,000 members the number of inpatient episodes is too small to analyze case mix in a meaningful way.

It is not at all unusual in the history of the evolution of quantitative techniques, both within the health care field and outside, to find premature pressure to make analysis relevant by linking basic research to immediate prescriptions for improvement. Short-sighted responses to these forces can lead, and have led, to measurement for measurement's sake and to the neglect of the sound foundations necessary for long-term credibility. It is to be hoped that the basic tools needed to extend the range of potential applied-analysis projects chosen by large institutional providers will be forthcoming. In the meantime, the following are two of the guidelines governing the selection of applied research projects at Kaiser-Permanente:

1. Keep the research issues simple and clearly framed with an emphasis on descriptive profiles of what exists now, or on historical trends. The only two Kaiser-Permanente projects that have ventured beyond descriptive analyses are the travel-time models used in facility-location analysis, and a probable-length-of-stay model incorporated in an optimal scheduling system for elective admissions. Otherwise, recommendations for change have been tentative, and stressed the use of pilot projects. Both the conceptual and operational designs of the pilots have relied heavily upon nonanalytic inputs from line staff and managers.

2. Concentrate on areas where significant differences appear to exist, so that the uncertainties introduced by less than desirable measuring rods are not critical. For the most part, this has led to a de-emphasis of such areas as outpatient provider manpower, quality of care, and health status outcomes.

For the foreseeable future, formal analysis within K-P will play a secondary, supporting role, and the judgment of intangibles will remain a key aspect of most major decisions. The decision makers within the program know the limits of the tools available, even if from time to time the analysts forget them. Any efforts to revise the current organization and practice of medicine must be led by the physicians immediately responsible and directly involved. Even within a formally structured group such as the medical group of K-P, policy can rarely be imposed from above and the hierarchical structure is somewhat of an illusion. This is rightfully so. Repeatedly, we have found that the autonomy of the seven medical centers in K-P has led to the evolution of differences in structure and administrative practice that are often the result of an understanding of special local conditions. However, as in any institution, lags can occur both in responding to changes in local circumstances, and in accepting innovations developed elsewhere. The issue in such circumstances is how to provide accountability in terms of broad measures of performance so that the autonomy is not abused, and equitable allocation of resources can be made. K-P is currently implementing two different performance-budgeting systems, one for its hospital operations and the other for the medical group, in an effort to improve the basic management controls to enhance local accountability. Many of the applied research projects described above have contributed to these systems, which are intended to lead to a more appropriate incentive structure for the local chiefs of service, department heads, and area administrators. This environment, combined with the ongoing natural experiments in administrative practice and operational structure, promises to make K-P an even more fruitful setting for applied research in the future.

References

Barnett, G. 1973. *COSTAR—Computer Stored Ambulatory Record*. Boston: Laboratory of Computer Science, Massachusetts General Hospital.

Fetter, R., and Mills, R. 1976. AUTOGRP: An Interactive Computer System for the Analysis of Health Care Data. *Medical Care* 14: 603–615.

―――, and Thompson, J. 1975. Case Mix and Resource Use. *Inquiry* 12: 300–312.

Greenfield, S., et al. 1978. Efficiency and Cost of Primary Care by Nurses and Physician Assistants. *The New England Journal of Medicine* 298: 305–309.

Luft, H. 1978. Why Do HMOs Seem to Provide More Preventive Services? *Milbank Memorial Fund Quarterly/Health and Society* 56 (Spring): 140–168.

Mechanic, D. 1978. Problems and Prospects in Health Services Research. *Milbank Memorial Fund Quarterly/Health and Society* 56 (Spring): 127–139.

Richter, S. 1978. Short-Range Planning in a Private Health Care System. Paper delivered at the Eastern Economic Association Meeting, Washington, D.C., April 1978.

Rubenstein, L., Hester, J., and Brannin, R. 1978. Long-Range Economic Planning in a Private Health Care System. Paper delivered at the Eastern Economic Association Meeting, Washington, D.C., April 1978.

Solon, J. 1967. Delineating Episodes of Medical Care. *American Journal of Public Health* 57: 401–408.

Somers, A. 1971. *The Kaiser-Permanente Medical Care Program: A Symposium*. New York: The Commonwealth Fund.

This work was completed while the author was Coordinator of Applied Research for the Southern California Region of the Kaiser-Permanente Medical Care Program.

Address correspondence to: Dr. James A. Hester, Executive Vice President, Alumni Association of the Massachusetts Institute of Technology, Room 10-110, Cambridge, Massachusetts 02139.

Dental Care and the
Health Maintenance Organization Concept

MAX H. SCHOEN

The principal dental diseases, caries and periodontal disease, affect almost the entire population and result in considerable pain and discomfort, with eventual tooth loss, if untreated. These disorders can either be prevented or their effects minimized through dental intervention so that intact functioning dentitions can be maintained.

Despite the fact that enough practicing dentists probably exist in the United States to achieve these results, the majority of the population lose all of their natural teeth if they live out their normal life spans. The solo-practice fee-for-service system, even with third-party payment, may reduce the difficulties somewhat but cannot solve the problem.

Prepaid dental group practice, either independently or as part of a general health care system, has the potential of virtually eliminating edentulism in populations for which it has responsibility. At present, it is possible to project costs and resource needs with sufficient accuracy to start viable entities. The "health maintenance organization" concept, therefore, applies to dental care.

This paper is a summary and synthesis of the ideas expressed by the author over a period of years with regard to the potential advantages and disadvantages of prepaid or capitation dental group practice as a vehicle for the delivery of oral health care. As such, it contains little that is new except for some updated references.

The current oral health status of the population of the United States is a result of the interaction of dental disease processes and their sequelae with dental treatment. Such dental care has been provided largely by solo practitioners charging fees for service and acting as an independent part of the health care system. A brief review of dental disease, oral health status, and treatment patterns is essential to any discussion of possible improvement in the delivery of care.

Dental Disease

The major disease categories which concern the dentist are: dental caries, periodontal disease, oral clefts and other lesser congenital or acquired deformities, and oral cancer. If left untreated, these

M M F Q / Health and Society / *Spring 1975*

diseases may result in loss of the teeth, facial disfigurement, and even, as in the case of cancer, death.

Two of the disorders, dental caries and periodontal disease, together with their sequelae, occupy almost all of the dentist's treatment time. If left untreated, they result in loss of the natural dentition. The process of ever-increasing severity is usually accompanied by considerable pain and discomfort and reduced ability to eat and enjoy a wide variety of foods.

Dental caries is both cumulative and irreversible. It is the most common chronic disease in the United States and attacks nearly everyone, commencing early in life shortly after the eruption of the deciduous teeth. It is a complex process involving bacterial infection and proceeds inward from the outer surface of the tooth (Young and Striffler, 1969).

At present, there are two major approaches to the prevention of dental caries. Fluorides, particularly if ingested throughout the period of calcification of the crowns of the teeth, can reduce the incidence of caries by up to 60 percent. The elimination of refined carbohydrates from the diet can prevent most caries by interfering with the bacterial conversion of sugars into demineralizing acids. More recently, pit and fissure sealants have been shown to be effective in preventing caries if applied to appropriate surfaces of the teeth on a regular basis.

Once caries is present in the tooth the decay must be removed and replaced by a suitable restorative material, since the enamel does not possess the capacity to repair itself. The longer the delay in treatment, the more severe the lesion. Therapy becomes more complex and time-consuming and eventually may be restricted to tooth removal and replacement.

Periodontal disease attacks the supporting structures of the teeth and increases in both prevalence and severity with age. Almost the entire population is affected to some degree by age 65. While dental caries is responsible for most tooth loss prior to age 35, periodontal disease becomes the leading cause after age 35 (Young and Striffler, 1969).

Even though much remains to be learned about the etiology of periodontal disease, it definitely has been established that a major factor is the accumulation of a complex matrix of hard and soft deposit (dental plaque) on the teeth, both above and below the gingival margin.

Most periodontal disease can be prevented or minimized by a combination of good home care to break up the accumulation of plaque and regular dental prophylaxis to remove to remove deposits left by the patient. Tooth loss can be prevented, even if the destructive process is fairly advanced, by a combination of home care (similar to that used for primary prevention) and treatment to reduce pocket depth and establish relatively normal contours of the teeth and supporting structures.

While there is considerable question as to whether malposed teeth and poor occlusion result in increased incidence of other dental disease, there is no question that poor facial appearance is considered undesirable in our society and may have serious psychological effects. Even though most orthodontic problems cannot be prevented, they can be treated. A recent study (National Center for Health Statistics, 1973) reported that 14.2 percent of all children had conditions for which treatment was highly desirable or mandatory. Another 22.4 percent had definite malocclusions for which treatment was classified as elective.

The treatment of oral malignancy generally is considered to be beyond the scope of dental practice, but its detection is not. About 3.4 deaths per 100,000 persons occur annually (Young and Striffler, 1969). Early discovery and therapy would reduce both mortality and the major disfigurement and loss of function which accompanies the radical surgery and radiotherapy necessary for late care.

In sum, oral disease is a curse which afflicts almost everyone, but which can either be prevented or minimized through a combination of environmental measures, appropriate personal behavior, and therapy. Therapy, by itself, while not too effective in primary prevention can prevent or minimize untoward outcomes.

In this regard dental care must be looked at in a different light than most medical care. Dentistry can be quite effective in maintaining dental health, but medicine is less effective in maintaining general health. Medical intervention in the chronic diseases such as heart disease and arthritis appears to have little effect on morbidity and mortality.

Current Treatment Needs and Patterns of Receipt of Service

Despite the existence of some 100,000 practicing dentists in the

United States and continuing educational campaigns about need for regular dental visits, appropriate home care, and good diet, the oral health status of the population is appalling. Some recent studies have reported the following:

—Over 20 million persons were edentulous in 1971. Of these almost two million had incomplete or no replacement and almost two million more never used the replacements they had. In all, about three out of every 10 edentulous persons thought they needed either new dentures or improvements on the existing appliances (National Center for Health Statistics, 1974a).

—The average dentulous adult had 17.9 DMF teeth in 1960–62. Of these, 1.4 were decayed (D); 9.4 were missing (M); and 7.0 were filled (F). At no age level was the percentage of filled teeth greater than those which were decayed or missing (National Center for Health Statistics, 1967).

—In 1960–62 two out of every five dentulous adults had a condition requiring an "early" visit to a dentist (National Center for Health Statistics, 1970).

—Children 6–11 years of age had an average of 1.4 DMF teeth per child in 1963–65—0.5 D, 0.1 M, and 0.8 F. The mean increased steadily with age and the number of erupted permanent teeth at risk (National Center for Health Statistics, 1971b).

—Over 25 percent of adults had oral hygiene levels ranging from barely adequate to injuriously poor (National Center for Health Statistics, 1965a).

—In 1965, the average 14-year-old white child visiting a dentist needed 0.44 permanent teeth extracted and already had 0.25 teeth missing (American Dental Association, n.d.).

—The average number of teeth requiring extraction in persons of all ages was 0.95 for males and 0.84 for females. The need for extractions was over 12 times as great for those who had last seen a dentist in over three years as among those who had had a previous visit in from 6–12 months (American Dental Association, n.d.).

—In general, unmet dental needs were greatest in the lowest socioeconomic groups and least in the highest, although even the persons in the highest strata still had considerable deterioration and unmet treatment needs.

There is some evidence that there has been an improvement over a number of years. For example, while the number of edentulous persons did not decrease in the 13-year period between 1957–58 and 1971, the percentage was reduced from 13.0 to 11.2 (National

Center for Health Statistics, 1974a). Extractions performed per person per year by private dentists dropped from 0.359 in 1950 to 0.280 in 1969 (Moen and Poetsch, 1970). This decreased tooth loss is hardly encouraging, since the rate of change is very slow.

That the concept that regular appropriate dental care can at least minimize the effects of dental disease, even if patients behavior cannot be modified enough for primary prevention, is not erroneous is borne out by the following facts. In 1960–62 the average DMF score for men with under $2,000 income was 15.3, while that for men with incomes over $10,000 was 19.0. However the number of decayed teeth was 1.8 and 0.9, respectively. In addition the number of missing teeth was 11.3 and 8.0 (National Center for Health Statistics, 1967). Therefore, while disease incidence and prevalence was higher in the upper-income group, tooth loss was less. Similarly, the percentage of edentulous persons age 65 and over was 58.5 for those with incomes under $3,000 and 35.2 for those with incomes over $15,000 (National Center for Health Statistics, 1974a). Comparisons for education follow the same pattern. These differences are associated with different patterns of use, with the higher socioeconomic groups having more "appropriate" use.

Indirect measures of the population's oral health status can be obtained from patterns of receipt of service. Some data from additional studies are:

—In 1973, 48.9 percent of the population visited a dentist at least once. The average number of dental visits per person was 1.6 (National Center for Health Statistics, 1974b).

—In 1963–64, 15 percent of the visits were for extractions and only 13.6 for prophylaxis (National Center for Health Statistics, 1965b).

—18 percent of the population accounted for 75 percent of dental office visits, while 10 percent accounted for 75 percent of dental expenditures in the early 1960s (Newman and Anderson, 1972).

—Use rates and service patterns favored the upper socioeconomic groups.

The change over the years appears to be slowly for the better. In 1963–64, 42 percent of the population had a dental visit, and the average number of visits was 1.6 (National Center for Health Statistics, 1966). In 1969 the respective figures were 44.9 percent and 1.5 (National Center for Health Statistics, 1971a). Over about a ten-year span the rate of use went up 7 percent and number of visits remained constant. From 1950 to 1969 examinations and pro-phylaxis almost doubled (0.221 to 0.418 and 0.210 to 0.384), but fill-ing rates remained about the same (0.990 to 1.069) (Moen and Poetsch, 1970). As mentioned previously the extraction rate dropped slightly. Another study (National Center for Health Statistics, 1965b) comparing 1957–58 with 1963–64 reported similar small improvements in the distribution of visits over a six-year in-terval. As with oral health status, the change in treatment patterns over a period of time, although improving, is relatively slight.

American dentistry prides itself as being the finest in the world, yet most persons who live out their normal life spans lose all their natural teeth. Clearly the current mode of delivery of dental care has not been able to accomplish the goal of maintenance of the dentition despite its technological achievements and the scientific knowledge to virtually eliminate tooth loss.

Manpower

It is possible that the organization of the delivery mechanism is not at fault, if resources as measured by personnel are inadequate. A pertinent question, therefore, is: "Is a ratio of approximately one practicing dentist per 2,000 population adequate?" If maldistribu-tion problems are put aside to simplify the problem, the ratio permits a full-time practitioner to spend almost one hour per person per year in treatment. Studies conducted over 20 years ago (Waterman and Knutson, 1954; Law et al., 1955) have shown that in non-fluoridated areas dentist man-hours per child per year (in-cluding prophylaxis time which could be spent by a hygienist) for maintenance care were 1.4 and 0.75 in two different communities. A more recent study (Ast et al., 1970) on younger children reported annual maintenance treatment time of around 20 minutes for a fluoridated community and 35 minutes for a non-fluoridated com-munity.

Pelton (1972) conducted a treatment program for university students and found that the dentist time required for an annual maintenance cycle could be reduced to less than one and a half hours. Prosthetic replacements were not included, but prophylaxis time was.

A study (U.S. Public Health Service, 1954) of a volunteer group who were members of Group Health Association found that 2.8 hours were needed for annual maintenance care, of which 0.9 hours were for prophylaxis and X-rays.

Even though some of these reports date back several decades and include several configurations of dental practice, none involving use of expanded duty auxiliaries, dentist chair time for maintenance care hovers in the vicinity of one hour, if treatment which can be provided by hygienists and assistants is excluded. Since even in a "maintenance" situation not all persons visit (or need to see) a dentist each year, the ratio of 1:2,000 is not very far removed from the ideal.

The discussion has omitted orthodontic care, but extrapolation from available information yields figures which also do not indicate a major manpower shortage. Orthodontists practicing with conventional use of auxiliaries can start about 100 full cases per year (estimate based on personal conversations). If about 25 percent of children are assumed to accept and receive orthodontic services (a larger percentage than those identified as having major needs), treatment would be commenced on about one million persons each year under a "maintenance" situation, since orthodontics needs to be performed only once in a lifetime and there are about four million children born each year. There are about 5,000 orthodontists in the United States, so they fall short of the 10,000 apparently needed to treat the one million cases. However, not all cases are "full" ones, and many orthodontists are now using expanded duty auxiliaries with consequent increases in productivity. In addition, general practitioners can treat minor cases, so the manpower discrepancy is not nearly as great as it would appear to be. In terms of dentist hours, using the "full" case figures, the 15 million treatment hours (100 cases completed in a 1,500-hour work year) would amount to less than one tenth of an hour per person per year when distributed over the entire population.

The ratio of dentists to population has hovered around the 1:2,000 figure for many years, so if the "maintenance" time mentioned previously was achieved with high utilization rates and low tooth-mortality rates, shortage of manpower is not a good explanation of the deplorable state of the nation's dental health. At best, "shortage" can account for only a small part of the problem.

Utilization Rates and Tooth Mortality

The studies previously cited as well as some others have shown that high annual utilization with associated low tooth mortality is achievable. The GHA study (U. S. Public Health Service, 1954), with volunteer participation, had total involvement by definition, and therefore was a very biased population. However, despite considerable need for dental care, annual need for all extractions was reduced to 0.1 teeth.

The Public Health Service projects (Waterman and Knutson, 1954; Law et al., 1955) in Richmond and Woonsocket dealt with the entire school population of these communities. About 6 percent used their own dentists, and 7 to 10 percent received no dental services. The programs were able to treat about 85 percent of all children and reduced extractions to 0.02 in the last series in Richmond and 0.03 in Woonsocket. New children entered the communities during the five- to six-year spans of the projects, and received services, so the results are understated.

Schoen (1965) has reported on a program achieving 85 percent annual utilization rates for a group of longshore children covered by a prepaid dental program. In the last year of a six-year longitudinal study tooth loss was reduced to zero. Another report (Schoen, 1967) on an adult population studied for five years produced data demonstrating tooth loss of less than 0.1 teeth per year and use rates of over 80 percent per year. Another program (Schoen, 1969) involving the same group practice reduced adult tooth loss from about 0.5 teeth in the first year to less than 0.1 in two subsequent years, while achieving use rates ranging from about 60 to 90 percent.

If the results of these various programs and projects are extrapolated to a lifetime, they demonstrate that tooth loss can be diminished to the point where edentulism is a rarity. The studies were not designed to review reduction in the incidence of disease, but even if primary prevention was not achieved, the goal of retention of the natural dentition and almost universal use of dental services was achieved. These results also appear to be better than those for the high socioeconomic strata of the population.

Population Responsibility

Up to this point it has been demonstrated that it is *possible* to provide dental care to population groups using resources which are not out of line with national averages and achieving, as a minimum, a major reduction in tooth loss. This performance is at variance with the picture for the country as a whole.

The author postulates that the factors common to all of these programs were an *organized practice system* and assumption of *responsibility for the oral health care of a given population.* Both of these are lacking in traditional solo-practice fee-for-service dentistry. This is true even if direct financial barriers are removed by some form of third-party payment. With the usual mode of practice there is no way to get each dentist to husband his valuable treatment time by using priorities and pacing. If each practitioner in a community chooses to perform large numbers of services, whether urgent or non-urgent, immediately essential or elective, on those patients who come to his office, often on a sporadic basis, there will not be enough resources to care for the dental health needs of the entire population. Also, as is evident from the data, sporadic use results in tooth loss and/or the need for more complex and time-consuming treatment (endodontics, crown and bridge) than is required for regular care. Even if a dentist attempts to establish a regular recall system, failure of a patient to return may or may not be due to a move from the geographic area and the dentist cannot know why he never sees the patient again. Lastly, the dentist has no direct knowledge or method of getting to those persons who may reside in his "service" area but do not request any treatment.

The dual requirement of an organized (and controlled) system and assumption of population responsibility is borne out by the report (Galagan et al., 1964) on the dental health status of children in Richmond and Woonsocket five years after the PHS programs stopped. The data show that the gains were largely wiped out. The achievements of the New Zealand dental nurse program are well known. However, a corollary is that the dental health of the population does not continue at the same level after they "graduate" from the school-based program (Redig et al., 1973).

Health Maintenance

A health maintenance organization is, by definition, an organized system for the provision of health care to an enrolled, and therefore well-defined, population. Everything about the HMO concept is, therefore, made to order for dental care, if the reasoning presented so far is correct. In fact, dentistry fits better than most medicine. The consequences of the common dental diseases *can* be prevented by regular health maintenance in an organized system accepting responsibility for a population.

It has been demonstrated that periodic visits to the dentist can reduce or even eliminate tooth loss. Further, it has been shown that organized systems with appropriate outreach can get a very high percentage of a given population to avail themselves of such service. The problems posed earlier in this paper are therefore reduced to proportions which can be managed by currently available resources.

At present, dentistry is not only practiced as a separate profession, but as a separate system. There is little relationship between dentists and the rest of the health care apparatus—even where prototype HMOs have existed for some time. For example, except for the Portland Region, the Kaiser-Permanante system does not provide dental care. Neither does HIP. While GHA has dentists on its staff, dentistry is not included as part of the general prepaid package. Group Health Cooperative of Puget Sound has a dental cooperative as a separate offshoot which provides care only on a fee-for-service basis.

Dental coverage as a fringe benefit whether through fee-for-service mechanisms or prepaid group practice has developed as a separate entity. Current HMO legislation (House of Representatives, . . ., 1973) is forcing a marriage, at least for the minimum basic and inadequate dental benefit: essentially a prophylaxis and topical fluoride treatment where water fluoridation is not in effect.

There are some good reasons why comprehensive dental care should be part of overall health care. The mouth is part of the body and should be treated as such (interestingly, many physicians and nurses probably visualize a body without the oral cavity while the dentist sees a mouth without a body). One-door health care applies to dentistry. It should be easier for an individual or family to identify with one system for its entire health care. Interaction between the different parts of the health care "team" is facilitated by close organizational relationships. Health education, preventive services, and care for persons with systemic disease can be coordinated for the benefit of all. The possibilities for joint outreach to those persons who do not use services appropriately or who do not practice preventive behavior are enormous. Why should attempts at diet control for caries prevention be separated from general dietary and nutritional counseling? Families with poor records on immunization probably are equally poor on regular and early children's dental care. Why not deal with the problems simultaneously?

One point, generally neglected, is that dentists really are "primary care" health providers and that the dental visit may be the most regular contact, or even the only one in a particular period, with the health system. As such, the visit may become the point of entry into care, if appropriate evaluation and screening are performed, and possible need determined. The dentist should be concerned with the general health status of the patient not just as it may impact upon dental treatment but as it affects the well-being of the individual. Integrating dentistry into the total system has the potential of enhancing interdisciplinary thinking and cooperation.

There is some doubt as to whether the dental record should be an integral part of the medical chart. Sheer bulk may create numerous problems. However, regardless of the mechanics, each type of health care provider should have available the information generated by the other therapists.

Unfortunately, this idea remains just that—an idea. Some of the organizations hoping to qualify as HMOs under the new act are getting into the dental field, but it still is too early to see whether the results will live up to the expectations.

Methodology for Estimating Costs and Resource Needs

Regardless of whether dentistry is part of a general health care maintenance organization or exists separately, certain general principles apply when costs and resource needs are estimated for a capitation group-practice program.

This particular approach has been developed in detail elsewhere (Schoen, 1974a; 1974b), but a summary will be presented here. Since fees for service are of no concern, the frequency and distribution of services are of no real consequence except as they affect resources. For a given population the essential factors are provider time and cost for given configurations of practice.

Simply stated, the annual cost for providing dental services can be expressed in the following formula:

$$R = T_D \times C_D + T_H \times C_H$$

where

R = annual cost
T_D = dentist time
C_D = cost per unit of dentist time (including dentist income)
T_H = hygienist time
C_H = cost per unit of hygienist time.

The formula can be used to estimate costs for a person, family, or group. The treatment-time factor appears to be affected by population stability and annual utilization rates (leading to different mixes of initial and maintenance care), and differences between adults and children. Specific age differences are not particularly important, since treatment time varies much less than distribution of services. Disease-attack rates are obviously a factor, but time estimates do not vary as much as incidence since a substantial component of time is diagnostic and preventive.

As stated, practice configuration affects time. The larger, more efficient dental team reduces treatment time, but at a somewhat increased cost per unit of time. The exact relationship between different mixes of personnel, facilities, and costs have not been determined as yet.

Since dental disease is chronic and much treatment deals with effects rather than disease itself, priorities and variable pacing of treatment can be established. These obviously affect time and cost, so estimates can be crude and still be successful. The organization controls use of resources, so the prophecy becomes self-fulfilling!

Clearly limits on either available dollars, or resources, or both affect program design. For example, if comprehensive dental care costs $20 per family per month and only $10 is available, changes must be made in order to have a viable plan. Assuming resources, in terms of personnel and facilities, are available, some method must be found to reduce costs to the prepaid portion of the program. One method is to impose surcharges to be paid by the patient for specific dental procedures. Since personal out-of-pocket payment tends to reduce use of elective services, and most dental care can be placed in that category, the savings on monthly premium are the sum of the patient direct payment and the reduced cost for lowered use of services. Such reduction in use is undoubtedly proportional to the amount of surcharge or co-payment, but the exact ratios for various populations are unknown as yet.

If the stated goal of preservation of the natural dentition is going to remain, great care must be taken in the imposition of surcharges. If possible, none should be imposed for preventive, early treatment and maintenance services so that periodic care is not discouraged. Proportionately heavier charges can be placed against extractions and replacements than against root canal and restorative procedures.

The impostion of a charge per visit, as opposed to a charge per service, even though common for outpatient medical care, can lead to serious problems in dentistry. Dental visits can vary considerably in content and time. Therefore, patients might object to the same charge for a five-minute procedure as for a three-hour procedure. Also if a program is in a financial bind, the visit charge places a temptation on the dentist to increase the number of sessions required to complete a case, despite the resulting loss of efficiency.

Another approach to reducing costs and, in this case, use of resources is to phase family members into treatment. Since initial care is both more expensive and time-consuming than maintenance care, starting with one family member (e.g., the employee or the child) in the first year and adding others each succeeding year reduces cost dramatically and levels out the need for personnel.

Lastly, benefits can be limited. Generally orthodontics is the first exclusion. Other limitations can be imposed by eliminating entire categories of service or restricting the conditions under which types of treatment are covered. For example, all prosthetic replacements can be excluded or just root-canal therapy for posterior teeth. The difficulty with exclusions is that they can have an adverse effect on the quality of care performed. If endodontics is not covered as a benefit, the large out-of-pocket cost can deter the patient from paying for the service. As a result an extraction is performed and the deterioration of the dentition is hastened. By and large, benefit limitations are not desirable.

A working formula is obviously more complex than the one presented here, but not overly so. It must include the factors for utilization rates, stability (initial versus maintenance care) and age (adult versus child). The base-line figure for provider time and cost is affected by efficiency and practice configuration, while premium levels can be modified by out-of-pocket payments.

With the limitations on the use of auxiliaries which still exist in most states, and current practice costs, a comprehensive dental care program for a reasonably stable population would cost about $200 per family per year, if the family size were about three. Such a program would include surcharges to cover dental laboratory costs and some payment for orthodontics. This estimate includes the costs for the initial year, by spreading them out over several years. Obviously no exact figure can be given without knowing the various population and dental practice characteristics described previously.

The annual cost for whatever coverage and benefit structure is decided upon should be added to the other HMO costs and then presented as a total "premium" if a full service HMO is contemplated.

Concerns and Problems

While examples have been presented which demonstrate the possibilities present in prepaid dental group-practice systems, they often do not live up to the potential. Some studies of paired populations, either in dual-choice situations or of similar populations locked into two systems, have shown that significant differences in general use rates or distribution of services are the exception rather than the rule. Simons (1967), in studying a dual-choice prepaid program, reported an annual use by adults of 38 percent for the group practice and 48 percent for the fee-for-service choice. The respective figures for children were 65 percent and 63 percent. Tumelty (1968), reporting on a three-way choice, found annual adult use to be 42 percent for the group practice, 42 per cent for the service corporation, and 32 percent for an insurance company. Figures for children were 52 percent, 55 percent, and 44 percent, respectively. Schoen (1969) compared plans in a dual choice for adults and found average annual use to be 74 percent for the group practice and 35 percent for the service corporation. In a non-dual-choice comparison involving members of the same industry in two adjacent counties, the group practice had an annual use of 33 percent, while a self-insured indemnity system has a use of 34 percent. A non-dual-choice group practice for a lower socioeconomic population without a comparison open-panel plan had a use rate of 41 percent. Annual use rates for children in a dual-choice program were 87 percent for the group practice and 66 percent for the service corporation. Schoen (1969) also studied extraction rates for the same populations. The average rates for maintenance years for adults were 0.16, 0.11, and 0.15 for the group practices and 0.12 and 0.15 for the fee-for-service systems. First permanent molar extraction rates for children for the entire period of an 11-year longitudinal study were 0.01 for the group practice and 0.00 for the service corporation.

In a report including additional non-paired populations, Schoen (1972) found little correlation between method of practice or method of payment on general use rates and little correlation between use rates and extraction rates. There did appear to be a relationship between third-party fringe-benefit payment and tooth loss, since extractions were reduced in any type of third-party system.

Unfortunately, controlled studies of utilization, distribution of services, outcomes, and so on, as they occur in different delivery systems, are few and far between or even completely absent. After many years all one can say is that the potential of a "dental health maintenance organization" is present, but does not appear to be carried out very often.

An additional problem is that of cost. The high-use plans described by Schoen (1967, 1969) have been competitive with the fee-for-service options available. Benefits have been the same as or somewhat better than the open-panel choice. However, dental health maintenance over a lifetime is probably more costly than total neglect. As an extreme example, total loss of teeth at an early age followed by either no replacement or only occasional replacement is less expensive in terms of either personnel time or dollars than annual maintenance care for an intact dentition that suffers from the incidence of some disease. Medi-Cal in California (California Department of Health Care Services, 1968) has approached the non-treatment extreme. There is no question that its cost for a reported annual use rate of under 20 percent is lower than it would be for a high-use maintenance program.

Since a substantial proportion of the American public still accepts tooth loss as an inevitable consequence of aging, and since quality in terms of preservation of the natural dentition is no less costly than neglect (or even more costly), dental health maintenance becomes hard to sell.

Another problem is the intergration of dentistry into some of the HMO prototypes now in existence. If comprehensive care is included in the basic package, the premium cost rises sharply. Unless group subscribers already have dental coverage as a fringe benefit, many persons might opt out of the prepaid plans into the fee-for-service choices usually available. If these members are covered for dental benefits through some separate mechanism, they may not wish to switch to the newly included dental portion of the HMO. Having one choice for the general medical plan and then another one for dentistry would solve that problem but would complicate administration enormously.

If the larger HMO systems offer a dental benefit as part of the basic package or even as an option, and a large percent of their subscribers choose it, they would have great difficulty in developing an "instant" dental system to match the medical one.

If dental benefits are voluntary, based on individual dues or premium payment, adverse selection is likely to occur. Those persons with large unmet dental needs either know they have them or would soon find out and then would sign up for a period long enough to cover initial treatment. They then could drop out until a new set of major needs developed. Even an annual lock-in would not cover for this experience.

Limiting dental coverage to the basic benefit mandated by the HMO act would reduce costs to pennies per family per month. However, the performance of this service to the exclusion of other dental care is of doubtful value, would probably be used by few persons, and would antagonize everyone. Patients would expect more or get a false sense of security, local dentists would criticize the service, and the HMO staff would have to face the outcry.

Even if the phase-in of dentistry can be accomplished, the organizational ties to the existing medical system must be carefully considered. Dentists must form an equal and autonomous unit within the HMO structure. Physicians should not be making dental decisions. If the dentists are part of the medical group, as opposed to a separate group, they should have at least the same representation on any boards as a major medical department such as internal medicine, pediatrics, or surgery. It must be remembered that most dentists are primary health care providers (only about 10 percent are specialists) and are probably about equal in number to physicians who provide primary care. If an HMO provides comprehensive dental care to its membership on the basis proposed in this paper, the dental section will be very large.

The relationships of dentists to physicians are not easily solved. As a result of the almost total separation of the two professions, they are covered by different licensing agencies and different state laws and regulations. The resultant legal complexities combined with the differences in organizational levels previously mentioned make it impossible to propose an "ideal" HMO model.

It is generally assumed that economies of scale would apply to larger dental group practices. Doherty (1972) has raised the question of whether this "axiom" really is true. While there are obvious savings in less duplication of equipment (e.g. fewer X-ray machines) and in discounts on bulk purchasing of supplies or even prosthetic appliances from the laboratory, these may be more than offset by the extra and more specialized personnel required to operate a complex practice.

This author has postulated that a group practice can make better use of expanded-duty auxiliary personnel than a solo practitioner. The solo dentist might have more difficulty in managing the larger team involved. Whether this is true or not remains to be seen. Some solo dentists, or those operating in groups of two or three, appear to be extremely productive and to be able to use the new "dentist extenders" very well (Redig et al., 1974). Whether any dentist, either in solo or group practice, will put increased productivity to use in the best interests of the patient is also an open question. If these "advances" are used to increase dentist income by producing more pieces of work without improving dental health or without reducing patient costs, then they are retrogressive. Unfortunately, it probably is true that HMOs will have to pay dentists the going rate however high it may rise. If this occurs, they will be no more effective in combating health care inflation than the medical groups have been.

The populations that need the HMO concept the most, those who have lower incomes and are poor, have no funds to pay the regular premiums. Unless a national health insurance plan becomes law and includes comprehensive dental care, there is little hope that such persons will be reached. Medicaid cannot be counted on, since its concern is lowest possible cost, which, as in the California example, can be achieved by low use and reduced service.

Conclusion

Despite the knowledge and ability to radically improve the dental health of the population of the United States, using the existing number of dentists, the current system has been unable to do so. If dental providers are organized into smaller controlled systems assuming responsibility for given population groups, these changes can be effected.

Many problems of organization and performance exist which must be solved in order to convert the possibility into reality. Studies of efficiency and effectiveness must be conducted with a view of arriving at the best approach.

Difficulties exist in the integration of dentistry into the HMO system, although it appears that the outcome would be worthwhile. A comprehensive national health insurance program, including dental health care, is a necessary ingredient.

Max H. Schoen, D.D.S., DR. P.H.
School of Dental Medicine
SUNY at Stony Brook
Stony Brook, New York 11794

References

American Dental Association
    n.d.   Survey of needs for dental care, 1965. Bureau of Economic Research and Statistics. Chicago: The Association.

Ast, David B., Naham C. Cons, Sydney T. Pollard, and Joseph Garfinkel
    1970   "Time and cost factors to provide regular periodic dental care for children in a fluoridated and non fluoridated area: final report." JADA 80 (April): 770–776.

California Department of Health Care Services
1968   Medi-cal Report No. 68-7, Sacramento, December.

Doherty, Neville J.G.
1972   "Production economics research and dental group practice." In Bailit,
          Howard L, Neville J.G. Doherty, and Charles Jerge (eds.), National
          Conference on Dental Group Practice, Proceedings. Farmington:
          University of Connecticut, School of Dental Medicine.

Galagan, Donald J., Frank E. Law, George E. Waterman, and Grace S.
Spitz
1964   "Dental health status of children 5 years after completing school den-
          tal care programs." Public Health Reports 79 (May): 445-454.

House of Representatives, U.S. Congress
1973   Health Maintenance Organization Act of 1973. Report No. 93-714,
          Washington.

Law, Frank E., Carl E. Johnson, and John W. Knutson
1955   "Studies on dental care services for school children—third and fourth
          treatment series, Woonsocket, R.I." Public Health Reports 70 (April),
          402-409.

Moen, B.D., and W.E. Poetsch
1970   "More preventive care, less tooth repair." JADA 81 (July): 25-36.

National Center for Health Statistics
1965a   Selected dental findings in adults by age, race and sex. Series 11, No.
          7. Washington: U.S. Government Printing Office, October.

1965b   Volume of dental visits, United States July 1963 June 1964. Series
          10, No. 23. Washington: U.S. Government Printing Office, October.

1966   Dental visits, time interval since last visit. United States—July
          1963–June 1964. Series 10, No. 29. Washington: U.S. Government
          Printing Office, April.

1967   Decayed, missing and filled teeth in adults. United States—1960-1962.
          Series 11, No. 23. Washington: U.S. Government Printing Office,
          February.

1970   Need for dental care among adults. United States—1960-1962. Series
          11, No. 36. Washington: U.S. Government Printing Office, March.

1971a   Current estimates from the Health Interview Survey. United
          States—1969. Series 10, No. 63. Washington: U.S. Government Print-
          ing Office, June.

1971b   Decayed, missing and filled teeth among children. United States.
          Series 11, No. 106. Washington: U.S. Government Printing Office,
          August.

1973   An assessment of the occlusion of the teeth of children 6–11 years. United States. Series 11, No. 130. Washington: U.S. Government Printing Office, November.

1974a   Edentulous persons. United States—1971. Series 10, No. 89. Washington: U.S. Government Printing Office, June.

1974b   "Profile of American health, 1973." Public Health Reports 89 (November-December): 504–523.

Newman, John, and Odin W. Anderson
1972   Patterns of dental service utilization in the United States: A nationwide social survey. Research Series No. 30. Chicago: Center for Health Administration Studies, University of Chicago.

Pelton, Walter J.
1972   "Dental health program of the University of Alabama in Birmingham: IX. A summary of seven years experience." AJPH 62 (May): 671–675.

Redig, Dale, Floyd Dewhirst, George Nevitt, and Mildred Snyder
1973   "Delivery of dental services in New Zealand and California." J. So. Cal. Dental Assn. 41 (April): 318–350.

Redig, Dale, Mildred Snyder, George Nevitt, and John Tocchini

1974 ⁻   "Expanded duty dental auxiliaries in four private dental offices: the first year's experience." JADA 88 (May): 969–984.

Schoen, Max H.
1965   "Effects of a prepaid children's dental care program on mortality of permanent teeth." JADA 71 (September): 626–634.

1967   "Group practice in dentistry." Medical Care 5 (May-June): 176–183.

1969   Observation of selected dental services under two prepayment mechanisms. Ann Arbor: University microfilms.

1972   "Program development in dental group practice—the quality and distribution of services." In Bailit, Howard L., Neville J.G. Doherty, and Charles Jerge, (eds.), National Conference on Dental Group Practice, Proceedings. Farmington: University of Connecticut, School of Dental Medicine.

1974a   "Methodology of capitation payment to group dental practice and effects of such payment on care." Health Service Reports 89 (January-February): 16–24.

1974b   Financing care in group practice. In Jerge, Charles R., William E. Marshall, Max H. Schoen, and Jay W. Friedman (eds.), Group practice and the future of dental care. Philadelphia: Lea and Febiger.

Simons, John H.
  1967   Prepaid dentistry—a case study. Berkeley: University of California—
          Institute of Industrial Relations.

Tumelty, Robert E.
  1968   Utilization and individual expenditures in three types of dental in-
          surance. Chicago: 19th National Dental Health Conference, American
          Dental Association.

U.S. Public Health Service
  1954   Comprehensive dental care in a group practice. Public Health Service
          Publication No. 395. Washington: U.S. Government Printing Office.

Waterman, G.F., and J.W. Knutson
  1954   "Studies on dental care services for school children—third and fourth
          treatment series, Richmond, Indiana." Public Health Reports 69
          (March): 247–254.

Young, W.O., and D.F. Striffler
  1969   The dentist, his practice, and his community. Philadelphia: Saunders.

The Pricing Behavior
of Medical Groups

RICHARD M. SCHEFFLER

This study discusses a model of the pricing behavior of medical groups. Using data collected, by a mail survey, from medical groups in North Carolina, an empirical test of the model is performed. The results suggest that the prices charged by medical groups are positively influenced by the per capita income of the county in which the group is located, and the per physician utilization of medical, technical, and office personnel. They also suggest that for groups in the sample, a non-physician manager and a non-salaried system of remuneration to member physicians are negatively related to the price of medical services. The results of this study also indicate that the managerial structure of group practice is an important area for further research.

Introduction

Improving the distribution and reducing the price of medical services are two of the major goals of our health care system. Difficulties in moving toward these objectives have produced increased pressure to alter the current system. One of the most frequent proposals is to increase the number of physicians in group practice. The American Medical Association (1971) reports that group physicians are presently 17.6 percent of the active non-federal physicians, and 19.9 percent of all physicians engaged in patient care, excluding interns and residents. Furthermore, there is an increased interest in group practice because the prepaid groups fit within the definition of Health Maintenance Organization (HMOs). The purpose of this study is to investigate the pricing behavior of medical groups.

After defining group practice, we discuss two important economic characteristics of group practice. In the next section we adopt Feldstein's "excess demand model" and expand it to include some important aspects of group practice—the size and type of group, utilization of non-physician personnel, type of manager, and the type of remuneration scheme used. An empirical test of this model, using data collected from medical groups in North Carolina, indicates that different managerial structures and pecuniary incen-

M M F Q / Health and Society / *Spring 1975*

tives to physicians are associated with variations in medical prices. The final section discusses some of the implications these findings have for social policy and points out needed areas for future research.

Defining Group Practice

The definition of group practice used by the American Medical Association (1971:4) is as follows:

> The application of medical services by three or more physicians formally organized to provide medical care, consultation, diagnosis, and/or treatment through the joint use of equipment and personnel, and with income from medical practice distributed in accordance with methods previously determined by members of the group.

Two important economic characteristics emerge from this definition. One is the joint use of equipment and personnel, which raises questions (Reinhardt, 1972; Scheffler, in press; Smith, et al , 1972; and Newhouse, 1973) related to the production function of medical groups. Of prime concern is the possibility that medical groups may be able to achieve certain economies of scale. Simply defined, economies of scale are achieved when, after all inputs are optimally adjusted to given rates of output, the unit cost of production can be reduced by increasing the rate of output (Reinhardt, 1972; Newhouse, 1973; Bailey, 1970; and Scheffler, 1974a). However, recent work by Kimbell and Lorant (1973), using a number of aggregate production functions and data collected on 1,181 groups containing 53,819 physicians in 1971, suggests that multispecialty groups exhibit decreasing returns to scale and that the optimal size for single-specialty groups is quite small, ranging from two to five doctors.

The second economic characteristic is the different income-sharing schemes used by groups and their effect on the group's economic behavior. There are three distinct types of income-sharing schemes used by medical groups: (1) fee for service, (2) salary, and (3) a percentage or point system. Under fee for service, physicians receive remuneration based on the volume of income generated for the group by their services. This system is identical to that used by solo practitioners. A salary system for group physicians means that each physician is paid a fixed sum, usually on an annual basis. Since income differentials are significant between different medical specialists, adjustments according to medical specialty are usually made. With the percentage or point system, physicians' remuneration is based on a number of considerations which may include years of practice, years with the group, specialty of the physician, investment in overhead, increasing the status of the group, the ability to attract new patients, the number of cases or patients treated by the physician, as well as other factors the group deems appropriate.

A Pricing Model for Physicians in Group Practice

We now turn our attention to the development of an empirical model of the pricing behavior of physicians in group practice. Following Feldstein (1970), we assume that physicians have discretionary power over their fees (i.e., they are price setters), and set them so as to maintain excess demand in the market for their services. In addition, our empirical model considers the effect of a number of important characteristics of the group. They include the composition of the medical specialties in the group, its size, the type of manager employed, and the income-sharing scheme which is used.

On a national scale (American Medical Association, 1971), in 1969 there were 6,371 medical groups; approximately 50 percent were single specialty, 37 percent were multispecialty, and the remaining 13 percent, general practice. One basic difference between these groups is that multispecialty groups provide a wider range of medical services than general-practice and single-specialty groups. It is possible that pricing policies may vary with the number of different medical services sold by the group. Therefore, we have included a dummy variable in the empirical model to test for any price differences between multispecialty, as compared to single-specialty and general-practice groups.

The relationship between the size of the medical group and medical care prices is an important public policy concern. If larger groups are able to lower their prices to patients, then recent policies to stimulate the growth of groups would have justification. Since physicians are clearly the most important factor of production, we include the number of physicians in the group as a proxy measure for size.

Another characteristic which may affect the pricing behavior of medical groups is their management structure. The type of manager employed by the group indicates a difference in the managerial structure of the group (Scheffler, in press), e.g., the manager may be a physician or a non-physician. Both types of managers, in order to justify their salaries, should be concerned with reducing costs. Their effectiveness in lowering costs may differ, however. In order to test for the effect of the type of manager used by the group, we include a dummy variable to measure whether the group is managed by a physician or a non-physician. Our expectation is that non-physician managers, because of their specialized skills, may be able to lower costs and thus permit the group to set lower fees.

The final economic characteristic to be considered is the type of income sharing scheme of the medical group. Although the variety of income sharing arrangments is large (as described earlier), our data permit us to consider only the difference between salaried and non-salaried schemes. A predetermined salary scheme may provide no incentive for physicians to improve their productivity, or to behave in a manner which would reduce costs.[1] Alternatively, a fee-for-service or point system may provide an incentive. A dummy variable is included to examine the relationship between the type of income-sharing scheme and the price of the medical services sold by the group.

The Data

Data were collected via mail survey of medical groups in North Carolina during 1972. Appendix A contains a copy of the questionnaire utilized. Some 80 medical groups were surveyed, and 61 responses were received, a figure which represents approximately 40 percent of the groups in North Carolina in 1969 (American Medical Association, 1971).

Table 1 presents the mean and the standard deviation of a number of variables derived from the survey results. Using the number of physicians as a measure of size, we observe that most groups are small. Groups in the survey vary from three to 26 physi-

---

[1]Newhouse (1973) has found that cost sharing by groups also increased average costs.

TABLE 1

Survey Results of Medical Groups
in North Carolina: 1972 [a]

	Mean	Standard Deviation
Number of full-time doctors in the group	5.44	5.15
Medical personnel per physician	1.08	0.47
Technical personnel per physician	0.26	0.24
Office personnel per physician	1.44	0.67
Presence of non-physician manager	0.48	0.51
Heterogeneous groups	0.35	0.48
Fee-for-service remuneration	0.05	0.23
Salary remuneration	0.47	0.50
Percentage or point system of remuneration	0.35	0.48

[a] There is a total of 61 groups in the sample.

cians, with a mean of 5.44 physicians and a standard deviation of 5.15 physicians. On the national level (American Medical Association, 1971) we find that in 1969, 95.3 percent of all medical groups had from three to 15 physicians, and that these groups employed 68.8 percent of all group-practice physicians. Therefore, we may conclude that an analysis of groups in this size range of our sample covers a significant portion of medical groups in the United States. Of interest is the fact that 36 of the 61 groups used a salaried system of remuneration. Of the remaining 35 groups, six used a fee for service, and 29 a percentage or point system.

Data on the employment of non-physician personnel per physician indicate that our sample of medical groups in North Carolina has characteristics similar to medical groups in the United States as a whole. In order to facilitate a comparison of non-physician medical personnel with national data, we have combined all categories of technical and medical personnel per physician in our sample into one category. This produces a ratio of 1.34 non-physician medical personnel per physician, which is similar to the national figure of 1.30. The number of office personnel per physician was 1.30 for the nation sample (American Medical Association, 1971) of medical groups also, as compared to 1.44 for groups in North Carolina. Thus, we conclude that the utilization of non-physician personnel by the groups in our sample is comparable to that found for the aggregate of medical groups in the United States.

In order to study the pricing behavior of medical groups, price data were collected on the customary price for three different medical services. Previous studies have used the price of an office visit as the unit of analysis. The unit is unsatisfactory, however, because an office visit is a heterogeneous output. Our approach was to select three basic medical services which are quite common and represent a significant portion of the volume of medical services. The services used were: (1) an initial complete physical examination, (2) a blood count, and (3) a set of chest X rays. These services have the additional characteristic of representing services which utilize different and distinctive production processes. Physical examinations usually require physician and non-physician medical personnel, a blood count may be produced with a physician; and X rays are more efficiently produced with technical personnel. Although disaggregation on the service level is an improvement in output measurement, it still has inherent problems. Each service is in fact the sum of a number of medical procedures that are separate and distinct. Some groups may set prices and bill for each individual service, while others do not. For example, a physical examination may involve laboratory tests. The group could include the laboratory tests in the price of the physical or bill for it separately. Different billing procedures make the collection of any price data a difficult task. However, with these caveats in mind, price data by service type still appear useful for study purposes.

Empirical Results

Using the data described above, our price equation for medical groups was specified in the following manner:

P_i = $f(Y, S, H, A, T, O, M, R)$, where $i = 1, 2, 3$, and
P_1 = price of physical examination
P_2 = price of blood count
P_3 = price of X rays
Y = per capita income of the county where medical group is located

S = number of full-time physicians in the group

H = type of group, a binary variable; one represents a multi-specialty group, and zero a general-practice or single-specialty group

A = number of medical personnel per physician

T = number of technical personnel per physician

O = number of clerical personnel per physician

M = type of manager, a binary variable; one represents a physician manager, and zero a non-physician manager

R = type of remuneration scheme used by the group, a binary variable; one represents a salaried group, and zero a non-salaried group

Estimates were made using ordinary least squares and may be found in Table 2. A table of first-order correlations between independent variables is found in Appendix B.

For both physical examinations and blood counts, there is a statistically significant positive relationship between prices and per capita income. However, because of the unavailability of county health insurance data, the estimate of the per capita income variable may be biased. To the extent that health insurance and per capita income are positively related, the bias is in an upward direction. The statistically insignificant result for X rays probably reflects the fact that this medical service is priced more uniformly than the other two. This is further evidenced by the smaller coefficient of variation for the price of X rays defined as the standard deviation divided by the mean (.23, as compared to .52 and .35 for physical examinations and blood counts, respectively). A relationship that is also of interest is the responsiveness of fees to income. One measure of this responsiveness is the so-called income elasticity of fees. [The elasticity at the mean for a linear equation $Y = a + bx$ such as one used here is equal to $b(\bar{x}/\bar{y})$.] For physical examinations and blood counts, the elasticity at the mean was found to be approximately .57 and .28. Newhouse (1970) found estimates that ranged from .7 to .9, which appear comparable to ours. Fedlstein's results (1970) include an insurance variable and, as expected, are somewhat smaller; they ranged from .09 to .21 depending on the specification.

Turning our attention to the size of the group, we find that size did not have a statistically significant effect on the price of the

TABLE 2

Estimates of Price Equations

	Income per Capita Y	Number of Doctors S	Medical Personnel per Physician A	Technical Personnel per Physician T	Office Personnel per Physician O	Prevalence of Non-physician Manpower M	Non-salaried System of Remuneration R	Type of Group H	Constant	R^2	No. of Cases
Physical examination, P_1 $\bar{X} = 23.12$ $\sigma = 11.85$	.005 (.723)	.091 (.221)	4.585 (2.581)	24.344 (2.910)	5.605 (1.905)	-4.408 -(1.943)	-2.194 -(2.266)	3.481 (.836)	-15.330	.524	61
Blood count, P_2 $\bar{X} = 5.32$ $\sigma = 1.98$	.003 (3.815)	.205 (1.007)	.651 (1.875)	4.922 (2.501)	.234 (.517)	-2.184 -(2.093)	-1.841 -(1.544)	.435 (.456)	-4.698	.540	60
X rays, P_3 $\bar{X} = 15.10$ $\sigma = 3.47$	-.000[b] (.000)[b]	.068 (.454)	2.141 (1.883)	4.482 (1.704)	0.557 (.645)	-.263 -(.148)	-1.181 -(.477)	-1.628 -(.802)	11.575	.450	58

[a] Using a one-tail test. "t" values of 1.67 or greater are significant at the 10-percent level.

$\bar{X}$ = mean σ = standard deviation

[b] Zero values due to rounding

medical services considered. Alternative specifications were also tested, including one with a size-squared term. The results produced estimates that were not statistically different from zero. If this relationship is representative of all medical services, then policies to stimulate the growth of medical groups may not be helpful to reducing medical prices. Because our sample contains groups that average 5.44 full-time physicians, the reader is cautioned that this result may not be as applicable for very large groups.

The empirical results for the three medical services tested indicates that the specialty composition of the group, H, does not have a statistically significant effect on price. Without further empirical work for other medical services, however, we should be careful not to generalize this result.

The relationship between the price and the utilization of non-physician personnel by group practices produced an interesting result. For the medical services analyzed, increases in the per physician utilization of (1) medical personnel, A, (2) technical personnel, T, and (3) office personnel, O, are associated with increases in price. These results, however, may not apply to physician assistants (Scheffler, 1974b), who are being trained to carry out many of the medical tasks previously performed exclusively by the physician. Feldstein (1970) found a similar relationship and suggested that this result may reflect quality differences in the services provided. These quality differences are probably due to the fact that these medical personnel complement the production of medical services and are not used as physician substitutes, and thus their impact on productivity may be quite small. Bailey (1970:270) points out that ". . . the addition of paramedical personnel does not directly affect physician productivity rates but may result in the substitution of paramedical time for physician time spent on certain tasks which are extraneous to patient visits." Although increases in quality may be desirable, the resulting price increases should not be overlooked.

Of considerable interest is the statistically significant negative coefficient found for the type of manager, M, in the equation for the price of physical examinations and blood counts. This suggests that groups with a non-physician manager set lower prices. Furthermore, the magnitudes appear substantial, a $2.19 difference for physical examinations and $1.85 for blood counts. One explanation for this finding is that managerial efficiencies in medical groups are a real possibility. Perhaps one of these efficiencies is the likelihood that a non-physician manager is more concerned with billing and collection methods which reduce costs, in order to justify his salary to the group. Another possibility is that we are observing some evidence of economies of scale. Since larger groups are more likely to be able to employ a specialized non-physician manager, they are subsequently able to benefit from the resulting management efficiency (Scheffler, in press). Because of limitations of the data, it is not possible to separate these two effects.

Our results indicate that in groups where physicians are paid using a non-salaried system, the prices for physical examinations and blood counts are reduced. The coefficient for X rays had the predicted negative sign but was not statistically different from zero at conventional levels. These findings are consistent with our a priori expectation that salaried physicians may not have the financial incentive to increase their productivity. Additional evidence related to the effect of incentives is provided by Newhouse (1973). He suggests that the physician behaves inefficiently in group practice because he does not have to bear the financial consequences of his decisions and that this inefficiency is an increasing function of the size of the group. An empirical test of this theory by Newhouse concluded that groups with cost-sharing agreements have higher costs of production.

Conclusions and Social Policy Implications

Generally, we have found that the pricing behavior of the sample of medical groups tested is comparable to Feldstein's results (1970) for all physicians in private practice. Other findings related to the characteristics of medical groups were important in explaining price differentials among groups. Of considerable interest is the type of manager and the remuneration system used by the group. Both results suggest policy recommendations that have the potential for reducing price of medical care delivered by medical groups.

Perhaps one of the most neglected areas of research in the health services industry is the management structure. Medical care delivered by any mode of practice requires managerial skills. Even the solo practitioner must devote some of his time to managerial functions. These functions become more complex for group practices, clinics, and hospitals, and thus they require important organizational decisions. Moreover, the efficiency of these models of practice depend, to some degree, on the successful performance of managerial functions. The empirical findings in this paper suggest that groups which utilize non-physician managers are associated with setting lower medical prices. Although there may be a number of reasons for this relationship, it certainly indicates the potential importance of the management input. Current proposals to stimulate group practice should consider the difficulties in providing the management skills required for the operation of group practices. Furthermore, additional attention should be given the entire question of managerial structure of group practice.

The results of this study strongly suggest that the income-sharing scheme used by the group will influence the economic behavior of the member physicians. Although the link between the productivity of the physician and prices set by the group has not been established in this paper, it is likely that an incentive system increases productivity and thus permits the group an opportunity of setting lower prices. Nevertheless, it is clear that the type of income-sharing scheme used by the group is an important economic characteristic of group practice.

Two other results deserve further discussion. For the sample of groups tested, the size of the group was not statistically significant in explaining variations among prices. If this relationship is correct for group practices as a whole, then policies to increase the size of medical groups may have little effect on the prices charged to patients. The other important result of this paper suggests that utilization of non-physician personnel is complementary to the production of medical care by the group. This result implies that both the quality and the prices of medical services are related to the increase in non-physician personnel. Measures to increase quality are useful; however, any policy that has the potential for increasing prices warrants very careful examination.

There appears to be a strong case for prudence in providing government funds in order to stimulate the development for group practice. At risk is the possibility that such a policy, without the proper safeguards, will contribute to increasing cost of medical care. It is hoped that this paper has identified some important factors that should be investigated before further stimulus is given to the growth of group practice.

Richard M. Scheffler, PH.D.
Department of Economics
The University of North Carolina at Chapel Hill
Chapel Hill, North Carolina 27514

References

American Medical Association
1971   Survey of Medical Groups in the United States, 1969. Chicago.

Arrow, Kenneth J.
1963   "Uncertainty and the welfare economics of medical care." American Economic Review (December): 941–973.

Bailey, Richard M.
1968   "A comparison of internists in solo and fee-for-service group practice in the San Francisco Bay Area." Bulletin of the New York Academy of Medicine 44 (November): 1293–1303.

1970   "Economies of scale in medical practice." Pp. 255–273 in Klarman, Herbert (ed.), Empirical Studies in Health Economics. Baltimore: The Johns Hopkins Press.

Berry, R. E., Jr.
1970   "Product heterogeneity and hospital cost analysis." Inquiry 7 (March): 67–75.

Boan, J. A.
1966   Group Practice. Ottawa: The Queen's Printer.

Davis, Karen
1971   "Relationships of hospital prices to costs." Applied Economics 4: 115–125.

Donabedian, A.
1969   "An evaluation of prepaid group practice." Inquiry 6: 3: 3–27.

Feldstein, Martin
1970   "The rising price of physicians' services." Review of Economics and Statistics 7:2 (May).

Garbarino, Joseph W.
1959   "Price behavior and productivity in the medical market." Industrial
        and Labor Relations Review 13 (October): 3–15.

Graham, F. E.
1972   "Group versus solo practice: arguments and evidence." Inquiry 60:2
        (June).

Kessel, Reuben
1958   "Price discrimination in medicine." Journal of Law and Economics
        (October): 20–53.

Kimbell, Larry J., and John H. Lorant
1973   "Physician productivity and returns to scale." Human Resources
        Research Center, University of Southern California. (Mimeographed).

MacCall, U.
1966   Group Practice and Prepayment of Medical Care. Washington, D.C.:
        Public Affairs Press.

Monsma, G. N., Jr.
1970   "Marginal revenue and the demand for physicians' services." Pp.
        145–160, in Klarman, Herbert (ed.), Empirical Studies in Health
        Economics. Baltimore: The Johns Hopkins Press.

Newhouse, Joseph
1970   "A model of physician pricing." Southern Economic Journal 37 (Oc-
        tober): 174–183.

1973   "The economics of group practice." The Journal of Human Resources
        8:1 (Winter).

Rafferty, John A.
1971   "Patterns of hospital use: an analysis of short-run variation." Journal
        of Political Economy 79:1 (January/February): 154–165.

Reinhardt, U. E.
1972   "A production function for medical services." Review of Economics
        and Statistics (February).

Scheffler, Richard M.
in   "Further considerations on the economics of group practice: the
press   management input." The Journal of Human Resources.

1974a   "Productivity and economies of scale in medical practice." Rafferty,
        John A. (ed.) Health Manpower and Productivity New York: D.C.
        Heath.

1974b   ''The market for paraprofessionals: the physician assistant.''
         Quarterly Review of Economics and Business 14:3 (Autumn): 47–60.

Smith, Kenneth R., Marianne Miller, and Frederick L. Golladay
1972   ''An analysis of the optimal use of inputs in the production of medical
         services.'' Journal of Human Resources 7:2.

APPENDIX A

Sample Questionnaire for Medical Groups

1. Name_____

    Address_____

    _____

2. How many doctors practice in association with your group? _____

    Full time?_____Part time (less than 20 hours/week)? _____

    Estimate of full-time equivalents. _____

    Please distribute totals by type:

    a. Generalists   _____

    b. Medical Specialists   _____

        (including pediatrics, psychiatrics)

    c. Surgical Specialists   _____

3. If your group is a single-specialty group, indicate type: '

    _____

4. Physician remuneration is by (circle):   a. individaul fee-for-service,

    b. salary, c. percentage split, d. point system allocation (if so,

    indicate major determining factors:_____

    _____)

5. The business organization of your group may be classified (circle):

    a. partnership,   b. association,   c. corporation,   d. foundation.

6. This questionnarie is being completed by (circle): a. professional business

    manager, b. administrator/director, c. financial manager, d. ad-

    ministrative practicing physician, c. physician, f. group-member liaison

    with professional management firm, g. member of professional manage-

    ment firm, h. other

    (specify) _____

7. What educational degree(s) do you hold? a. none, b. associate

degree, c. B.S. or B.A., d. M.B.A., e. M.A., f. Ph.D., g. J.D., h. M.D.

How many years of group directorship experience have you had? _____

8. Which of the following establishes operation policies or planning for the group? a. the business manager(s) or director(s), b. a policy or planning committee, c. physician-partners of the group, d. other
(specify) _____

9. If a policy committee exists, enumerate composition of such by profession:
   a. physicians/surgeons _____
   b. administrators _____
   c. others (specify) _____

10. For what reason was the most recently acquired physician recruited?
   a. general community needs, b. community demand for an additional specialist, c. replacement, d. decision to expand the size or operations of the group, e. other
   (specify) _____

11. Indicate the customary charge for the following services:
   a. chest X ray (p.a. and lat.) _____
   b. blood count _____
   c. complete physical examination
      (excluding proctoscopic exam) _____

12. If you use the Relative Value Scale, what is your charge for a single unit? _____

13. Enumerate group-employed personnel other than physicians and surgeons:
   a. directors, assistants _____
   b. clerical staff _____
   c. physicians' assistants _____
   d. registered nurses _____
   e. practical nurses _____
   f. lab technicians, pharmacists _____
   g. custodial personnel, aides _____

14. As a group practice manager or director, list several of the more complex problems you have had to face (on reverse).

15. Additional comment: _____
    _____
    _____
    _____

APPENDIX B

Matrix of Simple Correlation Coefficients
Between Independent Variables

	Y	S	A	T	O	M	R	H
Per Capita Income (Y)	1.00							
Number of M.D.s (S)	0.06	1.00						
Medical Personnel per M.D. (A)	0.18	0.51	1.00					
Technical Personnel per M.D. (T)	0.05	0.11	0.84	1.00				
Office Personnel per M.D. (O)	0.18	0.50	0.01	0.46	1.00			
Presence of Nonphysician Manager (M)	-0.08	0.15	0.08	0.24	0.41	1.00		
Non-salaried System of Remuneration (R)	-0.12	0.18	0.04	0.31	0.05	0.01	1.00	
Type of Group (H)	-0.02	0.21	0.12	0.03	0.21	0.58	-0.14	1.00

Prepaid Group Practice
and the
New "Demanding Patient"

ELIOT FREIDSON

Based on an extensive field study of the practitioners in a large, prepaid service contract group practice, this paper discusses how a prepaid service contract and closed-panel practice brings a new dimension into doctor-patient relations and how physicians respond to it. Unable to manage "unreasonable" demands for service by use of a fee-barrier or encouragement to "go elsewhere," as in traditional, solo, fee-for-service practice, they were particularly upset by a new type of "demanding patient" who claimed services on the basis of contractual rights and threatened appeal to higher bureaucratic authority. Modes of dealing with such patients are briefly discussed.

The future dimensions of medical practice in the United States are beginning to emerge now, both through the steady increase in prepaid insurance coverage for ambulatory care, and through the pressure on physicians to work together in organizations. But what will be the impact of those changes on the people involved, and on their relationships with each other? What will the doctor-patient relationship be like? There can be little doubt that prepaid medical care insurance plans will, by changing the economic relationship between doctor and patient, also change many ways in which they interact with each other. And there can also be little doubt that when physicians routinely work in organizations where they are cooperating rather than competing with colleagues, other elements of their relationships with patients and colleagues will change.

Obvious as it is that change will occur, we have rather little information relevant to anticipating its human consequences. We have fairly good estimates of the economic consequences of those changes in the organization of medical care, and we have hopeful evidence on how the medical quality of care might be affected, but between the input and output measures there is only a black box: we have little information on how the human beings in medical practice produce the results which are measured, on the quality of their experience in practice, and on the characteristic

MMFQ / Health and Society / *Fall 1973*

ways they try to manage their problems at work. Without knowing
something about that, it is rather difficult to anticipate how doctor-
patient relationships will change and what problems will be em-
bedded in them.

This paper is an attempt to provide some information about
how the participants in a medical care program which anticipated
present-day trends responded to each other and to the economic
and social structure of practice. The data upon which I shall draw
come from an eighteen-month-long field study of the physicians
who worked in a large, prepaid group practice. Most of the primary
practitioners (internists and pediatricians) worked on a full-time
basis in the medical group, and most of the consultants worked
part-time, but all fifty-five of them were on salary, officially employees of the institution. Their medical group contracted with
an insurance organization to provide virtually complete care to
insured patients without imposing on them any out of pocket
charges. In studying the physicians of the medical group, a very
large amount of observational, documentary, and direct evidence
was collected in the course of examining files, attending all staff
meetings, listening to luncheon-table conversations, and carrying
out a series of intensive interviews with all the physicians in the
group. The research obtained a systematic and comprehensive
view of how the group physicians worked and what their problems
were. Because of a lack of space here, however, only a summary
of findings bearing on a single issue is possible.

The Administrative Structure of the Group

To understand practice in the medical group, it is necessary to
understand the framework in which it was carried out. The group
did not have an elaborate administrative structure, since it lacked
clear gradations of rank and authority and had rather few written,
formal rules. It was not organized like a traditional bureaucratic
organization. The few rules which were bureaucratically enforced
all dealt in one way or another with the *terms* of work—with how
and what the physician was to be paid, and the amount of time
he was to work in return for that pay. Ultimately, the terms of
work were less a function of the medical group administration

than of the health insurance organization with which the medical group entered into a contract. The absolute income available for paying the doctors derived primarily from the insurance contract, which specified a given sum per year per insured person or family, plus additional sums by a complicated formula not important for present purposes. The administration of the medical group could decide how to divide up the contract income among the physicians but had to work within the absolute limits of that income.

By the same token, critical aspects of the *conditions* of work stemmed more from the terms of the service contract than from the choice and action of the group administration. The most important complaint of the physicians about the conditions of work in the medical group was of "overload"—having to provide more services in a given period of time than was considered appropriate. Such "overload" was a direct function of the prepaid service contract, which freed the subscriber from having to pay a separate fee for each service he wished, and encouraged many physicians to manage patient demands by increasing referrals and reappointments.

It was around these externally formulated contractual arrangements that we found the administration of the medical group establishing and enforcing the firmest bureaucratic rules, perhaps because it had no other choice than to do so in order to satisfy its contract to provide services. The prepaid service-contract arrangement could be conceived of as purely economic in character —simply a rational way of *paying* for health care, which did not influence health care itself. But it was much more than that, since it organized demand and supply, the processes by which health care takes place. In fact, it was closely connected with many of the problems of practice in the group. This is not to say that it created those problems in and of itself. Rather, it gave rise to new possibilities for problematic behavior on the part of both patient and physician and prevented the use by both of traditional solutions. To understand its relationship to the problems of practice in the medical group, to the way the physicians made sense of their experience, and to the ways they attempted to cope with it, let us first examine the way the physicians responded to the differences they perceived between prepaid service-contract group practice and private, fee-for-service solo practice.

The Meanings of Entrepreneurial and Contract Group Practice

All of the physicians interviewed, including those who had left the group and were solo practitioners at the time of being interviewed, had at one time or another worked on a salary in the medical group. Thus, they reported on circumstances in which they could not themselves charge the patient a fee for the services they rendered. Their income was independent of the services they gave, just as the cost to the patient was independent of the services he received. The patient demanded and the physician supplied services on the basis of a prepayment contract which established a right for the patient and an obligation for the physician. Furthermore, the group was organized on a closed-panel basis, so that in order to obtain services by the terms of his contract, without out-of-pocket cost, the patient had to seek service only from the physicians working at the medical group, and no others.

Virtually all of the physicians interviewed had also had occasion to work on the traditional basis of solo, fee-for-service "private" practice. In that mode of organizing work and the marketplace, the physician makes a living by attracting patients and providing them with services paid for by a fee for each service. The physician's income is directly related to the fee charged and the number of services provided. He has no contractual relationship with patients. He must attract them by a variety of devices—accessibility, reputation, specialty, referral relations with colleagues—and maintain a sufficiently steady stream of new or returning patients to assure a stable if not lucrative practice. In theory, the patient is free to leave him for another physician, and relations with colleagues offering the same services are at least nominally competitive.

How did the physicians interpret these different arrangements and what did they emphasize in their experience with each? In the interviews, the prepaid group physician was often represented as helpless and exploited, with words like "trapped," "slave," and "servitor" used to describe his position. Since the contract was for all "necessary" services, however, it was hardly accurate to say that the physicians had to provide every service the patient demanded. They could have refused. But at bottom it was not really the formal contract which was the issue. Rather, the physicians were responding to the absence of a mechanism to which they were accustomed, a mechanism which, by attesting to the value of the physician's services in the eyes of the patient, and by testing the strength of the patient's sense of need, precluded the necessity of actually refusing. The physicians were responding to the absence of the out-of-pocket fee which is a prerequisite for service in "private practice."

The fee was seen as a useful barrier between patient and doctor which forced the *patient* to discriminate between the trivial and the important before he sought care. The assumption was that if the patient had to pay a fee for each service, he would ask only for "necessary" services, or, if he were too irrational or ignorant to discriminate accurately, he would at the very least restrict his demands to those occasions when he was really greatly worried. The fee served as a mechanical barrier which freed the physician of the necessity of having to refuse service and of having to persuade the patient that his grounds for doing so were reasonable. Since a fee operates as a barrier in advance of any request for service, it reduces interaction between physician and patient. In the prepaid plan, the physicians were not prepared for the greater interaction which the absence of a fee encouraged.

In addition to the service contract, there was also the closed-panel organization of the medical group. The physicians themselves were aware that some patients often felt trapped, since, in order to receive the benefits of their contract, they had to use the services only of a physician employed by the medical group. If he wanted to be treated by a particular individual in the group, he might nonetheless have had to accept another because of the former's full panel or appointment schedule. And when patients were referred to consultants, they were supposed to be referred to a specialty, not to an individual specialist. Some of the physicians themselves found this situation unsatisfactory because they were not personally chosen by patients, but were seen by patients because they happened to have appointment time free or openings on their panel, not because of their individual reputation or attractiveness.

Finally, there was the issue of group practice itself, of the constitution of a cooperative collegium rather than, as in entrepreneurial practice, an aggregate of nominally competing practitioners. In the latter case, the physician may be "scared that somebody would . . . take his patient away," or that the patient may "walk out the door and you may never see him again." Nevertheless, if he can afford it, the physician in fee-for-service solo practice can choose to refuse to give the patient what he asks for, and can even discourage him from returning. But in the group practice, the physicians did not generally have the option of dropping a patient with whom they had difficulty. The reason was not to be found in any potential economic loss, as in entrepreneurial practice, but rather in the closed-panel practice within which colleagues were cooperating rather than competing. When physicians form a closed-panel group, they cannot simply act as individuals, "drop" a patient who is troublesome, and allow him to go to a colleague, for if each of the group dropped his own problem patients, while he would indeed get rid of the ones he had, he would get in return those his colleagues had dropped, as his colleagues would get his. And so the pressure was to "live" with such patients and try to manage them as best one could— something for which the physician with ideological roots in private practice was poorly prepared.

From the view which the physicians presented, it seemed that the medical group involved them in a situation in which traditional safety valves had been tied down and the pressure increased. The service contract was thought to increase patient demand for services, while at the same time it prevented the physician from coping with that demand by the traditional method of raising prices. The closed-panel arrangement restricted the patients' demands to those physicians working cooperatively in the medical group, so the physicians could not cope with the pressure by the traditional method of encouraging the troublesome patient to go elsewhere for service. Confrontation between patient and physician was increased, and both participants explored new methods for resolving them. Indeed, the insurance scheme itself provided the resources for some of those new methods of reducing the pressure on demand and supply.

Paradigmatic Problems and Solutions

The basic interpersonal paradigm of a problematic doctor-patient relationship may be seen as a conflict between perspectives and a struggle for control or a negotiation over the provision of services. From his perspective the patient believes he needs a particular service; from his, the physician does not believe every service the patient wishes is necessary or appropriate. The content of this conflict between perspectives is composed of conceptions of knowledge, or expertise, the physician asserting that he knows best and the patient insisting that he is his own arbiter of need.

The conflict, however, takes place in a social and economic marketplace which provides resources that may be used to reinforce the one or the other position. In the case of medicine in the United States, that marketplace has in the past been organized on a fee-for-service basis, practitioners being entrepreneurs competing with each other for the fees of prospective patients. The fee the patient is willing and able to pay, in conjunction with the physician's economic security, constitute elements which are of strategic importance to private practice. If the physician's practice is well enough established, he can refuse service he does not want to give or does not believe necessary to give, even though he loses a fee and possibly a patient. On the other hand, if he desires to gain the fee and reduce the chance of "losing" the patient, he may give the patient the service he requests even if he believes it to be unnecessary. Like a merchant, he is concerned with pleasing his patients by giving them what they want, suspending his own notions of what is necessary and good for them in favor of his gain in income should he desire such gain.

The patient, on the other hand, has his fee as a resource (if he is lucky), and the freedom to turn away from the practitioner who does not provide him with the service he wants and pay it instead to the physician who does. He may take his trade elsewhere, but before he does he may introduce pressure by implying that if he does not get what he wants he will find someone else. In essence, the patient can play "customer" to the physician's merchant.

In contrast to these marketplace roles, there are those more often ascribed to doctor and patient by sociologists—that of expert consultant and layman. The layman is defined as someone who has a problem or difficulty he wishes resolved, but who does not have the special knowledge and skill needed to do so. He seeks out someone who has the necessary knowledge and skill and cooperates with him so that his difficulty can be managed if not resolved. In dealing with the expert, the layman is supposed to suspend his own judgment and instead follow the advice of the expert, who is considered to have superior knowledge and better judgment. When there are differences of opinion of such character that the patient cannot bring himself to cooperate, the *generic* response of the expert is to attempt to gain the patient's cooperation by persuading him, on the basis of evidence which the expert produces, that it would be in his interest to cooperate and follow the recommended course. To *order* him to comply, or to gain compliance by some other form of coercion or pressure, is a contradiction of the essence of expertise and its "authority." Analytically, expertise gains its "authority" by its persuasive demonstration of special knowledge and skill relevant to particular problems requiring solution. It is the antithesis of the authority of office.

As a profession, however, medicine represents not only a full-time occupation possessed of expertise which participates in a marketplace where it sells its labor for a profit, but more particularly an occupation which has gained a specially protected position in the marketplace and a set of formal prerogatives which grant it some degree of official authority. For example, the mere possession of a legal license to practice allows the physician to officially certify death or disability, and to authorize pharmacists to dispense a variety of powerful and dangerous drugs. Here, albeit in rudimentary form, we find yet a third facet by which to characterize a third kind of doctor-patient relationship that of the bureaucratic official and client. The latter seeks a given service from the former, who has exclusive control over access to services. The client seeks to establish his need and his right, while the official seeks to establish his eligibility before providing service or access to goods or services. In theory, both are bound by a set of rules which defines the rights and duties of the participants, and each makes reference to the rules in making and evaluating claims. In a rational-legal form of administration, both have a right of appeal to some higher authority who is empowered to mediate and resolve their differences.

In the predominant form of practice in present-day United States, the physician is more likely to be playing the role of merchant and expert than the role of official, though the latter is real enough and too important to be as ignored as it has been by sociologists and physicians alike. It is, after all, his status as an official which gives the physician a protected marketplace in which to be a merchant. Nonetheless, to be a true official virtually precludes being a merchant, so that only in special instances in the United States can we find medical practice which offers the possibility of taking the role of official on an everyday rather than an occasional basis.

The medical group we studied was just such a special instance, for it eliminated the fee and discouraged the profit motive, while setting up its physicians as official gatekeepers to services specified in a contract with patients, through an insurance agency with supervisory powers of its own. The contractual network specified the basic set of systematic rules, and established the official position of the physician. Under the rules, the physician served as an official gatekeeper to and authorizer of a whole array of services— not only his own, but also those of consultants who, even though "covered" in the contract, would not see a patient without an official referral, and those of laboratories, which do not provide "covered" tests without an official group physician's signature. In other reports of this study I show how the physicians were led to use their official powers to cope with problems of work, and how they exercised their role of expert. I also show how some railed against a situation which prevented them from using the more familiar techniques of the merchant to resolve their problems.

Here, however, I wish to point out that in the medical group the physician was not the only participant to whom a new role was made available. The situation, which left open the option of official and closed the option of merchant for physicians, also left open the option of bureaucratic client and closed the option of shopper or customer for patients. And when the patients acted as bureaucratic clients they posed different problems to the physician than they did when they acted as a customer, or as a patient: they asserted their rights in light of the rules of the contract. This untraditional possibility for patient behavior was one which upset the physicians a great deal and served as the focus for much of their dissatisfaction. Most of their problems of work stemmed ultimately from their relationships with patients and tended to be characterized in terms of the patient, so that it is important to understand the way the physicians saw their patients. Typically, work problems stemmed from patients who "make demands"; "the demanding patient" was seen to lie at the root of those difficulties.

Three Types of "Demanding Patients"

It is very easy to get the impression from this analysis that the work-lives of the group physicians were constantly fraught with pressure and conflict. Such an impression stems partially from the strategy of analysis I have chosen, a strategy which focuses on work problems rather than on the settled, everyday routines which stretch out on either side of occasional crises. Without remembering that most medical work is routine rather than crisis, one could not understand how physicians manage to get through their days. Indeed, the kinds of medical complaints and symptoms which are most often brought into the office were such that the daily routine posed a serious problem of boredom to the practitioners. Furthermore, most patients were not troublesome. As members of the stable blue- and white-collar classes, most knew the rules of the game, respected the physicians, and were more inclined than not to come in with medically acceptable (even if "trivial") complaints.

Nonetheless, the fact of routine, even boredom, would be difficult to discern in the physicians' own conversations. They did not talk to each other, or to the interviewers, about their routines; they talked about their crises. They did not talk about slow days, but about those when the work pressure was overwhelming. They rarely talked about "good" patients unless they received some unusual letter of thanks, card, or gift of which they were proud; they talked incessantly about troublesome or demanding patients. They almost never talked about routine diagnoses and their management, but talked often about the anomaly, the interesting case, or one of their "goofs." So the analytical strategy for reporting this study is not arbitrary, since it reflects the physicians' own preoccupations. It was by the problematic that they symbolized their work and it was in terms of the problematic that they evaluated their practice. Even though all agreed that "demanding patients" were statistically few in number, many who left the medical group ascribed their departure to their inability to bear even those few patients.

Most important for present purposes was the fact that, upon analysis of the physicians' discussion of "demanding patients," it was discovered that the most important type was a new one for them. They posed demands which the physicians were unaccustomed to dealing with, for the demands stemmed from the contractual framework of practice in the medical group and were generic to the role of the bureaucratic client rather than the customer or layman. Perhaps this was why they seemed so outrageous and insulting, for such demands treated the physicians as if they were officials rather than "free professionals." The distinction between that kind of demandingness and others was more often implicit than explicit in the physicians' talk when they were asked to characterize demanding patients. The tendency, however, was to distinguish one kind of demanding patient as dictatorial and another as essentially the opposite—eternally supplicant.

Of the two kinds of demanding patients, one would be familiar to the informed reader as the ambulatory practice version of the "crock" met in complaints by medical students and the house staff in the clinics of teaching hospitals. The crock was the person who played the respectful patient role, but presented complaints for which the physician had no antibiotic, vaccine, chemical agent, or technique for surgical repair. All the physician could provide for such complaints was what he considered "palliative" treatment rather than "cure." He neither learned anything interesting by seeing some biologically unusual condition nor felt he accomplished successful therapy. And he worried that he might overlook something "real."

Clearly, this kind of demanding patient was irritating because he had to be babied rather than treated instrumentally and because the doctor had to devote himself to "treating people [whom he considers to be] well, or have the same kind of anxieties we all have." Furthermore, he confronted the doctor with failure: he "can never be reassured. You know you are not getting anywhere with him and you just have to listen to him, the same chronic minor complaints and the same business." "I'm just not satisfied with my results, and the patient just keeps coming back, worse than ever."

In light of the distinctions I made earlier, it should be clear that this kind of demanding person was not playing either the role of bureaucratic client or that of customer. The role of the helpless layman was adopted, which did not contradict the role the physician wished to play. The problem was that the nature of the complaints was such that the medical worker could not play his role in a satisfying way—he could not really help, and his advice that there was no serious medical problem was refused.

The other kind of demanding patient was quite different, however, for he did not ceaselessly *beg* for help so much as *demand* services on the basis of his economic and contractual rights. Such rights do not, of course, exist in fee-for-service solo practice, but the analogue in such practice would be the demanding customer. Such a person is more likely to shop around from one physician to another rather than stick to one and demand his service. Given the structure of fee-for-service solo practice, we should expect in it rather less confrontation with demanding customers, though the physicians did tell stories about some who openly threatened to take their business elsewhere if they did not get what they wanted. Rare as such confrontation was, when it did occur, it was described with the same shock and outrage as was observed in the physicians' stories about demanding contract patients.

The "power of the contract" which one physician spoke of implied correctly that some patients, playing the role of bureaucratic client, threatened to and on occasion actually employed the device of an official complaint. They could complain either to the administration of the medical group or to an office established by the insuring organization to receive and investigate complaints. After all, if one has a contract, one also has the right to appeal decisions about its benefits. And naturally, the more familiar and effective with bureaucratic procedures the patients were, the more were they able to make trouble. The seventeen physicians who generalized about the social characteristic of demanding patients yielded in sum a caricature of the demanding patient as a female schoolteacher, well educated enough to be capable of articulate and critical questioning and letter writing, of high enough social status to be sensitive to slight and to expect satisfaction, and experienced with bureaucratic procedures. In the physicians' eyes, they were also neurotically motivated to be "demanding."

Also specially nurtured in the framework of the prepaid group practice—contrary to the ideal of bureaucracy but faithful to its reality—was the use by the bureaucratic client of "pull" or political influence to reinforce his demands and gain more than nominal contract benefits. Analogous to political influence in the free medical marketplace is the possession of wealth or prestige, making one a desirable customer who may refer his friends to the physician. Another form of "pull" lies in having connections with an especially influential and prestigious medical colleague. Both types of patients gain special handling in solo practice. In the medical group, however, "pull" was more related to influence in those segments of the community engaged in negotiating insurance contracts. There were occasional instances when a demanding patient was also an important member of a trade union, or had friends in high political places. Managing such patients was particularly difficult for the administration, since it was unable to protect its own staff in the face of such political influence.

Managing Demanding Patients in the Future

In this paper I have assumed that a prepaid service-contract medical group has important characteristics which will become more common in the future and which, therefore, allow us to make plausible and informed anticipations of the problems of medical practice in the future. On the basis of extensive interviews with physicians who worked in such a medical group, I suggested that a new kind of problem of management was posed to them by the social and economic structure of their practice. Ostensibly, the problem was the familiar and traditional one of the "demanding patient." Looking more closely at the usage of that phrase, however, led to the conclusion that there was more than one kind of "demanding patient." Indeed, on the basis of the physicians' discussions of their problems, I suggested that there were three types of demanding patients, each posing a different problem of management and a different challenge to medical self-esteem.

Virtually unmet in the medical group (but mentioned by the physicians) were those who acted like demanding customers by insisting on either obtaining the services they wished or of taking their business (and fees) elsewhere. Such a strategy is of course generic to entrepreneurial practice, and most effective with weakly established practitioners in a highly competitive medical market. The second type of demanding patient was the traditional "crock," what a spokesman for Kaiser-Permanente once called "the worried well." Such a patient persisted in seeking consultation for complaints which the physicians felt were trivial and essentially incurable. They were a more serious problem in the medical group than they were reported to be in fee-for-service solo practice because their demands could not be reduced by the imposition of a fee barrier or by suggesting that they go elsewhere for service. The third type of demanding patient was new and particularly disturbing to the physicians—the patient who demanded services which he felt he had a right to under the terms of his prepaid service contract and who had recourse to complaining about the deprivation of his rights to the bureaucratic system of appeal and review.

In the future, with prepaid group practice far more common, we should expect new problems in the doctor-patient relationship as that new kind of demanding patient is met with by more physicians. Insurance coverage in the future may be such as to maintain some kind of fee barrier (as in prepaid plans which now impose small charges for house calls), but the barrier will be less than that to which physicians were accustomed in fee-for-service practice and will be less effective in discouraging demandingness. In addition, since he will be working cooperatively with colleagues in group practice, the physician will be less able to simply "drop" his demanding patients. Unable to use money or evasion to cope with his relationship to problem patients, the physician will have to use other methods. What options are open to him?

Just as the structure of fee-for-service solo practice produces the possibility of using mechanical financial solutions, so does the structure of prepaid service-contract practice also produce the possibility of using mechanical solutions. The mechanical solutions observed in the medical group studied lay in providing all services covered by the contract which were not inconvenient to the practitioner—office visits, referrals, and laboratory tests. (The house call was not convenient, and was resisted strongly.) But whereas the former solutions were traditional and so regarded as "natural" and "reasonable," the use of the latter was regarded as "giving in," and treated with resentment and concern. Both are, analytically, equally mechanical, an equally passive reflex to the organization of the system of care.

The consequences of passive response to the new conditions by which patient demand will be structured are already clear. In the face of rising services and costs, strong administrative, financial, and peer-review pressures will force the physician to limit his "giving in" and restrict the supply of demanded services. But how exactly can the physician limit services, and what kind of interaction will go on between him and his patient under such circumstances? I cannot provide empirical evidence from my study because in the medical group there was rather little organized pressure to limit services. The physicians could "give in" when they chose to. But the logic of my analysis would lead me to expect that when there is pressure to limit service to demanding patients in a structure like that of the medical group, the structure taken by itself provides the opportunity for doing so on the bureaucratic grounds of the official authority of the physician as a gatekeeper to benefits. He can simply refuse the patient, standing on the official position which the structure provides him.

But it need not be that way. While the prepaid service-contract group practice virtually precluded the adoption by physician and patient of a merchant-customer relationship, and allowed the adoption of an official-client relationship which was precluded in private solo practice, it did not *force* the practitioners to manage their problems that way. Some chose to adopt the interactional strategy which is an inherent possibility in medical practice no matter what the historical framework in which it takes place—the strategy of the expert consultant who relies neither on his position in the marketplace nor on his official position in a bureaucratic system but on his knowledge and skill. Some physicians were persuaded that if they invested extra attention and energy in "educating" their patients and developing a relationship of trust they would ultimately have fewer "management" problems. To cope with suspicion on the part of the patient they initially provided services on demand in order to show that they recognized the legitimacy of the patient's contractual rights, and that they were not motivated to withhold services from them. At the same time, however, they tried to explain to the demanding patient the grounds for their judgment that the services were medically unnecessary. They undertook, in other words, to persuade and demonstrate, and avoided mechanical solutions to the problem of demandingness. The social, moral, and technical quality of the medical care of the future will depend on whether medical practice will be organized in such a way as to encourage such a positive mode of responding to patient demands, or whether it will, like traditional practice, be merely a fiscally and technically functional structure which does not take cognizance of the human qualities of those it traps.

E. Freidson
Rm. 308, Sociology
19 University Place
New York University
New York, N.Y. 10003

Abridged version of a chapter of Eliot Freidson, *Doctoring Together* (Chicago: Aldine Publishing Company, forthcoming). Copyright © 1974 by Eliot Freidson. All rights reserved. The study reported here was partially supported by USPH grants RG-7882, GM-07882, CH-00025, CH-00414, and HS-00104.

Medical Malpractice: Some Implications of Contract and Arbitration in HMOs

CARL M. STEVENS

Department of Economics,
Reed College

M OST MALPRACTICE CLAIMS ARE PROCESSED BY the tort-law system, which includes, in addition to the decision rules embodied in the law and the process by which these rules are applied, the settlement-negotiation process, which disposes of 90 percent or so of claims without resort to trial and 95 percent or so of claims without a finally adjudicated outcome. In recent years, in the context of the medical malpractice "crisis," the tort system has been the subject of considerable study, evaluation, and adverse criticism, a good bit of which has advocated abandoning the whole fault-finding approach in favor of some form of no-fault approach (American Bar Association, 1976; Institute of Medicine, 1978; State of New York, 1976; Schwartz, 1976; Havighurst and Tancredi, 1973; Havighurst, 1975; O'Connell, 1975).

One response to alleged failures of the tort system has been to urge the superiority of contract in this domain. In what follows, I suggest that health maintenance organizations (HMOs) afford a peculiarly appropriate institutional setting for developing a contract-based approach to medical malpractice. Indeed, it may be argued that only by explicitly contracting on provider liability and related performance standards can the parties to HMOs fully exploit the inherent advantages of this kind of delivery system.

Although most medical malpractice claims have been and are dis-

Milbank Memorial Fund Quarterly/*Health and Society*, Vol. 59, No. 1, 1981
© 1981 Milbank Memorial Fund and Massachusetts Institute of Technology
0160/1997/81/010059-30 $01.00/0

posed of by the tort-law system of dispute management, for many years a few such claims have been disposed of by arbitration systems. Recently there has been some move toward more arbitration of such claims, although the volume of arbitration in this domain is still modest.[1] In what follows, I will suggest that arbitration (rather than trial) is the appropriate adjudication process for disposition of contract-based malpractice claims against HMOs. More generally, in the design of dispute-management systems, evaluation of the relative merits of different theories on the basis of which claims might be asserted requires that these be considered in the context of the adjudication modes to be associated with them. And, in turn, evaluation of the relative merits of different adjudication modes requires that these be considered in the context of the theories that provide the basis for asserting the claims to be adjudicated.

HMOs and the Contract Approach:
Initial Considerations

Usually, claims against providers charge negligent conduct, the plaintiff claims that the defendant provider has committed a tort. At the

---

[1] According to the Research Institute of the American Arbitration Association (AAA), fourteen states between 1975 and 1979 enacted statutes specifically authorizing medical malpractice arbitration, viz: Alabama, Alaska, California, Georgia, Illinois, Louisiana, Maine, Michigan, North Dakota, Ohio, South Dakota, Vermont, Virginia, and Puerto Rico. Courts in all states enforce some agreements to arbitrate medical malpractice disputes, for the most part under modern general arbitration laws. The AAA further reports that there are fifteen state-wide or local private programs for malpractice arbitration, four in California, two each in New York and Washington, and one each in Illinois, Massachusetts, Minnesota, New Mexico, Pennsylvania, Virginia, and Wyoming.

As of July, 1979, the AAA's Medical Malpractice Research Data Base included 205 closed cases that entered arbitration after 1970 in fourteen states under ten different formal arbitration plans and various ad hoc arrangements. Seventy-five percent of these cases were processed under two state-wide programs—the private California Hospital and Medical Associations' program, and the statutory Michigan program (both administered by AAA). Although the Kaiser-Permanente (K-P) health plans in California (and elsewhere) have had arbitration systems for several years, no K-P cases are included in the AAA data set. In addition, the AAA has identified individual provider plans in nine states (American Arbitration Association, 1979). Heintz (1975, 1979) has reported extensively on the Southern California Arbitration Project.

same time, the provider-patient relationship is ordinarily considered to be based on contract, expressed or implied, such that, theoretically, if not frequently in practice, many malpractice claims could be cast in terms of breach by the provider of a provider-patient contract (Waltz and Inbau, 1971:40). It has been urged that contract law might afford a superior basic theory of medical malpractice. In a perceptive discussion, Epstein makes the case for contract, pointing out, in part:

> The typical malpractice case raises issues of both tort and contract law. The physical injury suffered by the patient is quite sufficient to place the tort element in sharp relief. The contractual element in medical practice is borne out by the simple fact that the physician does not conscript unwilling persons to be his patients. When malpractice cases are treated as though they raise only tort issues, there is the unmistakable tendency to treat the judicial rules as the inflexible commands of positive law. It becomes, therefore, a natural if unfortunate tendency for courts to overlook the possibility, indeed the desirability, of having the rules that they have laid down varied by the agreements between the parties. Where the situation is looked upon as contractual, the basic rules governing the relationship between physician and patient are best understood as approximations of the rules which the parties themselves would choose to govern their own relationship.... And within the contractual orientation, we encourage the parties by private means to develop a set of individuated responses of the sort precluded by the rigid form of the tort law.... There are of course problems with private agreements and there are imperfections in the marketplace.... Yet it is not possible to dismiss contract solutions and a market orientation simply by pointing to these problems. For while it is easy to say that contract rules shall be disregarded, it is very difficult to fashion public standards, be they judicial or legislative, that function better than the contract rules they replace. (Epstein, 1976:93–95)

In making the case for contract, Epstein remarks upon arbitration only in passing, expressing his view that arbitration is consistent with his theme that contract solutions to medical malpractice problems are in general superior to administrative solutions.

With the decentralized, fee-for-service delivery system, and although there is a contract implied by the parties' relationship, there will usually be no formal, explicit contract between provider and patient. The HMO-type delivery-financing system, on the other hand, does feature an explicit contract between the parties. This kind of delivery system features a very distinctive provider-patient relationship in which the HMO contracts with members to arrange the provision of a stipulated bundle of health care services in exchange for periodic dues payments by the members. (Under conventional health insurance, on the other hand, the insurer contracts only to pick up some or all of the tab for services utilized by the insured, leaving it up to the insured to find a provider of the services as best he can.)

As matters now stand, HMO membership contracts do not spell out the HMO's duty to the member with respect to proper performance of the substantive terms of the membership contract (i.e., in terms analogous, say, to definition of the provider's duty afforded by legal negligence rules). However, as Curran and Moseley have pointed out, a contract approach to malpractice claims seems natural in the HMO context:

> Contractual liability, however, seems particularly appropriate in the HMO context. Although there is an express contract between the member patient and the HMO which may not contain specific assurances of high quality care, these terms may usually be implied. The HMO, after all, has agreed to meet the member's every health need up to well-defined limitations and to furnish an acceptable physician for these purposes, and whether that physician is considered an agent of the HMO or the HMO an agent of the physician it would not be unreasonable for the member to infer a guarantee that high standards of quality will be met. (Curran and Moseley, 1975:75)

There is one major problem in the contract approach to performance standards in the medical services sector generally to which the HMO form of delivery system may be regarded as responsive. The general case for freedom of contract (namely, that generally the parties are wiser about their own affairs than are others, including government regulating through its legal institutions) may seriously be questioned if the parties are in some essential way unequal, such that one may opportunistically take advantage of the other. For the usual run of economic transactions, competition in the marketplace, providing the marketeers with alternatives, is supposed to take care of this. In the medical marketplace, however, competition operates only weakly. Moreover, as has frequently been emphasized, there is a large inequality in the amount of information possessed by the patient and by the provider, such that the latter may have a substantial advantage. How might the contracting patient cope? In other domains the "collective contract" has been regarded as affording an answer. For example, Wellington, after considering a number of noncontract alternatives to the admittedly frail individual contract of employment, remarks:

> The drawbacks to these alternatives to contract ... and the values which support the freedom of contract doctrine make the case for collective bargaining an appealing one. If the union bargains for the worker, perhaps the contract between union and employer can be treated according to the usual freedom of contract dogma.... The collective contract simply is less likely to be unfair to one of the parties than an individual contract, and it is more likely to reinforce important societal values than its alternatives. (Wellington, 1968:37)

Similarly, the members of an HMO, although not in any usual sense "organized" *qua* members, do comprise a collectivity in their dealings with the HMO. Indeed, their substantive contracts (those spelling out the services to be delivered in exchange for periodic dues payments) are in a real sense "collective agreements." Most members of HMOs are group members in consequence of employment-related health plans—the same terms apply to all members of the group, and the employer (and union, if any) are parties to the contract.[2] Contract terms spelling out the HMO's duty to the members with respect to standards of care (proper performance of the substantive terms of the membership contract) would, like the substantive terms themselves, be part of a collective agreement. Bovbjerg (1975:n.63, 1395) has alluded to the possibility of HMO members bargaining about care standards, commenting that "an HMO's subscribers, at least as a

---

[2] That these circumstances may warrant distinguishing HMO provider-client contracts has been recognized: "The primary feature of *Wheeler* that distinguishes it from *Madden* is that *Madden* involved a prepaid health plan (Kaiser), and *Wheeler* involved St. Joseph's Hospital, a nonprepaid facility. The *Wheeler* court assumed that the plaintiff in *Madden* was represented by her employer in bargaining with Kaiser concerning the inclusion of the arbitration agreement in the contract for group medical services. Therefore, both parties had equal bargaining power. The patient in *Wheeler,* on the other hand, was 'negotiating' with the hospital by himself" (Bukata, 1978:n.35, 406).

group, may well be able to bargain over the general style of their medical care, including, for example, what facilities are to be provided and whether physician assistants are acceptable." He also pointed out that "the extent to which agreements on risk reduction between provider and patient or enrollee ought to influence or supersede malpractice standards is an important, difficult, and seldom considered question" (Bovbjerg, 1975:n.119, 1412).

Contract Terms: General Considerations and Barring Claims Based on Tort Theories

Generally speaking, a major advantage in moving from the tort system to a contract system *cum* arbitration is that the latter would facilitate development of definitions of the provider's duty, and facilitate development of ways to manage disputes about compliance with that duty that would prove superior for both provider and consumer to those featured by the tort system. Thus both stand to gain from their bargain on this score and this is the spirit that should inform the devising of contract terms. (Although both stand to gain from their cooperation, there may also be a competitive element, i.e., there may be room for difference of opinion about the terms on which they shall cooperate.) Pursuant to this, the parties to HMO performance-standards contracts would best serve their mutual interests by explicitly barring claims based on liability for negligence as defined in tort law. In addition to advantages in principle, such a bar has a practical aspect. From the point of view of the HMO, development of performance-standards contracts to spell out the provider's duty to the members might entail an unacceptable increase in exposure, unless such contracts could also bar claims that in effect contend that the provider has committed a tort as conventionally defined. That is, without such a bar, the provider would confront all of the exposure historically confronted on tort account, plus additional exposure in consequence of other terms of the contract.[3]

---

[3] These considerations raise the question of whether provider-client performance-standards agreements *cum* arbitration legally may preclude claims based on public rights. Parties to such agreements legally may give up their rights to trial by jury in a court of law. But giving up the right of access to a particular forum is not the same thing as giving up a cause of action. More

Social Functions of the Law of Negligence

The law of negligence has been supposed to serve not only the private interests of plaintiffs who may sue in tort but also important social functions, e.g., as by promoting efficient rates of resource allocation to accident prevention. Suppose that the parties (as suggested foregoing), deeming it to their mutual advantage, agree to bar claims based on negligence so defined. They might in this way serve their own private interests. But, might they not at the same time deny service to the public interest in the social functions of the law of negligence? The answer to this question depends partly upon how effective the conventional negligence rule may be expected to be in securing the social benefits attributed to it. If it is not very effective, then, in any event (i.e., whatever the contract terms the parties may substitute for it), not much will be lost on public-interest account by abandoning it. This, it may be argued, is indeed the case. From the point of view of service to its supposed social functions, the law of negligence suffers from a number of technical problems that have not been adequately remarked.[4] Moreover, as will be pointed out, parties to HMO performance standards contracts are in a good position to respond to some of these problems.

The general common law rule mandates that a physician (or other provider) has the obligation to the patient to possess and employ such reasonable skill and care as are commonly had and exercised by reputable, average physicians in the same general system or school of practice in the same or similar localities. Owing in part to the vague-

---

particularly, is the concept of negligence as defined in tort law a "vested common law cause of action" such that a statute authorizing voluntary agreements to give up the right to assert claims based on this cause of action would be unconstitutional? Fortunately, it would appear that statutes can constitutionally authorize the execution of such agreements (Amicus Curiae Brief on Behalf of the California Hospital Association in Support of Petitioners, 2nd Civil No. 51239, 31 et seq.). We may note that under workers' compensation and no-fault auto laws, plaintiffs give up the right to sue in tort and this appears to pass constitutional muster (O'Connell, 1975: Appendix 5).

[4] Various dysfunctions (private and social) of fault-finding litigation under tort law have effectively been exposed (see, e.g., Havighurst, 1975; O'Connell, 1975). I restrict my attention here mainly to a few technical problems that seem to me to warrant additional attention.

ness of this negligence concept (as applied operationally in particular cases), many students and practitioners believe that the Learned Hand formulation of the negligence standard affords a more useful approach. Thus, according to Posner:

> It is time to take a fresh look at the social function of liability for negligent acts. The essential clue, I believe, is provided by Judge Learned Hand's famous formulation of the negligence standard— one of the few attempts to give content to the deceptively simple concept of ordinary care.... In a negligence case, Hand said, the judge (or jury) should attempt to measure three things: the magnitude of the loss if an accident occurs; the probability of the accident's occurring; and the burden of taking precautions that would avert it. If the product of the first two terms exceeds the burden of precautions, the failure to take those precautions is negligence. (Posner, 1972:32)

Thus, under the Hand rule, the expected costs of accidents are to be weighed against the costs of avoiding them. If an injurer has failed to take accident-avoidance steps that would have entailed costs less than the expected costs of the accident, he has been negligent and bears the cost of the accident. The victim, on the other hand, would bear the costs of those accidents "not worth avoiding"—i.e., such that the costs of avoidance are greater than the expected cost of the accident. A social-function advantage claimed for this rule is that it establishes incentives that should, in principle at least, contribute to minimizing the total costs of accidents and accident prevention.[5] In this sense, proponents contend, the rule helps to achieve efficient rates of resource allocation to the various economic activities.

Schwartz and Komesar (1978) have urged the appropriateness of the Hand formulation for analysis of the function of the law of negligence in the context of medical malpractice. They suggest that, since in practice not all untoward events can be prevented, the Hand rule be modified to define negligent behavior as the failure to invest resources in accident prevention up to a level that equals the expected saving in accident cost.

---

[5] The Hand rule, per se, seems to be silent on the matter of what role, if any, is to be assigned to contributory negligence. Calabresi and Hirschoff (1972) have pointed out that the addition of a modified contributory negligence rule would improve the theoretical efficiency of the Hand rule.

Critical in the evaluation of any negligence rule, or, more generally, any liability rule, is not only the theoretical efficiency of the rule, if properly implemented, but also the probability that, in practice, the rule can properly be implemented.[6] The Hand rule leaves a good bit to be desired from this point of view, particularly in the context of existing medical malpractice institutions.[7]

However, the Hand rule (at least as modified by Schwartz and Komesar) in the domain of medical malpractice confronts a number of conceptual problems that run deeper than what properly might be characterized as implementation problems, per se. One such problem is how to operationalize the concept of "failure to invest resources in accident prevention." Some mishaps, e.g., those owing to incomplete diagnostic workups, might seem to fit this paradigm in a fairly natural way—as, say, failures to invest enough provider time. However, the paradigm would not seem naturally to comprehend some categories of claims that, most would agree, might appropriately be asserted pursuant to a negligence rule. For example, to characterize mishaps owing to lack of provider knowledge or lack of provider skill or expertise as instances of *that* provider's "failure to invest resources" would surely strain the meaning of that concept in many such cases. Such mishaps might be comprehended as failure of the medical services *system* to invest enough resources, e.g., in the selection and training of providers. Negligence law and the dispute-management procedures associated with it address incentives to the parties and prospective parties to negligence actions, namely, the consumers of services and the individual providers of those services (as well as counsel for these parties and insurers). The decision-making process that determines a medical services-system parameter, such as the rate of resource investment in the selection and training of providers, is a complex, multiparty process. Included among these parties are the medical schools and their associations (e.g., the Association of American Medical Colleges), the physicians and their associations (e.g., the

---

[6] A point emphasized by Calabresi and Hirschoff (1972), who propose a formulation they regard as more likely than the Hand formulation, in practice, to accomplish accident-prevention cost minimization.

[7] Schwartz and Komesar (1978) afford a discussion of some of these implementation problems. They compare what they regard as the "ideal" negligence signal called for by the Hand formulation and the negligence signal generated in the "real world."

American Medical Association), the hospitals and their associations (e.g., the American Hospital Association), the specialty boards, the state and federal legislators who provide funding for medical education, and various additional parties. These parties are not, as such, prospective parties to negligence actions claiming provider malpractice. That is, most of the decision makers who, collectively, are important for determining the rate of resource allocation to selection and training of physicians and, hence, to this aspect of accident prevention, are insulated from the incentives afforded by administration of the law of negligence in accord with the Hand Rule (or, indeed, any other rule). These considerations mean that, at least in the medical services sector, to contend, as do Schwartz and Komesar (1978:3), that "the Learned Hand Rule serves to assure that resources are being efficiently allocated ... by establishing procedures that minimize the total cost incurred by accidents and accident prevention" is to make a claim that is dubious at best, even at the level of the theoretical efficiency of the rule.

How might a remedy for the foregoing problem be found within the context of the law of negligence? In rather abstract principle, one approach that would be responsive to this problem would be for plaintiffs in malpractice actions to bring not only professional-services suits against physicians but also what might be thought of as product-liability suits against, say, the medical schools and residency programs responsible for selecting, training, and professionally motivating the physicians who turn out to be defendants. To characterize this approach as responsive, in principle, to the problem helps to elucidate the nature of the problem. But this approach can scarcely be regarded as a practicable solution. In what sense can medical schools and residency programs, say, be expected to guarantee the knowledge, skill, and professional responsibility of each of their "products"? It is true that such training programs must be accredited. The nature of and rationale for the accreditation process would seem to imply that these training programs ought to be able to guarantee that each physician possess some minimum level of knowledge, skill, and professional responsibility at the time of exit from the program. But, for events and circumstances beyond that exit point, these programs can assume no responsibility.

There probably is no solution to this problem strictly within the context of administering the law of negligence. A more hopeful approach would seek some institutional bridges such that the outcomes of individual malpractice cases would provide information to other agencies, which would then take appropriate action on the basis of the information. Some such arrangements do exist (although not, so far as I know, addressed to problems in training programs).

For example, a big factor affecting the management of malpractice suits in California is the Board of Medical Quality Assurance.[8] All recoveries against providers in excess of $3,000 are reported to the board, which may then elect to investigate the circumstances of the case. Investigation by the board is mandated when the total of recoveries against a provider is in excess of $30,000. If the board finds something amiss, the sanctions available to it include restriction or limitation of a physician's practice to certain types of procedures or, in an extreme case, revocation or suspension of a provider's license. Pursuant to the problem here being considered, the purview of such a board could be extended. The board could review all cases in which there were recoveries against physicians, to determine whether there was any tendency for the physicians involved in misadventures to be the product of certain training programs or certain kinds of training programs. If the record revealed such tendencies, the board could investigate these programs. In principle, a possible outcome of such investigation could be a recommendation by the board that an increased allocation of resources to these training programs would be an investment in accident prevention that would be worth the cost in terms of accidents averted. An investigation or trial would be required to determine whether, in practice, one might anticipate any useful yield from adopting such procedures. What can be said is that, in principle, such procedures would provide a more general link between the outcomes of malpractice actions and decisions to invest in (some aspects of) accident prevention than can now be provided by the law of negligence as it is administered.

An assessment of the social significance of following a Hand-type negligence rule suggests an additional, important technical issue. This turns on how the "cost" of accidents is to be measured. One approach

---

[8] Established by the Medical Injury Compensation Reform Act of 1975 (MICRA) to replace the former Board of Medical Examiners. The board's Division of Medical Quality is directed to take action against any certificate holders guilty of "unprofessional" conduct, with "incompetence" identified as a form of unprofessional conduct.

would be to appeal to the performance of the malpractice system and reckon as the cost of any given kind of accident plaintiffs' actual average recovery. This measure would be directly relevant for the management of, say, a self-insured delivery system making decisions about how much to invest in accident prevention. It would not, however, necessarily be relevant from the point of view of the social function of the negligence rule. In selecting an appropriate measure of accident costs, it is important to keep in mind that consumers in the aggregate pick up the tab for accident costs and the costs of accident prevention—by incurring the costs (monetary and psychological) of accidents, by paying health insurance premiums and taxes, and by making out-of-pocket payments for services. (Damages assessed, premiums to insure liability, and prevention costs are, from the provider's point of view, costs of doing business that will be reflected in the price of the product.) The question to which the negligence rule must generate the correct answer is whether any given investment in accident prevention is worth the cost to consumers. That is, the relevant evaluation standard for investment in accident prevention is whatever it is worth to consumers, *ex ante* the occurrence of any of various mishaps to reduce the risk that they will experience the mishaps.[9] It would appear that only by chance would the *ex ante* accident evaluation correctly be measured by *ex post*-accident recoveries generated by the medical malpractice dispute-management system. The costs represented by plaintiffs' recoveries do, of course, have some relevance for decisions about investment in prevention. The malpractice system will generate some rate of recovery by victims, and consumers in the aggregate will pay this tab.

If an additional dollar in prevention will save more than a dollar in accident costs, rational consumers will want to invest the dollar

---

[9] This same standard is the relevant one for evaluating efficient rates of resource allocation, not only to accident prevention, per se, but also to any life-saving, morbidity-reducing activity, e.g., the medical services sector as a whole. For discussion of this see Schelling (1966). As Schelling points out, it may be difficult for consumers to establish their own preferences with confidence on this score. The problem is that, even given good technical data relating investment in life-saving and morbidity-reducing activities to risk reduction, the consumer would still typically confront the problem of evaluating the worth of small reductions in very small probabilities of the occurrence of untoward events—the very prospect of which may evoke high levels of anxiety.

in prevention. But this investment decision is based upon only a subset of the factors the consumer will want to take into account, and this subset of factors may well not be decisive for the preferred rate of investment in prevention. Suppose that any given consumer wants to invest at a given rate to reduce the risk that he, or members of his family, or his friends (or others in his utility function) will, say, suffer brain damage owing to anesthesia accidents. That preference is based on the consumer's evaluation of the expected disutility of the untoward event, an evaluation that is made independently of whatever rate of recovery the extant malpractice system happens to be generating for victims of these particular accidents—and that rate of recovery will only by chance motivate the rate of investment in prevention the consumer would elect on the basis of his more fundamental risk-aversion preferences.

It seems likely that consumers' *ex ante*-accident risk-aversion preferences would call for a higher rate of investment in prevention than would be warranted on the basis of *ex post*-accident recoveries generated by the extant malpractice system. This is so because for various reasons the extant system probably tends to undercompensate victims in the aggregate. For one thing, a significant number of meritorious claims are never asserted. Also, according to data published by the National Association of Insurance Commissioners (NAIC), indemnities paid for incidents with economic loss (past and anticipated medical expense, past and anticipated wage loss) of $100,000 and over are less on average than the economic loss itself, i.e., there is no compensation for the real costs of pain and suffering. These data show, however, that indemnities paid for incidents with small economic loss are in excess of that loss—a result one might expect for very small claims where the parties are likely to settle for an amount that is largely determined by what it is worth to avoid the cost of adjudicating the claims (National Association of Insurance Commissioners, 1977).

If the extant malpractice system were to generate recoveries that would warrant a higher rate of investment in accident prevention than would be motivated by the consumers' more fundamental, *ex ante* preferences, the former will presumably determine the investment rate.

Much more could be said about the social efficiency of the law of negligence. The foregoing analysis has been intended only to direct attention to a couple of technical points that mean that, even at the level of theoretical efficiency, the law of negligence is unlikely to achieve the resource allocation benefits sometimes attributed to it. Moreover, the analysis points to a fundamental advantage for consumers in contracting with providers on performance standards. Rather than relying on administration of the law of negligence to determine efficient rates of investment in accident prevention, consumers would be wiser to negotiate such rates with providers. Consumers could, in this way, directly map their *ex ante*-accident risk-aversion preferences into the decision. In the decentralized, fee-for-service delivery setting, there may be no very feasible way to accomplish such negotiations. It is a peculiar advantage of organized delivery systems such as HMOs that it would appear feasible to take more or less systematic account of consumers' risk-aversion preferences in making decisions about investment in prevention. Thus, for example, HMO members might, through suitably selected representatives or agents, negotiate with HMO management the decision about prevention programs and strategies to be adopted, weighing the cost of such programs (reflected in the dues the members pay) against what the reduction in risk is worth (as best this might be estimated). In practice, such negotiations would probably be addressed not just to accident prevention, per se, but more generally to the overall quality of delivery system performance as this might be affected by such factors as the supply of physicians and other health manpower and facilities to be afforded per member.[10]

Contract Terms: Some Further Considerations

Some students appear to contend that there is one appropriate social function of liability rules, namely, to promote economic efficiency. The fact is, however, that malpractice institutions based on such rules,

---

[10] Although my discussion has focused on medical malpractice, the points on the law of negligence likewise may be relevant to the case of product liability. Markets for some products may permit the consumer to bargain with producers by choosing among a number of models, each featuring a different rate of investment in accident prevention and each a different price reflecting the investment rate. In medical services markets, however, to bargain on this score with providers, consumers will probably have to negotiate, i.e., rather than play take-it-or-leave-it in the marketplace.

and the dispute-management systems associated with them, in practice discharge a number of different social functions. Among these is the compensation of victims. In consequence, they have a distributional impact, transferring income from consumers in the aggregate to the victims. For this function, the malpractice system should be responsive to canons of equity and justice (not just to canons of economic efficiency).

The problem of achieving distributional equity is a peculiarly vexing one in the context of the extant malpractice system, in part because of the way the system structures the decision-making process. Eligible victims recover for economic loss and pain and suffering in amounts determined by adjudicators (judges, juries, arbitrators) or by settlement negotiations. Perhaps there would be general agreement that equity requires that victims be made whole for economic loss. But what is an appropriate recovery for pain and suffering (a rubric that is supposed to comprehend all of the disutility suffered by the victim other than economic loss)? One answer is to accept as the appropriate recovery on this score whatever recovery is yielded by the proper decision-making process (e.g., trial by jury, or arbitration, or—as in most instances—settlement negotiations). Given the recovery rate, whatever "tax," levied on consumers in the aggregate, was necessary to finance it would likewise be regarded as appropriate. That is, the tax loading (on prices of services) would simply follow, given independent determinations of appropriate recoveries.

This approach, it may be argued, leaves a good bit to be desired, because it does not come directly to grips with the fact that gains for persons in their roles as victims mean losses for persons in their roles as nonvictims, such that an appropriate decision-making process should *simultaneously* take account of these distributional effects. What kind of decision-making process can achieve this?[11] Trial by jury (or

---

[11] In a recent study sponsored by the California Medical Association (CMA) and the California Hospital Association (CHA), a systematic attempt was made to define and measure the prevalence of "potentially compensable events" in a sample of California general hospitals. These events were defined in a way suitable to inform the design of various models of patient-disability (more or less no-fault) compensation systems (Mills et al., 1977). An actuary's analysis of the data developed by this study concluded that the cost in California of a no-fault system would run between $700 million and $1.5 billion per year. But, if we assume an efficient dispute-management system, as the proponents of no-fault contend such a system would be, most of the

by judge, or by arbitrator) is not well suited to accomplish this. Even if one makes the assumption that these adjudicators strive to perform as effective, responsible agents representing the interests of both victims and consumers in the aggregate, it would remain to explain how, in fact, they are able validly to represent these competing interests. It is the peculiar advantage of an HMO delivery setting, on the other hand, that it does afford the institutional context for a properly structured decision-making process addressed to this distributional question. The members of the HMO are, at once, prospective victims who will benefit from whatever rates of recovery might be agreed upon and those who will, in the aggregate, finance the recoveries. Thus each member can simultaneously take account of the competitive utility implications for these two roles in arriving at preferences about appropriate rates of recovery—and, given that the members can reach some agreement, they can negotiate the result with the HMO.

Whatever mix of principles (e.g., economic efficiency, equity) the parties resort to to inform the drafting of their performance-standards contracts, the process of selecting particular contract terms may be assisted by considering various suggestions that have been made about the definition and administration of liability concepts in this domain. For example, they might adopt a straightforward no-fault approach, following the lead of the California Medical Insurance Feasibility Study, which took the view that, to the extent possible, compensation in a no-fault system should not be predicated upon whether or not the disability was preventable. With this approach, they might make no attempt to build into the liability system, per se, incentives to reduce the rate of mishaps.

Alternatively, they might try an approach along the lines suggested by Havighurst's "medical adversity insurance" (MAI) concept. According to Havighurst (1975:1249), "the central tenet of the MAI scheme is that financial incentives supplied by liability rules can be

---

total premium expense should be simply an income transfer, i.e., from nonvictims to victims. It is not at all clear how large an income transfer of this kind would be regarded as appropriate by consumers in the aggregate. It should be kept in mind, however, that even a very generous income transfer to victims would entail only a relatively small loading on each individual's cost of health care.

a major guarantor of good-quality medical care." Pursuant to this, he suggests that "if experience rating could not be expected as a spontaneous development, a possible means of creating quality-assurance incentives in an MAI program ... would be simply to impose a share of the cost of each claim directly on the responsible providers through some kind of deductible or coinsurance requirement" (Havighurst, 1975:1251). Adapting this approach to the HMO context would mean that each physician member of the medical group would be at some direct financial risk. MAI is essentially a no-fault scheme, but it embodies the concept of "liability without fault," a notion that, as Havighurst observes, physicians and others have some trouble getting used to.

O'Connell (1975) has put forward the concept of "elective" no-fault liability. Under this scheme, providers would be authorized unilaterally to elect no-fault for themselves and their patients, i.e., if a provider so elected, patients would be barred from suits in tort. He anticipates constitutional challenges to this approach, remarking, "Perhaps to some the most disturbing constitutional feature ... is that private persons ... are allowed unilaterally to alter the common law rights of those they insure" (O'Connell, 1975:206). The answer to this problem is for both parties to elect no-fault, i.e., by explicitly contracting on no-fault if they deem it to their mutual advantage. If, as O'Connell holds, patients (and product customers) are really better served by no-fault, then contract is the natural way to get it.

The parties might abjure the no-fault route, staying within the framework that defines liability by reference to customary standards of care. There would still be room for innovation, e.g., along the lines suggested by Bovbjerg. As matters stand, negligence in HMO practice is defined by reference to customary standards of care developed on the basis of experience in the health services sector generally, which is dominated by the fee-for-service delivery mode. Bovbjerg argues that the application of this standard may tend to inhibit efforts by HMOs to develop innovative, more efficient delivery systems. He urges that HMOs be given legal authorization to substitute "HMO custom" as the standard of care against which to measure liability (Bovbjerg, 1975:1408–1409). He points out that his suggestion would in effect allow the subgroup of medical practitioners in HMOs to set their own malpractice standards. Statutory authorization would be required for HMOs to impose such standards unilaterally. Such authorization presumably would not be required for HMOs and their members explicitly to contract on such standards.

In addition to the foregoing, the parties to performance-standards contracts in HMOs could consider any of various other possibilities. The general point, exemplified by the foregoing suggestions, is that there is a rather rich mix of contract provisions among which the parties might choose in negotiating a package that best accommodates their mutual interests.

Arbitration of Malpractice Claims Against HMOs

I now develop the proposition that arbitration (rather than conventional litigation) is the superior adjudication mode for managing those disputes that arise pursuant to performance-standards contracts in HMOs—particularly if the full potential of the contract approach is to be realized.[12]

Arbitration has been a feature of various HMO (e.g., the Kaiser-Permanente Health Plans) malpractice-dispute management systems. For example, the Amendment to Group Medical and Hospital Services Agreement of the Kaiser Foundation Health Plan of Oregon provides, in part:

ARBITRATION OF CLAIMS

A. *Claims Subject to Arbitration.* Any claim arising from alleged violation of a legal duty incident to this Agreement shall be submitted to binding arbitration if the claim is asserted: (1).... (2) On account of death, bodily injury, disease or ailment allegedly arising out of the rendition of, or failure to render, services under this Agreement, irrespective of the legal theory upon which the claim is asserted.

---

[12] I should make it clear that I do not undertake in this essay a *general* assessment of the relative merits of arbitration and the trial in the domain of medical malpractice. To do so would not only require a very large amount of space, but it would also divert attention from the particular points I want to make—namely, those concerned with the relations between contract and arbitration. There has been much controversy over medical malpractice arbitration, both in the literature and in the field. I have discussed this controversy at some length elsewhere (Stevens, 1979).

The membership contracts of the Kaiser Foundation Health Plans in California contain similar arbitration provisions.

A common objection to voluntary agreements to arbitrate medical malpractice claims is that, in many cases, they may not be really voluntary on the part of the patient. When the patient presents to the provider seeking care, it is argued, he may well be somewhat confused by the unfamiliar situation and he may, moreover, be anxiety-ridden, preoccupied with his medical condition, such that he is unable to reflect in a self-serving way on the relative merits of adjudicating any disputes that might subsequently arise in one way rather than another way. Under these circumstances, it is argued, the patient may unwittingly become party to an arbitration agreement. It may be remarked that precisely these same circumstances might result in the patient's unwittingly failing to become party to an arbitration agreement. Generally speaking, of course, individuals are made better off, not worse off, by an increase in the number of alternatives freely available to them. It requires some special argument to reach the conclusion that the law should not *permit* the choice of arbitration. The problem is to devise suitable hedges against the possibility of unwitting agreement to arbitrate or unwitting agreement not to arbitrate.

Thus, for example, California's Code of Civil Procedure Section 1295 provides in part:

(b) Immediately before the signature line provided for the individual contracting for the medical services must appear the following in at least 10-point red type:

NOTICE: BY SIGNING THIS CONTRACT YOU ARE AGREEING TO HAVE ANY ISSUE OF MEDICAL MALPRACTICE DECIDED BY NEUTRAL ARBITRATION AND YOU ARE GIVING UP YOUR RIGHT TO A JURY OR COURT TRIAL, SEE ARTICLE 1 OF THIS CONTRACT.

In addition, the patient may rescind the agreement to arbitrate by written notice within thirty days of signature.

The HMO form of delivery system affords an inherent advantage from the point of view of this problem. The clients agree to arbitrate when they become members of the organizations, as part of their overall membership contract. In the usual case, at the decision point they are well and going about their ordinary business, not preoccupied with the anxieties of illness. Those who have argued that arbitration agreements in HMOs should not be allowed because, since they are a condition of membership in the health plan, they smack of adhesion, have distracted attention from the real significance of such arbitration agreements. The clients are not, after all, forced to choose membership in an HMO. They have a choice, the HMO delivery system *cum* arbitration or some other type of delivery system *cum* actions in tort. They can choose the "package" that seems to them, on balance, the best. The "package" approach is predicated on the notion that the procedure for managing disputes about performance standards is and ought to be regarded as an integral part (along with the delivery system) of the "health care services systems" to which individuals may attach themselves. There is a fundamental reason why this way of looking at the matter is sound. As emphasized earlier in this essay, the choice of contract rather than tort as the legal-theory basis for asserting malpractice claims may have important consequences for the performance of the health services system *qua* delivery system (e.g., appropriate rates of investment in accident prevention and, more generally, quality assurance). Similarly, the procedures adopted for managing malpractice disputes may have an important bearing on the quality of the overall provider-patient relationship. It would be an error to suppose that the choice of dispute-management procedure is neutral to the performance of the delivery system component of the health care services system of which both are a part.

The association of arbitration and contract-based claims is natural. The parties to a contract establish by mutual assent the substantive rules to govern their relationship: these rules are not imposed by the outside authority of public law. Likewise, their agreement to arbitrate disputes over interpretation and application of their contract has a consensual basis, agreement by the parties upon their own dispute-management process. In short, the contract creates private rights that may appropriately be adjudicated by resort to private tribunals.

For the parties to performance-standards contracts in HMOs, the evolution of a formal grievance procedure that would set up steps before arbitration would greatly facilitate the administration of their contracts.[13] Under such a procedure, a grievance would be a claim

---

[13] I have discussed this matter elsewhere (Stevens, 1974). My discussion in the text draws on my earlier treatment. For a general discussion of grievance

by the member that there had been a violation of the performance-standards contract and, if the claim were disputed, it would be processed through one or more steps at each of which the parties and their representatives would attempt to reach a resolution of the problem. Failing resolution, the claim would go to arbitration. Thus, under a formal grievance procedure, arbitration of a malpractice claim would be the final step in a multistep dispute-management process.

It should be pointed out that grievance procedures as thus far developed in HMOs are for the most part not intended to process malpractice claims; these are processed through more conventional procedures. Rather, extant HMO grievance procedures are in the main addressed to administrative matters such as dues payments, the services to which members are entitled, and so on. The American Arbitration Association (AAA) has developed a grievance procedure for processing malpractice claims in organized delivery settings, which includes arbitration as the final step (Ladimer, Solomon, and House, 1979). Invoking the AAA procedure, however, does not depend upon the existence of explicit contracts on performance standards such as those advocated in this essay.

A special feature of the relation of arbitration to contract to which I wish to direct attention is that the arbitration of contract disputes is frequently more than just a matter of contract administration; it can also be a matter of contract-making. Indeed, for some of the potentially most important terms of performance-standards contracts, there will be no way other than by administering the contract under arbitration and accompanying grievance procedure to develop an acceptable contract. The most parsimonious way to make this point is by resort to a collective bargaining analogue (Stevens, 1974).

Most collective bargaining agreements provide (in the so-called management-rights clause) that the management may discipline or discharge employees "for due cause"—with this concept being nowhere explicitly defined in the agreement. If an employee feels that management has violated this contract clause, he may grieve. The outcome of many grievance arbitrations, in many contexts, over many years has clothed the concept of "due cause" with operational meaning—a meaning that might be said to reflect the "common law" of the

procedures including arbitration in HMOs see Ladimer, Solomon, and House (1979). In general, these authors adopt a systems perspective in which they evaluate arbitration as part of a larger system of dispute management, of which it is but one component.

workplace, those customs of the workplace that generally are regarded as equitable and viable. There really is no other way in which satisfactory meaning can be ascribed to the "due cause" concept in this context. Administering the collective contract under the grievance procedure, for this kind of subject matter, is very much a matter of contract-making.

Turning to the medical care sector for an analogue, we may remark that among the potentially most important terms of explicit contracts on performance standards will be language addressed to the provider's duty of "full disclosure" in the therapeutic relationship. ("Full disclosure," which imposes a more demanding duty of communication on the provider than that imposed by the traditional "informed consent" doctrine in most jurisdictions, is a controversial issue in the provider community. The general statements about it in the text, sufficient for present purposes, do not engage this controversy.) The general idea comprehended by the duty of full disclosure can readily be set out, viz: the provider shares with the patient information about the (differential) diagnosis of his condition, about the treatment alternatives available (including no treatment), and the probabilities (as best these can be estimated) of risks and benefits associated with each. The therapeutic decision becomes a genuine two-party decision. The informed consumer elects the preferred regimen in light of his own preferences over the possible outcomes and in light of his own risk-aversion propensities. It may be argued that a properly complied-with duty of full disclosure can go a long way toward improving the quality of medical care, and it may also diminish the number of malpractice claims. Brittain, one of a group of physicians and physician-attorneys who examined in depth a consecutive series of more than 1,000 malpractice claims, has reported:

> As strange as it may seem to many physicians, only a few malpractice suits are initiated specifically because of the damages which the patient will later claim. To the contrary, a majority of malpractice suits are brought because of patient or patient-family anger over something totally peripheral to the event leading to the claimed damages. This may be an excessive bill, or, more commonly, a misunderstood bill, hostility, inattentiveness, abruptness, or any one of many other human characteristics which would cause any of us to turn hostile.... The second most frequent reason why patients consult attorneys about potential medical liability is real

or alleged "surprise.".... The law is clear that at least for elective procedures, it is the patient who has the right to decide on whether to be treated or not. Truly "informed" patients are rarely surprised. (Brittain, 1978:19)

Albeit the general idea comprehended by full disclosure can readily be set out, realistically the parties must recognize that in the actual administration of the standard there will be problems and legitimate exceptions to literal compliance with the standard. For one thing, some patients in some circumstances may not want to be as fully informed as literal compliance might urge. Also, in some situations, full disclosure might, in the professional judgment of the provider, have a negative medical impact. Also, there are problems with communication in this domain, both because of the sometimes technical nature of what must be communicated and because the patient's anxiety and fear may impede his comprehension. What is the answer? One answer would be simply to abandon any effort to administer such a standard. But the potential importance of full disclosure may be regarded as too great to accept this solution. Alternatively, the parties might attempt to draft contract language in sufficient detail explicitly to take account of all contingencies. But this is not really a practical solution. The best solution is to leave the contract language setting the duty of full disclosure rather general in nature, and to permit consumers who feel that the duty has not been complied with to grieve. We might anticipate that (as with the "due cause" analogue) arbitration awards would clothe the concept of "full disclosure" with operational meaning—a meaning that would be sensitive to and would reflect the realities and the equities of the provider-patient relationship. Parties to continuing relationships agree to arbitrate, rather than litigate, their contract disputes, in part because they seek a forum with this kind of capacity to contribute constructively to the making of their contract.

In the domain of labor relations, the parties, with their collective agreements, grievance procedures, and arbitration, have constituted a pervasive system of "industrial jurisprudence." Rather than resorting to the public law and its institutions for the enforcement of contracts, the parties have created their own system of private law for these purposes—and, I again emphasize, it is a system with various complementary parts. Similarly, in the domain of organized, medical care delivery systems, the parties with their performance-standards contracts, grievance procedures, and arbitration could constitute an analogous system of "private medical care jurisprudence." And this private system, as I have elsewhere remarked, could well develop an expertise, sensitivity, and dispatch in the handling of malpractice and related matters scarcely to be anticipated under formal litigation at public law (Stevens, 1974). The development of such a system should be recognized as one of the major potential advantages of organized delivery settings such as HMOs.

As I hope the discussion in this essay has suggested, the implications of contract and arbitration in organized delivery systems such as HMOs are very far reaching. A medical services system delivers medical services and achieves medical outcomes in the context of a somehow structured provider-patient relationship. From the point of view of the utility experienced by consumers in consequence of participating in the system, it is the whole package that counts. In the decentralized, fee-for-service practice setting, the provider-patient relationship is in important part structured by negligence (and other liability) rules, conventional settlement negotiations, and the prospect of trial. On the other hand, in organized delivery system settings, the provider-patient relationship might, as has been suggested herein, in important part be structured by explicit contracts on performance standards, formal grievance procedures, and arbitration. This system is more likely than is the conventional system to serve the interests of the parties.[14]

Private Adjudication of Public Rights

I have suggested in this essay that arbitration is peculiarly appropriate for the adjudication of contract-based malpractice claims—peculiarly appropriate, that is, for the adjudication of private rights. Does this imply the other side of the coin—namely, that arbitration is not appropriate for the adjudication of public rights (e.g., tort negligence rules)? This is an important question for the design of optimal medical malpractice dispute-management systems. And, given the increasing

---

[14] See Ladimer, Solomon, and House (1979) for a discussion that urges this same conclusion.

resort to arbitration in this domain and the character of various arbitration provisions, it is far from an academic question.

Some arbitration provisions are very broad, in the sense that they will accommodate claims irrespective of the legal theory upon which the claim is asserted, e.g., the Kaiser Health Plan provision cited earlier in this essay, and the State of Michigan arbitration statute. For example, Sec. 5140 (1), Act No. 140 (State of Michigan Public Acts of 1975) provides:

> The provisions of this chapter shall be applicable to the arbitration of a dispute, controversy, or issue arising out of or resulting from injury to, or the death of, a person caused by an error, omission, or negligence in the performance of professional services by a health care provider, hospital, or their agent, or based on claimed performance of such services without consent, in breach of warranty, or in violation of contract.

The Michigan statute, however, is restrictive in a special way. Section 5043 (1) (b) provides: "The prevailing standard of duty, practice, or care applicable in civil action shall be the standard applied in the arbitration." This provision would appear to mandate the private adjudication of public rights. More generally, the argument in this essay would suggest that such a restriction is unfortunate in that it ties the hands of parties to performance-standards contracts in HMOs, such that they may be precluded from realizing the advantages of designing their own standards to reflect their own peculiar preferences.

Proponents of arbitration contend that broad scope is necessary if arbitration is to be a really effective alternative to litigation such that the maximum benefits of arbitration are to be realized. That is, proponents of arbitration generally see no reason why the alleged benefits of arbitration (e.g., lower cost, more expeditious disposition of claims) should be peculiar to claims asserted under some theories but not other theories. Nevertheless, it may be argued that the arbitration of public rights, those established by public law, does raise questions of propriety in a way that the arbitration of contract disputes does not. In the malpractice domain, the proliferation of arbitration schemes represents a kind of invasion by private tribunals of legal turf historically presided over by public tribunals. This development, over the longer term, might lead to some displacement of public law and public legal theories by private law and private legal theories—a result that, this essay has argued, would be of benefit to the parties. This development might also lead, however, to private construction and application of public law—a result that may have untoward implications for the development of public law. Consideration of some recent developments in labor law may help to inform judgment about this matter.

Recent developments in labor law have seen an invasion, by public law and public tribunals, of turf long presided over by private law and private tribunals (the reverse of the situation with malpractice disputes, where private tribunals have been the invaders).

Historically in this country, the "web of rules" to govern in the workplace has largely been fashioned by the collective bargaining system, relatively few terms and conditions of employment being determined by external public law. In recent years, however, there has been an increasing tendency to substantive federal regulation of the terms and conditions of employment, including Title VII of the Civil Rights Act, the statutory provision that has resulted in most of the private-law/public-law jurisdictional conflict in this domain. Most collective bargaining agreements include antidiscrimination provisions. In some instances, these provisions are virtually identical with or incorporate Title VII by reference. In this case, the grievance arbitrator in a discrimination case, although interpreting and applying the collective agreement as usually instructed by that agreement, will also find himself or herself in effect or explicitly interpreting and applying federal law. Is this appropriate? There is opinion in the labor-relations community that this is not appropriate (Feller, 1976a, 1976b; Edwards, 1977). In Feller's view, the labor arbitrator should stick to his last, should confine his attention to the contract; otherwise, the whole system of private industrial jurisprudence and arbitration as part of it will be threatened:

> Deference to arbitral competence was and is difficult to achieve. And I suggest it will be impossible to maintain if arbitrators extend themselves and regard arbitration as the tribunal in which broader policies than those contained in the agreements themselves are to be enforced.... My view is that the profession and the process are best protected to the extent that the process is regarded as a specialized one rather than a generalized one." (Feller, 1976a:110–111)

Edwards is in agreement with Feller's view that arbitrators should not take on public-law issues, but contends:

> At issue here is not whether arbitration will suffer if arbitrators go beyond collective bargaining agreements in settling disputes.... At issue is the private development of public law. Where arbitrators decide issues of public law, two major problems arise. The first is that they may be wrong. The second is that their errors, if honored by a public tribunal out of deference to arbitration, may distort the development of precedent. (Edwards, 1977:90)

Similar concerns have been voiced in other arbitration contexts, viz:

> Arbitration is power, and courts are forbidden to look behind it. The protection of awards against judicial interference and, under that umbrella, of the development of organized arbitration as a rule maker have established "judicial powers" other than those provided by federal and state constitutions. It is not possible to maintain any legally established policy or order ... if courts abdicate their power in favor of private tribunals serving private interests. (Hessen, 1965:64)

Obviously, labor relations and medical malpractice relations represent very different kinds of institutional situations—e.g., disputes with entirely different topical content, and a very different legal context as this engages the relation of private tribunals to public law. Nevertheless, the issues raised are relevant to the arbitration of medical malpractice disputes. Some medical malpractice arbitration schemes, such as the Michigan statue cited earlier, put the arbitrator in the business of adjudicating public rights established by public law. Are concerns such as those expressed by Feller, that the arbitration system will lose viability if it is extended to the adjudication of public rights, relevant in the domain of medical malpractice? Or, are concerns such as those expressed by Edwards and Hessen, namely, that the private development of public law may have untoward consequences, relevant in this domain? In the extensive debate over the merits of arbitrating malpractice disputes, these questions get very little attention. In my view, these concerns are relevant to an evaluation of the merits of medical malpractice arbitration and do cast doubt on the propriety of arbitrating public rights. By themselves, however, they cannot be regarded as decisive for the choice between arbitration and litigation. To fully inform this choice, a number of additional factors, namely, all of those upon which the quality of justice yielded by these dispute-management systems depend, must be taken into account.

References

American Arbitration Association, Research Institute. 1979. Executive Summary of Final Report to the National Center for Health Services Research, Department of Health, Education, and Welfare: *Health Dispute Resolution: Methods and Case Experience*, 1–13. New York: American Arbitration Association.

American Bar Association. 1976. *Interim Report of the Commission on Medical Professional Liability*, 1–68. Chicago.

Amicus Curiae Brief on Behalf of the California Hospital Association. 1977 (September). In the Court of Appeal, Second Appellate District, State of California, Division One. 2nd Civil No. 51239.

Bovbjerg, R. 1975. The Medical Malpractice Standard of Care: HMOs and Customary Practice. *Duke Law Journal* 1975:1375–1414.

Brittain, R.S. 1978. Preventing Malpractice Claims. *Hospital Tribune* 12 (November):19.

Bukata, D.C. 1978. California Medical Malpractice Arbitration and Wrongful Death Actions. *Southern California Law Review* 51:400–428.

Calabresi, G., and Hirschoff, J.T. 1972. Toward a Test for Strict Liability in Torts. *Yale Law Journal* 81 (May):1055–1085.

Curran, W.J., and Moseley, G.B., III. 1975. The Malpractice Experience of Health Maintenance Organizations. *Northwestern University Law Review* 70:69–89.

Edwards, H.T. 1977. Arbitration at the Crossroads: The "Common Law of the Shop" v. External Law. *Arbitration Journal* 32 (June):65–95.

Epstein, R.A. 1976. Medical Malpractice: The Case for Contract. *American Bar Foundation Research Journal* 1976 (1):87–149.

Feller, D.E. 1976a. The Impact of External Law upon Labor Arbitration. In *The Future of Labor Arbitration in America*, 83–112. New York: American Arbitration Association.

———. 1976b. The Coming End of Arbitration's Golden Age. In Dennis, B.D., and Somers, G.G., eds., *Arbitration-1976: Proceedings of the 29th Annual Meeting of the National Academy of Arbitrators*, 97–126. Washington, D.C.: Bureau of National Affairs, Inc.

Havighurst, C.C. 1975. Medical Adversity Insurance: Has Its Time Come? *Duke Law Journal* 1975:1233–1280.

———, and Tancredi, L. 1973. Medical Adversity Insurance: A No-Fault Approach to Medical Malpractice and Quality Assurance. *Milbank Memorial Fund Quarterly/Health and Society* 51 (Spring):125–168.

Heintz, D. 1975. An Analysis of the Southern California Arbitration Project, January 1966 through June 1975. Research Report Series, National Center for Health Services Research, Department of Health, Education, and Welfare.

Heintz, D. 1979. Medical Malpractice Arbitration: A Viable Alternative. *Arbitration Journal* 34 (December):12–18.

Hessen, J. 1965. Arbitration: The Credit Executive's Ally. Cited in Lazarus, S., et al., *Resolving Business Disputes: The Potential of Commercial Arbitration*. New York: American Management Association.

Institute of Medicine, National Academy of Sciences. 1978. *A Policy Analysis: Beyond Malpractice: Compensation for Medical Injuries.* Washington, D.C.: National Academy of Sciences.

Ladimer, I., with Solomon, J.C., and House, S.G. 1979. *Democratic Processes for Modern Health Agencies.* New York: SP Medical and Scientific Books, distributed by Halsted Press.

Mills, D.H., Boyden, J.S., and Rubsamen, D.S. 1977. *Report on the Medical Insurance Feasibility Study.* Sponsored jointly by the California Medical Association and the California Hospital Association. San Francisco: Sutter.

National Association of Insurance Commissioners. 1977. *Malpractice Claims* 1 (May). Milwaukee: National Association of Insurance Commissioners.

O'Connell, J. 1975. *Ending Insult to Injury: No-Fault Insurance for Products and Services.* Champaign: University of Illinois Press.

Posner, R.A. 1972. A Theory of Negligence. *Journal of Legal Studies* 1:29–96.

Schelling, T.C. 1966. The Life You Save May Be Your Own. In Chase, S.B., ed., *Problems in Public Expenditure Analysis.* Washington, D.C.: Brookings Institution.

Schwartz, D.H. 1976. Societal Responsibility for Malpractice. *Milbank Memorial Fund Quarterly/Health and Society* 54 (Fall):469–488.

Schwartz, W.B., and Komesar, N.K. 1978. Doctors, Damages, and Deterrence: An Economic View of Medical Malpractice, R-2340-NIH/RC. Rand Corporation.

State of New York. 1976. *Report of the Special Advisory Panel on Medical Malpractice.* State of New York, January.

Stevens, C.M. 1974. Voice in Medical-Care Markets: "Consumer Participation." *Social Science Information* 13 (June):33–48.

————. 1979. Medical Malpractice Settlement Negotiations: Some Implications of Substituting Arbitration for the Trial. (Unpublished.)

Waltz, J.R. and Imbau, F.E. 1971. *Medical Jurisprudence.* New York: Macmillan.

Carl M. Stevens

Wellington, H.H. 1968. *Labor and the Legal Process*. New Haven: Yale University Press.

This work has been supported by the National Science Foundation Program in Law and Social Science. The author expresses his thanks to Prof. Clark C. Havighurst for helpful comments on an earlier draft.

Address correspondence to: Prof. Carl M. Stevens, Department of Economics, Reed College, Portland, OR 97202.

Index

449